EXHAUSTION
A History

Anna Katharina Schaffner

Columbia University Press   New York

Columbia University Press
Publishers Since 1893
New York   Chichester, West Sussex
cup.columbia.edu

Library of Congress Cataloging-in-Publication Data
Schaffner, Anna Katharina.
    Exhaustion : a history / Anna Katharina Schaffner.
    pages cm
    Includes bibliographical references and index.
    ISBN 978-0-231-17230-1 (cloth : alk. paper)
    ISBN 978-0-231-53885-5 (e-book)
1. Fatigue. 2. Social history. I. Title.

    BF482.S33   2016
    152.1'886—dc23   2015034503

♾

Columbia University Press books are printed on permanent and durable
acid-free paper.
Printed in the United States of America

c 10 9 8 7 6 5 4 3 2 1

COVER DESIGN: Julia Kushnirsky
COVER IMAGE: Monica Rodriques/Getty

We think of our own crisis as pre-eminent, more worrying, more interesting than other crises. . . . It is commonplace to talk about our historical situation as uniquely terrible and in a way privileged, a cardinal point in time. But can it really be so? It seems doubtful that our crisis . . . is one of the important differences between us and our predecessors. Many of them felt as we do. If the evidence looks good to us, so it did to them.

Frank Kermode, *The Sense of an Ending:
Studies in the History of Fiction*

CONTENTS

Acknowledgments   *ix*

Introduction   1

1. Humors   15

2. Sin   31

3. Saturn   52

4. Sexuality   72

5. Nerves   85

6. Capitalism   111

7. Rest   132

8. The Death Drive   150

9. Depression   169

10. Mystery Viruses   184

11. Burnout   202

Epilogue: The Future   233

Notes   *243*

Bibliography   *265*

Index   *277*

ACKNOWLEDGMENTS

I would like to thank the following friends and colleagues for their help in shaping this book at various stages in its development: Tim Binding, Peter Buse, Felicity Callard, Francesco Capello, Andreas Corcoran, David Corfield, Mary Cosgrove, Chris Dooks, Laurence Goldstein, Michael Greaney, Claudia Hammond, Katja Haustein, Ben Hutchinson, Annette Kern-Stähler, Jenny Laws, Gordon Lynch, Ayesha Nanthoo, Caitríona Ní Dhúill, Patricia Novillo-Corvalán, Anita O'Brien, Karla Pollmann, Ernst and Eva Schaffner, Wilmar Schaufeli, Natalia Sobrevilla Perea, Axel Stähler, Nuria Triana-Toribio, Verena Trusch, William Viney, Greta Wagner, Simon Wessely, Laura Williams, and Angela Woods.

Thanks are also due to the Wellcome Trust for funding a conference on exhaustion at the University of Kent.

Finally, I would like to thank my editor at Columbia University Press, Jennifer Perillo, for her belief in the project and for her invaluable feedback, as well as Shane Weller, as always, for everything.

EXHAUSTION

Introduction

On a wintry afternoon in February, an old man steps out onto a balcony. There are no clouds in the sky, but a chilly wind is blowing. The old man shivers and wraps his garments more tightly around his frail, delicate body. His hair is as white as his robes. His face is a landscape marked by toil and sorrow, and the dark shadows under his watery eyes are an unhealthy shade of purple. His head is bowed so deeply that his neck almost forms a right angle with his hunched back, and his hands are trembling. He tugs at the heavy golden ornament that hangs around his neck.

The moment he steps out onto the balcony, the chatter in the square below him dies down, to be replaced by an expectant hush. It costs the old man all his energy to perform the next task. He clears his throat and, slowly, like an ancient turtle, raises his head. He spreads his arms and blesses the crowd. Then, in a grating, broken voice, he begins to say his farewells.

The figure is not any old man. It is Pope Benedict XVI, who announced his retirement to an astonished world on February 11, 2013, in a statement composed in Latin, read at a gathering originally convened to consolidate the canonization of three new Catholic martyrs. He reported both physical and spiritual exhaustion and offered his advanced age and deteriorating physical strength as the primary reasons for his decision to retire. He spoke of the burden of an office that had become too heavy for him; he said that the world was changing and was doing so at a pace with which he could not keep up. The ship of believers, he concluded, needed a helmsman stronger than he, someone capable of steering it safely through the choppy waters of our age.

A few weeks later, on February 28, 2013, a helicopter whisked the pope away from the Vatican to Castel Gandolfo, the palace where pontiffs traditionally rest during the summer months. Later that day, from the palace balcony, he addressed a crowd of pilgrims and well-wishers for the very last time, thanking them for their sympathy. In April 2013, he retired to a monastery in the Vatican Gardens, where, he said, he hoped to spend his remaining days in peaceful seclusion, praying, meditating, and once again dedicating himself to his long-abandoned and much-loved piano playing. On his first day in retirement, the pope emeritus watched recordings of his own farewell ceremony on television.

On only one previous occasion in the history of the Catholic Church had a pope resigned voluntarily: the year was 1294, and the pope in question was Celestine V (formerly the hermit Pietro del Murrone), who had been in office for only five months. Like Benedict XVI so many centuries later, he cited exhaustion as the primary cause for his wish to retire: "Owing to the weakness of my body . . . , in fact the weakness of my entire person, I hereby resign from the glory and the honors of the papal office," he declared.[1] Yet in Celestine's case, too, age and waning physical strength were only secondary factors; far more important was his spiritual exhaustion, a weariness of the soul, perhaps even a crisis of faith. Celestine, known to suffer from low self-esteem, was also thought to have been incapable of coping with the taxing administrative tasks that came with the papal office. Benedict XVI's motives, in contrast, were much more disturbing: visibly affected by the news of the many sordid sexual and financial scandals uncovered within the inner sanctums of the Catholic Church during the last years of his papacy, he confessed in one of his final papal addresses that sometimes he felt as though God were sleeping.[2]

There is something decidedly unsettling about the fact that the most iconic and symbolically important spiritual figure of the

Western world—traditionally a beacon of unwavering faith and indefatigable service unto death—should have decided to hang up his papal mantle and to play the piano instead. Moreover, the former pope's resignation aptly illustrates the all-pervasive sway that the experience of exhaustion—both physical and spiritual—holds over our age. It certainly feels as though ours is the age of exhaustion, an age characterized above all by weariness, disillusionment, and burnout. A particularly virulent form of cultural pessimism, it seems, has come to dominate our discussions of politics, economics, ecology, and health care. The much-debated death of so-called grand narratives, and in particular the demise of political idealism that followed the collapse of the last Communist regimes in Europe, as well as the sad aftermath of the Arab Spring, have ushered in a new wave of political apathy, fed further by the ascendancy of opportunist party politics that have nothing to offer but the tired old mantra of economic growth.

Although there no longer appears to be a viable political alternative, the demise of capitalism has been proclaimed repeatedly after a recent succession of banking crises that are unprecedented in their severity and scale—but even these apocalyptic verdicts themselves appear weary and lackluster, as though they, too, were merely another symptom of our burned-out age.

In addition to the doubts about the sustainability of our current economic system, the very sustainability of our ecosystem continues to be called into question, the scientific evidence becoming ever stronger. The land, sea, and sky are being irreparably damaged by our careless habits of consumption.[3] The rain forest is being depleted; the ozone layer is shrinking at an alarming rate; the oceans are heaving with toxins and industrial waste; the ice caps and glaciers are melting; and carbon monoxide emissions are still high.[4] Moreover, a rapidly growing world population is on course to exhaust the planet's raw materials.[5]

It is hardly surprising, then, that these serious social, political, and environmental concerns, all of which center around the idea of exhaustion, should have an impact on the mental well-being of the individual. Major depression (which counts the symptoms of physical and mental exhaustion among its core indicators), chronic fatigue syndrome (CFS), and burnout are now frequently diagnosed ailments. Depression, in particular, has reached epidemic proportions—it is thought to affect more than one in ten people in the Western world at some period in their lives. The World Health Organization (WHO) estimates that more than 350 million people are affected by it globally.[6] Seventeen million people experience CFS worldwide, and more than 1 million people are currently diagnosed with CFS in the United States. The illness thus strikes more people than multiple sclerosis, lupus, and some forms of cancer.[7] Burnout features among the three most commonly diagnosed complaints in the workplace, after backache and stress. The number of popular self-help and scientific publications on burnout has grown massively in recent years, attesting further to its importance.[8] While not synonymous with exhaustion, all these syndromes include the core symptoms of physical and mental exhaustion.

There is no doubt that the specter of exhaustion shapes both public debates and lived experience in the early twenty-first century, chiming eerily with our weary zeitgeist. Is not ours the most exhausted age in history? And does the current epidemic of exhaustion not threaten the very future of the human animal? There are many who believe this to be the case.[9] Yet before simply assenting to this assessment of our times, there is another question that needs to be asked: What do we really mean when we speak of exhaustion? In spite of the ubiquity and the metaphorical potency of the term, and its many applications in medical, psychological, economic, and political debates, exhaustion is a slippery concept, one that borders on, and often overlaps with, various others. How can we define exhaustion, and how can we demarcate it from related ideas and diagnoses? Is exhaustion a state that we can quantify scientifically, or is it a wholly subjective experience? Is it primarily a physical or a mental condition? Is it predominantly an individual or a wider sociocultural experience? Is it really the bane of our age, something that is intimately bound up with modernity and its discontents, or have other historical periods also seen themselves as the most exhausted?

✳ ✳ ✳

Exhaustion can be understood not only as an individual physical, mental, or spiritual state but also as a broader cultural phenomenon. Physically, exhaustion manifests itself as fatigue, lassitude, lethargy, and weakness. It can be a temporary state (for example, as the result of exertion) or a chronic condition. It is the pathological forms of exhaustion that are the subject of this study, and, more specifically, those that are not obviously the result of an underlying and clearly diagnosable medical condition.

On an affective, emotional, and spiritual level, we can describe the symptoms of exhaustion as weariness, disillusionment, apathy, hopelessness, and lack of motivation. Exhaustion can also result in restlessness and irritability. Culturally speaking, exhaustion is often connected with the idea of "lateness," as a preoccupation with exhaustion tends to emerge in the context of the final stages of epochs and empires—for example, during the decline of the Roman Empire and the nineteenth-century fin-de-siècle—and it is in these cases associated with concepts such as ennui and decadence.

Medically speaking, exhaustion is related to various historical and current diagnostic categories, including melancholia, nervousness, neurasthenia, depression, chronic fatigue syndrome, and burnout. Yet these diagnoses are not simply synonymous with exhaustion: all combine the core physical and mental symptoms of exhaustion with a range of other symptoms. Sometimes exhaustion is seen as the consequence of other symptoms; sometimes it is thought to be their cause. In one way or another, however, the key symptoms of exhaustion feature at the very heart of all of these fatigue syndromes. Moreover, there is nothing "natural" about the groupings of diverse symptoms into specific disease categories. History shows that disease entities are subject to continuous change, and especially in the field of mental health.

The ancient humoral conception of melancholia, for example, was originally based on the idea that its primary symptoms were fear and causeless sorrow, but other frequently discussed symptoms include lassitude, weariness, misanthropy, and pessimism. Neurasthenia is a notoriously baggy label, a catch-all diagnosis that draws together a staggering range of symptoms, including not just nervous weakness and various indicators of physical and mental exhaustion, such as lethargy, apathy, irritability, and restlessness, but also phobias, digestive complaints, dry hair, and cold feet. While major depression is defined as being characterized by low mood, feelings of guilt, self-hatred, and loss of interest or pleasure, it also counts lethargy, lack of motivation, fatigue, physical slowing, and low energy among its core symptoms. Finally, emotional exhaustion, a cynical attitude toward the people with whom one works or the institution with which one is affiliated, and reduced personal accomplishment are the three core markers of burnout. Burnout has also been defined in terms of a waning of engagement.[10]

It is certainly striking that we rarely find discussions of states of exhaustion in their pure form in the medical and psychiatric literature but tend to encounter them embedded in more complex symptom clusters, the constellations and names of which, and of course their accompanying etiological narratives, are prone to change. This book explores in detail the specific symptoms with which exhaustion is combined in both past and present fatigue syndromes, and what these combinations can tell us about the underlying assumptions of the theorists of these conditions more generally.

As exhaustion is already a metaphoric concept in its own right, it is helpful to look more closely at the origins of the word and the reasons for its continuous allure. Metaphors matter, in medical as in all other debates.[11] They shape the way we picture what is happening inside us—just think of terms such as "burned out," "highly strung," "thin-skinned," "nervous," "drained," and "overloaded." They can help us to form visual and linguistic representations of our inner life, suggesting links between concepts to illustrate shared qualities, or to gesture toward something we cannot yet fully understand. They are also often shaped by ideological assumptions, as in the phrase "nervous bankruptcy" (introduced by George M. Beard, the inventor of the neurasthenia diagnosis), which suggests that nerve force is a limited quantity that needs to be managed as wisely as one's monetary assets. It also indicates that whoever experiences it has carelessly wasted a precious reserve through unwise decisions or a dissolute lifestyle.

The etymological roots of exhaustion suggest the act of drawing out or using up a limited supply: the English term derives from the Latin *exhaurire*, composed of the prefix *ex-* (out) and *haurire* (to draw). According to the *Oxford English Dictionary*, the noun "exhaustion" includes the following meanings:

> 1. The action or process: a. of drawing out or forth, esp. air; b. of emptying of contents; the condition of being emptied; c. spec. (Steam-Engine) the discharge of waste steam from the cylinder . . . ; 2. The action or process of consuming or using up completely . . . ; 3. a. The state of being exhausted of strength, energy, etc.; extreme loss of strength; b. the draining (anything) of valuable properties; the condition of being so drained.

"To exhaust" means to draw off or out, to consume or empty something in its entirety, to account for or utilize the entire quantity of something, and "to drain (a person, kingdom, etc.) of strength or resources, or (a soil) of nutritive ingredients; hence, to weary out, enfeeble extremely." The French *épuiser* (literally, "to draw out") and the German *erschöpfen* (to scoop out something of a liquid nature) are akin to the English "exhaustion" in both their literal and their metaphorical range of associations. They, too, evoke imagery related to air and liquids, such as a person drawing out final rasping breaths on a deathbed, a well that is being emptied of its water, or a stretch of land that is drained by persistent overcultivation. Exhaustion generally suggests the vampiric depletion or harmful consumption of a limited (and usually nonrenewable) resource, which leaves an originally well-functioning person, object, system, or terrain in a weakened or dysfunctional state. Above all, the figurative associations of the term make explicit the notion that energy reserves are both precious and limited in nature: they can be run down by wastage or overexertion, or else by parasitic external forces.

Finally, exhaustion can of course also be defined negatively by what it is not and what a person afflicted by it lacks: its conceptual opposites include, above all, energy but also vitality, strength, optimism, engagement, and care for the future. While Western cultures are clearly preoccupied with theorizing pathologies centering on the depletion of energy, it is interesting to note that, apart from the prosaic calorie-intake model, there are currently no scientifically accepted models of human energy available in Western medicine. Explorations of the workings of human energy are largely relegated to the domain of esoteric speculation. In the psychoanalytic tradition, too, Sigmund Freud's and his successors' theories of the life drive, and of drive energy more generally, remain curiously vague.

Many Eastern medical traditions, in contrast, are based on widely accepted models of human energy, such as *prana* and the chakras in the Indian tradition, *qi* in the Chinese tradition, and auras and energy fields in shamanic cultures. In Western models from the past, too, there have been concepts of human or life energy: Galen, for example, writes of the "animal spirits," the Stoics analyzed "pneuma," and the vitalist tradition in medicine held that living organisms are fundamentally different from inanimate ones because they are powered by a nonphysical energy that has been variously described as the *élan vital*, the vital spark, or the soul. Yet curiously, our own age, albeit so anxious about the loss of human energy, lacks a clear concept of it.

✳ ✳ ✳

Exhaustion is commonly understood as a specifically modern affliction, irrevocably bound up with the rise of capitalism and new technologies. The marriage of man and modernity, many commentators argue, is both unhappy and unnatural, constituting a permanent drain on our energy reserves. They tend to suggest that in the past, when life followed a more serene rhythm, regulated by the seasons and nature, rest was more plentiful, and stress as we know it did not exist—ignoring, of course, the fact that other stressors related to health and personal safety abounded, and that physical labor was much more taxing without the aid of the many technological inventions on which we can draw today.

In late-eighteenth- and early-nineteenth-century medical theory, exhaustion was above all construed as both an individual and a broader cultural reaction to various features of modernity, including urbanization, industrialization, and bureaucratization; the faster, technologically enhanced pace of modern life; the specific stresses of sedentary "brain work"; secularization; the dissolution of stable social hierarchies and the (largely theoretical) possibility of social mobility; and the psychological repercussions of capitalist competition.

The more recent literature on depression and burnout also embraces the idea that exhaustion has never been a more pressing problem and that there is something unique to our times that is responsible for the epidemic of depression, fatigue, and burnout.[12] The rapid spread of burnout, for example, is blamed on radical changes in the organization and value of work. These include the transformation of an industrial into a service economy, the subjectivization of work, as well as the adverse effects of globalization and resulting economic uncertainties, such as ever fiercer competition and more precarious work arrangements. Even more important is the ubiquity of new information and communication technologies, such as the Internet, e-mail, Twitter, social networks, and cell phones, which no longer allow us properly to disconnect and to relax, blurring the boundaries between work and life and thus causing chronic stress.

However, while there is no doubt that the increased preoccupation with exhaustion coincided with the rise of modern capitalism, this book shows that exhaustion and its various symptoms have also been a serious concern in other historical periods. The experience of exhaustion, a curiosity about its effects, and the desire to understand its origins are *not* unique to our times. In fact, many historical periods have seen themselves as the most exhausted. Most commentators on fatigue-related syndromes have tended to paint equally apocalyptic scenarios, claiming that the specific conditions of their own age are by far the worst. A common denominator in those discourses is the presentation of their age's sufferings as greater than those of their ancestors: thus commentators nostalgically glorify the past while criticizing specific aspects of the present. They also frequently tend to complain about and to pathologize social changes, arguing that external demands on the individual have increased, while the available energy has remained the same or even decreased.

Yet how can we explain not only the historical changes in the etiological explanations of exhaustion-related syndromes but also the changes in the perception of the dominant symptoms of exhaustion? In certain periods, for example, theorists and also patients may emphasize primarily its physical symptoms, while in others the focus might be on its mental or spiritual ones. The medical historian Edward Shorter argues that throughout history, patients have unconsciously chosen to exhibit psychosomatic symptoms that doctors deem "legitimate" and that are in harmony with the medical paradigms of their time. In the Middle Ages, for example, when people believed in the reality of demonic possession, individuals would enact the symptoms of possession and respond positively to exorcism rites. The biological models that dominated medical thinking for most of the nineteenth century, in contrast, focused mainly on organic and hereditary causes of illnesses. When the these models were gradually replaced by psychological explanatory ones, the convulsive fits, paralyses, and other highly theatrical motor symptoms that hysterics had produced gave way to less dramatic sensory symptoms—above all, fatigue.[13] Shorter argues that the unconscious mind is influenced by the surrounding culture and is able to adapt to current medical models of "legitimate" and "illegitimate" medical symptoms. Medical discourses thus shape the production of specific symptoms, in that they provide culturally determined templates of legitimate illness behavior on which the unconscious draws: "The unconscious mind desires to be taken seriously and not be ridiculed. It will therefore strive to present symptoms that always seem, to the surrounding culture, legitimate evidence of organic disease. This striving introduces a historical dimension. As the culture changes its mind about what is legitimate disease and what is not, the pattern of psychosomatic illness changes."[14]

Shorter's model is thought-provoking and explains some of the dynamics that drive the rise and fall of so-called fashionable diseases. It does not, however, allow for exchanges that work the other way around: medical discourses, too, are influenced by and respond to wider sociocultural developments. Technological innovations, sociocultural changes, dietary fashions, and transformations of the world of work, for example, affect patients' lived experience and the development of physical and mental responses in a more immediate manner and may then feed back into the medical realm. The exchanges among culture, lived experience, and medicine work in a complex fashion, and this book aims to pay close attention to the multidirectional cross-traffic between these domains.

* * *

This study explores the forgotten history of exhaustion, from classical antiquity to the present day. It analyzes the protean syndromes in which the symptoms of exhaustion have been embedded and the many different narratives that have been constructed to theorize its origins. In the past two thousand years, exhaustion has been explained as a product of humoral or biochemical imbalance, as a psychological or somatic ailment, as a viral disease or a dysfunction of the immune system, as a spiritual failing or the result of planetary movements, as a reaction to loss and a desire to return to a death-like state of repose or as a broader cultural response to a faster pace of life and transformations of economic and social structures.

Narratives about the causes of exhaustion tend to vacillate between organic and mental explanatory models. Above all, these narratives illuminate the ways in which the interactions between mind and body, inside and outside, the individual and society, and the cultural and natural environments has been imagined at particular historical moments. Some theories privilege holistic models, in which body, mind, and society are assigned equal significance; some focus exclusively on biology; some on the psyche; and some on the social and physical environment. Moreover, many of them touch on ethical questions pertaining to agency and willpower: Is the care for the self the responsibility of the individual, the community, or the state? Are we theoretically able to pull ourselves out of exhaustion-related states via willpower alone?

The different etiological narratives of exhaustion have, of course, resulted in radically different suggestions for its cure: therapeutic recommendations include a diverse range of dietary regimes; bloodletting, emetics, and the application of leeches; the prescription of tonics and stimulants; the infamous "rest cure"; occupational and exercise therapy; hydro- and electrotherapy; the talking cure; psychopharmacological medication; cognitive behavioral therapy (CBT); mindfulness meditation; and reforming occupational health legislation in order to protect citizens' work–life balance.

There is much we can learn from past theories of exhaustion that can help us make sense of our own experience of exhaustion today. Almost by default, historical analyses render apparent the relativity of our own attitudes and values, which we often tend to experience as absolute truths. Furthermore, there is something soothing about the knowledge that ours is not the only age to have wrestled with the demon of exhaustion.

This study explores the sociohistorical causes that determine and shape the preoccupation with exhaustion in different historical periods. Given that exhaustion is triggered by a combination of mental, physical, and social factors, it is a condition that tends to be related to specific social and cultural changes in both medical and popular debates. Frequently, theories of exhaustion are presented in conjunction with what essentially constitutes cultural criticism: a shifting regime of sociocultural changes are often not only represented as illness-enhancing factors but pathologized in their own right. Exhaustion, moreover, is tied to some of our core values: productivity and activity. When these values gain renewed importance at particular historical moments, the fear of exhaustion and the number of medical and popular publications that reflect on it tend to rise. Exhaustion is thus the flip side of some of our dominant cultural values, and it rises and falls in conjunction with these.

However, in addition to these historically specific reasons for increased anxieties about exhaustion, there are some important transhistorical psychological factors that determine an ongoing interest in the phenomenon. Most important, exhaustion is related to some of our darkest primordial fears: decay, illness, aging, waning of engagement, death. We all have felt the effects of exhaustion—hopefully only occasionally, as a consequence of a hard day's work or an overindulgence in pleasure—but some of us are familiar with its more frequent, even chronic forms. Exhaustion is a familiar concept, one that is close to home, and the boundaries between its normal and its pathological manifestations are not as stable as we might assume. Unconsciously, we may fear that we, too, could all too easily find our engagement waning, our apathy and hopelessness reigning, and the awareness of the insignificance of our actions in the wider scheme of things and our inevitable physical decline becoming acute.

Finally, exhaustion is bound up with two contradictory desires: the concept chimes with us because, on the one hand, we all long for rest and the permanent cessation of exertion and struggle. A part of us wishes to return to an earthly paradise, from which work is banished—a state that resembles childhood, in which we are relieved of all responsibilities, and where everything revolves around pleasure. Yet, on the other hand, work is crucial not only for our survival but also for the shaping of our identity. It is bound up with self-realization and autonomy. In our age, moreover, work is particularly overdetermined: boundaries between public and private selves, between work and leisure, and profession and calling, are becoming ever more blurred.

* * *

This study draws on many sources in order to describe the changing faces of exhaustion. Among these are medical studies and, from the nineteenth century on, texts from the "psy" subjects—psychiatry, psychoanalysis, and psychology. Medical discourse forms part of the wider culture, however, and the medical imagination draws on other discourses, including philosophy, theology, the arts, popular culture, and literature.

Works of fiction, in particular, can grant us precious experiential insights into how particular physical conditions and affective and emotional states may feel. One of the many strengths of literary works is that they can give us access to the minds, experiences, and perspectives of others—for example, characters prone to exhaustion who might have experienced the world in a way that is radically different from, or else surprisingly similar to, our own. Read in conjunction with medical texts, fictional accounts can illustrate and bring to life abstract ideas, and reflect both on their specific subjective-experiential and on their wider ethical consequences. Importantly, though, fictions also form culture—they do not just mirror certain historical dynamics, values, and medical paradigms but also help to create, to complicate, and to question them. Medicine frequently draws on knowledge developed in the fictional realm, just as literary works draw on medical ideas. This book pays particular attention to the exchanges among the medical, the literary, and the popular imagination, as these have the power to shape and illuminate one another.

The boundaries between text and context are often difficult to maintain in a cultural history that traces a concept as metaphorically suggestive as exhaustion, which has been theorized and deployed in numerous disciplines and conceptual frameworks. But that is not necessarily a bad thing. In order properly to understand the many historical transformations of the idea of exhaustion, an interdisciplinary view that considers medical, sociohistorical, and aesthetic developments as interconnected processes is essential.

Finally, this study is arranged broadly chronologically, with a few exceptions where breaks with a linear narrative were deemed necessary. Each chapter is also dedicated to a specific discipline, including humoral medicine, theology, astrology, sexology, biology, economy, psychoanalysis, biochemistry, and sociology, as well as to a specific theme: "Humors," "Sin," "Saturn," "Sexuality," "Nerves," "Capitalism," "Rest," "The Death Drive," "Depression," "Mystery Viruses," "Burnout," and "The Future."

1

Humors

Recent biomedical theories of depression, and of the symptoms of physical and mental exhaustion that are associated with it, center primarily on chemical imbalances in the brain. They are based on the assumption that pathological low mood states are connected to neurotransmitter deficiencies. Since the 1980s, biomedical depression research has concentrated predominantly on the mono-amines norepinephrine and serotonin, and the enhancement of selective serotonin reuptake inhibitors (SSRUI).[1] Serotonin is a molecule that transports signals between the synapses in the brain and that regulates emotions, reactions to external events, and physical drives. Low serotonin levels are generally seen as a symptom of depressive moods, but there is still considerable debate as to whether they are also their cause. SSRUIs were first sold under the trade name Prozac in 1987, and Prozac rapidly became a block-buster prescription drug. It is still the most frequently prescribed antidepressant to date.

Yet the idea that an imbalance of specific substances in the body causes states of low mood–related exhaustion is not at all new. Indeed, it is to be found in ancient humoral theory. Hippocrates first introduced humor theory to medicine in the fifth century B.C.E., and the Greek physician Galen of Pergamum (129–ca. 216) further developed the idea. Galen's version of humor theory was so influential that it remained the dominant medical paradigm until the advent of modern medicine in the nineteenth century.[2] One of the central tenets of this theory is the importance of a balance among the four bodily fluids, or humors: blood, yellow bile, black bile, and phlegm. Within this framework, all illnesses—be they chronic or acute, mental or physical—can be explained by the relative excess or insufficiency of one or more of the four humors. According to Galen, each humor is also associated with specific qualities and with one of the four elements: blood is aligned with warmth and moisture, and the element air; yellow bile with warmth, dryness, and fire; black bile with coldness, dryness, and earth; and phlegm with coldness, moisture, and water. Furthermore, each of the humors is also related to a particular temperament— blood is associated with the sanguine, yellow bile with the choleric, black bile with the melancholic, and phlegm with the placid temperament. Humor theory functions thus to explain not only acute and chronic physical and mental disturbances but also long-term character traits and psychological dispositions.

The balance among the humors was thought to be precarious— it could easily be upset by a surplus or deficit of particular fluids, which could be caused by infections, inflammations, unwise dietary choices, and intemperate lifestyles, as well as by grief and sleeplessness. Acute diseases were mainly associated with disturbances in the quantities of blood or yellow bile, while chronic diseases were generally related to a deficiency or an excess of phlegm or black bile. Consequently, the most common cures administered by physicians until the modern period entailed bloodletting, emetics, the application of leeches, blistering, and purging—all designed to evacuate the body of a humoral excess and thereby to reestablish an equilibrium among the bodily fluids.

In Galen's writings, we encounter exhaustion primarily in the guise of lethargy, torpor, weariness, sluggishness, and lack of energy. Moreover, all these were thought to be typical symptoms of melancholia, which thus features some of the key symptoms of physical and mental exhaustion among its core indicators. Melancholia is a complicated disease entity, the exact definition and symptoms of which were subject to change through the centuries.

For a long time, melancholia's defining features were considered to be causeless sorrow and fear, but they were always accompanied by a range of other symptoms, among which the symptoms of physical and mental exhaustion feature prominently. Like neurasthenia, the diagnosis often encompasses a plethora of associated complaints, ranging from irritability, restlessness, mania, hallucinations, and paranoia to misanthropy and self-loathing.[3]

One of the most persistent myths surrounding the condition is the supposed link between a melancholic disposition and exceptionality, artistic inclinations, and "brain work." It can be traced all the way back to Aristotle (or one of his followers), who wonders in *Problemata* 30 (ca. 350 B.C.E.): "Why is it that all men who have become outstanding in philosophy, statesmanship, poetry or the arts are melancholic, and some to such an extent that they are infected by the diseases arising from black bile, as the story of Heracles among the heroes tells?"[4] Yet in the Middle Ages, melancholia was redefined in a theological context as acedia, with a particular focus on forms of lethargy, torpor, and lack of motivation, which were considered sinful diseases of the will and a sign of bad faith, as it was assumed to be within the power of the individual not to yield to these "demonic" temptations, which entailed contempt for the divine nature of God's creation.[5] In the early modern period, melancholia was revalorized and once again associated with creativity, genius, and scholarship, and it was celebrated as the natural inclination of sensitive and emotional men in the age of Romanticism.[6] The nineteenth century saw the advent of biological medical models and psychiatric classificatory systems, and melancholia was explained in purely organic terms.[7] In the twentieth century, Sigmund Freud introduced the idea that melancholic self-loathing is a reaction to the loss of a love object and a form of narcissistic aggression turned masochistically against the self.[8] Currently, cognitive behavioral theorists understand some forms of depression, melancholia's twentieth-century successor, as the result of distorted cognitive process and faulty reasoning.[9] Yet in spite of the eclectic diversity of explanatory models of melancholia, almost all accounts mention the physical and mental symptoms of states of exhaustion as either associated or primary symptoms.

Aristotle's and Galen's highly influential descriptions of the causes and symptoms of melancholia were to shape substantially all that followed. Galen explicitly theorizes exhaustion symptoms as belonging to the melancholic symptom cluster. The most important physician of the Roman era, trained in Platonic, Aristotelian, Stoic, and Epicurean systems of thought, Galen became court physician to the emperor Marcus Aurelius in Rome. He was a prolific writer and added his own empirical findings to past writings on medical subjects, in particular to Hippocrates's teachings.[10] In *On the Affected Parts* (composed after 192 C.E.), one of his most important treatises and originally written in Greek, Galen argues that a surplus of black bile triggers melancholia. He distinguishes between two types of melancholia. In the first kind, the entire blood supply of an individual becomes atrabilious, the melancholic humor thickening and slowing the blood, rendering the patient lethargic, slow, and prone to stupor.[11] (Interestingly, a general slowing of the patient's movement and speech and the impairment of cognitive faculties are still considered behavioral signs of depression.)[12] Galen proposes that as a result of the denser texture of the black-bile-infected blood, it either does not reach the brain at all, as it travels more slowly and is often obstructed on the way, or else damages the brain's functions by clogging up its pathways. The cure for this kind of melancholia entails bloodletting, so as to purge the excess of bilious fluids from the body and to reinvigorate the sluggish bloodstream.

The second kind of melancholia Galen describes in *On the Affected Parts* originates in the stomach and can be caused by inflammation, indigestion, heartburn, and certain types of food. To fight these disturbances in the fluid economy, the body attempts to burn the excess of melancholic humors accumulating in the stomach. However, the ashes of the burned black bile rise to the brain in the form of a black vapor that subsequently clouds the sufferer's judgment and feelings: "As some kind of sooty and smoke-like evaporation or some sort of heavy vapors are carried up from the stomach to the eyes, equally and for the same reason the symptoms of suffusion occur, when an atrabilious evaporation produces melancholic symptoms of the mind by ascending to the brain like a sooty substance or a smoky vapor."[13]

Ostensibly figurative expressions still in use, such as "clouded judgment" and "black mood," are thus rooted in what in ancient medical theory was actually thought to be the case: the assumption that the brain and its cognitive and affective functions were literally clouded and dulled by black vapors. (Interestingly, a strand in current depression research focuses on the role of negative attention and memory biases in the thought processes of the depressed, that is, the selective and often exclusive attention to and memory of negative information, which can be considered as forms of clouded judgment.) Galen emphasizes the literal link between darkness and melancholia elsewhere, too: not only is the color of the melancholic humor explicitly designated as black, but a certain type of person is more prone to becoming melancholic—that is, "lean persons with dark complexion, much hair and large veins."[14] (Other twenty-first-century avenues of depression research involve the search for defective genes that predispose certain individuals to depression and for other definitive biological markers of the condition.) Moreover, the inherent qualities of black bile, coldness and dryness, are of course primarily associated with dead matter, organic life being defined by warmth and moisture.

In addition to more or less predetermined temperamental and physiognomic qualities, external circumstances and lifestyle choices can trigger melancholia. Like many other theorists writing on exhaustion syndromes, Galen is keenly interested in diet and compiles a long list of forbidden foods that can bring about atrabilious reactions. Among the potentially melancholia-inducing and energy-draining fare he counts

> meat of goats and oxen, and still more of he-goats and bulls; even worse is the meat of assess and camels, since quite a few people eat these as well as the meat of foxes and dogs. Above all, consumptions of hares creates the same kind of blood, and more so the flesh of wild boars. [Spiral] snails produce atrabilious blood in a person who indulges in them, and so

do all kinds of pickled meat of terrestrial animals, and of the beasts living in water, it is the tuna fish, the whale, the seal (phoke), dolphins, the dog shark and all the cetaceous species [related to the whale].

He also warns against the consumption of cabbage, sprouts prepared in brine, lentils, and "wheatbreads made from bran."[15] Furthermore, he advises against the consumption of heavy and dark wine in large quantities, as well as aged cheeses. Other controllable lifestyle factors aggravating melancholic symptoms such as lethargy, weariness, and a dark mood can be lack of exercise and not enough sleep. (Again, physical exercise and a balanced diet are still thought to be important in the treatment of depression.)

While Galen emphasizes that every melancholic is unique, reacting differently to a surplus of black bile in the system, he agrees with Hippocrates's basic definition of melancholia's two key symptoms: "Fear or a depressive mood (dysthemia) which lasts for a long time render [patients] melancholic [that is, atrabilious]." All his melancholic patients, Galen writes, exhibit fear or despondency. One of them, for example, is afraid that "Atlas who supports the world will become tired and throw it away and he and all of us will be crushed and pushed together."[16] This is a particularly telling fantasy of catastrophe, which betrays a timeless fear about the calamitous consequences of the waning of engagement, the inevitable decline of our physical and mental powers, and the inescapability of death. Galen's melancholic patients also generally "find fault with life and hate people," many tiring of life altogether and wishing to die.

Galen believes in the Hippocratic and Platonic idea of the division of the soul into three faculties: the rational, the spiritual, and the desiderative. Unlike Plato, he also believes that each of these faculties is seated in a particular organ: the rational part is thought to be located in the brain, the spiritual in the heart, and the desiderative in the liver.[17] Moreover, Galen proposes that the soul is embodied and that it is directly affected by bodily processes: "All of the best physicians and philosophers agree that the humors [krâseis] and actually the whole constitution of the body change the activity of the soul."[18] He does not conceive of the soul as an autonomous entity but repeatedly emphasizes that it is a "slave to the mixtures of the body" and that the body thus has the ability to deprive the soul of its energy:[19] "So one is bound to admit, even if one wishes to posit a spare substance for the soul, at least that it is a slave to the mixtures of the body: these have the power to separate it, to make it lose its wits, to destroy its memory and understanding, to make it more timid, lacking in confidence and energy, as happens in cases of melancholy."[20]

The idea that physical processes essentially determine the soul, moods, and even specific behaviors starkly contrasts with later medical thinking, which frequently divides phenomena into those that pertain either to the mind or to the body, and which leaves little room for theorizing the complex interactions between the two entities. (There are parallels here to the arguments of researchers who believe in the purely biomedical origins of depression, that is, the idea that chemical processes in the brain, the "mixtures of the body," are the exclusive determiners of our moods.) Galen draws on the authority of Plato to support further the idea that the bad humors of the body commonly cause diseases of the soul:[21]

When the humours of sharp and salty phlegm, or any other bitter and bilous humours, wander about the body without finding any path of exit, but are churned around and mix their spirit with the motions of the soul and are blended with it, they cause all kinds of diseases of the soul, great and small, few and many, in accordance with the three places of the soul to which they are brought, multiplying the kinds of ill-temper and low spirits, of bravery and cowardice, of forgetfulness and ignorance.[22]

Irritability, low mood, difficulty concentrating, and cognitive impairments are symptoms of exhaustion that frequently appear in other syndrome-clusters, too—for example, in later discussions of acedia, neurasthenia, and depression.[23]

According to Galen, melancholic exhaustion thus originates at a physical, almost proto-biochemical level and only in a second step proceeds to adversely affect the mind and the spirit by slowing or blocking the movement of the blood or by literally clouding the spirit. The causes of exhaustion symptoms such as weariness, lethargy, and torpor, as explained in the humoral framework, then, are essentially physiological in nature: it is the body that adversely affects the mind, and not, as twentieth-century psychosomatic theorists would argue, the other way around. Consequently, Galen also believes that doctors rather than philosophers should be charged with the improvement of the intellectual and moral qualities of the soul.[24]

Yet curiously, there appears to be no room in Galen's model for the notion that purely mental processes can influence bodily reactions and result in physical symptoms—for example, that faulty reasoning and irrationally pessimistic interpretations of phenomena and experiences may become manifest in a physical lack of energy. Although Galen very briefly mentions "excessive worrying" and grief as potentially melancholia-enhancing phenomena, he never theorizes further how these psychological factors might actually interact with and affect the physical body.

While the humoral model of melancholia offers a theory of the ways in which the body affects the spirit, it centers on the idea that the mind and soul are pure and pristine, and that it is the body that acts as the corrupting force. But might not the mind also affect the body in a comparable way? Galen does not comment on this possibility. In contrast, many twenty-first-century biomedical researchers investigating the chemical makeup of depressed brains admit that they are not at all certain whether reduced serotonin levels are a consequence of depression or its cause. This matter is still essentially considered an unresolved chicken-and-egg question.

❊ ❊ ❊

Both during and since the age of classical antiquity, the exact nature of the interrelation between the mind and the body has been the subject of ongoing speculation, and it is very far from having been resolved by modern science. In the Hellenistic period, the Greek writer Apollonius of Rhodes (b. ca. 295 B.C.E.) depicts in his epic poem *Argonautica* a mind–body model that seems to be the exact opposite of Galen's. While Galen grants the body absolute supremacy over the mind, Apollonius focuses instead on the potent influence of the mind over the body, showing how mental states affect physical energy levels. His epic is a hymn to positive thinking and the power of mind over matter, and his underlying psychomedical assumptions are much closer to twentieth- and twenty-first-century psychosomatic theories than to Galen's one-way humoral model.

The *Argonautica*, telling the myth of Jason and the Golden Fleece, is a classic quest narrative. Written in dactylic hexameters and modeled on the epics of Homer, this Hellenistic poem tells of the many challenges that Jason and the Argonauts have to overcome on their perilous sea voyage, the aim of which is to secure the fleece of a golden-haired winged ram from the faraway kingdom of Colchis. Jason is dispatched on the strenuous mission by the "chilling command of a wicked king," Pelias, who was warned by an oracle to beware of a man wearing only one sandal.[25] This man turns out to be Jason, who arrives at court one day having lost one of his shoes. He obeys the king's orders, puts together a crew, and heads for the waters of the Black Sea. They overcome numerous obstacles on their journey and, with the help of the Colchian princess Medea, who is well versed in the art of sorcery, successfully manage to complete a series of seemingly impossible challenges posed by her father, Aietes, king of Colchis, who does not want to give up the Golden Fleece. Aietes charges Jason with yoking two fire-spitting bulls, to plow the land and sow serpents' teeth, from which spring a race of horrible earth-born warriors whom he has to defeat in battle. Although Jason succeeds in this task with the help of Medea's tricks and potions, it becomes apparent that Aietes does not intend to honor his side of the deal, forcing the Argonauts to seize the Golden Fleece at night and to flee. They take Medea with them. Eventually, after much hardship and the loss of a number of their comrades, the Argonauts arrive safely back home in Iolkos in Greece.

Hellenistic culture saw the waning of Greece's political and military powers and the rise of the Roman Empire. In keeping with the declinist cultural mood and a general focus on human weakness in the third century B.C.E., Apollonius repeatedly shows Jason and his men being overcome by despair, grief, and hopelessness during their voyage.[26] Here, a pervasive atmosphere of cultural decline and political apathy, as well as strong instances of personal despair and hopelessness, form the basis of powerful examples of all-consuming exhaustion in its broader sociopolitical as well as individual-experiential manifestations. Jason's helplessness contrasts starkly with the resourcefulness of his Homeric counterpart Odysseus: while the Homeric hero is described as *polymechanos* (resourceful, with many resources), Apollonius calls Jason *amechanos* (resourceless, without resources).[27] Jason, who is also neither of divine parentage nor blessed with any particular talents or skills, is thus from the outset (and by epic standards) characterized by a deficit, as a man who lacks the genealogical, emotional, and intellectual assets essential for the completion of his arduous mission. Jason is prone to despondency when faced with loss, death, and the many seemingly impossible challenges with which he has been tasked. Again and again, he sinks into the sand or falls to his knees, head in hands, overcome by exhaustion, and weeping bitterly over his fate.

The *Argonautica* is essentially a story of overcoming despondency, of battling with the demons of mental and physical exhaustion, and of not losing hope in the face of extreme adversity. Numerous scenes illustrate the ways in which hope and despair affect morale and the physical energy levels of the crew. From the very start, Jason's moments of helpless despondency are legion: while the other Argonauts guzzle sweet wine and exchange entertaining stories at the beginning of their voyage, for example, "the son of Aison pondered upon everything helpless and absorbed, like a man in despair." When the crew accidentally leaves Herakles and Polyphemos behind on the way to Colchis, "the son of Aison was so struck by helplessness that he could not speak in favour of any proposal, but sat gnawing at his heart because of the grim disaster which had occurred." He frequently delivers pessimistic speeches to his men, bewailing the doomed nature of their mission and complaining about the burden of responsibility that is weighing on him:

I have erred; my wretched folly offers no remedy. When Pelias gave his instruction, I should have immediately refused this expedition outright, even if it meant a cruel death, torn apart limb from limb. As it is I am in constant terror and my burdens are unendurable; I loathe sailing in our ship over the chill paths of the sea, and I loathe our stops on dry land, for all around are our enemies. Ever since you all first assembled for my sake, I have endured a ceaseless round of painful nights and days, for I must give thought to every detail. You can speak lightly, as your worries are only for yourself. I have no anxiety at all for myself, but I must fear for this man and that, for you no less than for all our other companions, that I shall be unable to bring you back unharmed to Greece.[28]

Overwhelmed, anxious, paranoid, and unable to experience pleasure, he repeatedly wishes that he had chosen death instead of embarking on the quest for the Golden Fleece.

Jason reacts to the deaths of his comrades with prolonged periods of despair. Here, despair is manifest primarily as hopelessness, as a lack of faith in a better future resulting in apathy, both of which are symptoms of exhaustion. When a white-tusked boar kills one of the Argonauts, for example, the crew buries him without delay, "but then they sank down where they were on the shore in helpless despair, wrapped themselves in their cloaks, and lay still without thought for food or drink. Their hearts were depressed with sorrow, because all hope for a successful return seemed very far way." The refusal of nourishment and a paralytic cessation of activity—which are also listed among the behavioral symptoms of twenty-first-century depression—are recurrent motifs in the epic. The Argonauts would have wallowed in their distress and delayed their journey indefinitely, had not the goddess Hera put boldness into the hearts of some of the men. They pass on her message by motivating their companions with hopeful speeches. Ankaios, for example, asks: "How can it be to our credit to ignore the challenge we have undertaken and to sit idle in a foreign land?" Immediately, Peleus's heart "lifts in joy," and he responds: "My poor friends, who do we grieve to no purpose? Nothing will come of it. We may suppose these men to have perished as their allotted fate decreed, but we have many steersmen among our number. Therefore let us not hold back from making the attempt: cast grief aside, and stir yourselves to your task!" Yet Jason's view of the future continues to be somber. He predicts "disaster for us no less grim than what has befallen those who have died, if we neither reach the city of deadly Aietes nor return again through the rocks to the land of Hellas. Here a miserable fate will hide us from men's view, without glory, growing old and useless."[29]

When Aietes tasks the Argonauts with yoking the fiery bulls and fighting the earth-born warriors, the crew's first reaction is once again to succumb to paralysis and inaction, a proleptic form of exhaustion: "To everyone the task seemed impossible; for a long time they sat in silence, unable to speak, and gazed at each other, depressed by the hopelessness of their wretched plight." Whenever they find themselves stranded somewhere, they are ready to give up their mission. Trapped in a vaporous landscape near the stream Eridanos, for example, the men "desired neither food nor drink, nor did their minds have any thought of delights. The days they spent worn out and exhausted, weighed down by the foul smell which rose from the small branches of the Eridanos. . . . As they wept, their tears were carried on the waters like drops of oil."

On their return journey, they find themselves cut off near the borders of Libya, in a particularly treacherous gulf with stagnant shallows. They can see only endless stretches of sand. Once again, they are seized by hopelessness when they disembark from their ship to explore the shore, for they "could see no source of fresh water, no path, no herdsmen's yard far off in the distance; everything was in the grip of perfect calm." In tears, the steersman declares to his distraught companions: "[W]e have lost all hope of continuing our voyage and of returning home safely." Everyone agrees with the despairing man, and despondency spreads like wildfire among the crew:

All their hearts went cold and the colour drained from their cheeks. As when men roam through a city like lifeless ghosts, awaiting the destruction of war or plague or a terrible storm which swamps the vast lands where cattle work; without warning the cult statues sweat with blood and phantom groans are heard in the shrines, or in the middle of the day the sun draws darkness over the heavens and through the sky shine the bright stars: like this did the heroes then wander in aimless distress along the stretches of the shore. Soon the gloom of evening descended upon them. They threw their arms around each other in sorrowful embrace and wept as they took their leave; each would go off alone to collapse in the sand and perish. They separated in all directions, each to find a solitary resting-place. They covered their heads with their cloaks and lay all night long and into the morning, with no nourishment at all, waiting for a most pitiful death.[30]

All the members of the crew would have perished with their task uncompleted had not once again some benign goddesses with an interest in their fate taken pity on the men. They suggest to Jason a way out of his dilemma and whisper words of encouragement in his ear: "Rise up, and no longer groan in distress like this! Stir your comrades!" Immediately powerfully energized, Jason jumps up and shouts "like a lion which roars as it seeks its mate through the forest." His companions, "their heads lowered in despair," listen to his speech. He succeeds in rekindling their hope and convinces the crew to carry their boat for twelve whole days and nights through the sandy deserts of Libya. Although "suffering grievously under its weight," they eventually reach Lake Triton, from which they continue their journey by boat.[31]

It is usually the gods who encourage the Argonauts to continue their quest and who urge them not to lose faith. Triton, the sea god, for example, tells them: "Go joyfully, and let no wearying grief come over you—your limbs burst with youth to meet the challenges ahead." It is the divine agents who manage to reenergize the men when they have lost all hope—hopelessness being, of course, one of the primary mental and spiritual symptoms of extreme exhaustion.

While mental despair paralyzes the men and prevents them from taking action, there are also numerous references to physical exhaustion in the epic and to the extreme hardships of the journey. The Argonauts enter various different harbors "completely worn out by their efforts," the relentless and vigorous plying of their oars rendering them "worn out and exhausted." Exhaustion also figures frequently in the extended epic similes deployed by Apollonius, often to indicate the time of day. Time is measured by the degree of physical weariness of laborers, which is given a negative slant: "At the hour when a gardener or a ploughman, hungry for supper, is glad to return from the fields to his hut and, filthy with dust, squats down on his weary knees in the entrance to pour curses on his belly and stare at his worn hands, at that hour the heroes reached the land of Kios near Mount Arganthoneion and the mouth of the Kios."[32]

Another simile also links physical weariness to time of day, but in a positive manner, referring to a good, satisfying kind of exhaustion that is temporary in nature and the result of physical exertion: "At the time when only the third part of the day which began at dawn is left, and exhausted labourers call for the swift arrival of the sweet hour at which they can release the oxen, then the field had been ploughed by the tireless ploughman, though it was four measures great, and the bulls were released from the plough."[33]

Exhaustion, then, is one of the key themes in the *Argonautica*, its reach extending even to the level of figurative devices. Moreover, the epic provides a powerful model of the ways in which body and mind may interact. The examples cited demonstrate how hopelessness (an attitude or a state of mind) directly affects the crew's ability to tackle the challenges they encounter. Following divine or human pep talks, as a result of which their outlook becomes more positive, they tap into hidden energy resources and develop superhuman strengths: the men are suddenly able to carry the Argo across the Libyan desert for twelve days and nights, while when their outlook was bleak they could do no more than lay apathetically in the sand, awaiting death. These episodes illustrate the powers that faith, confidence, and optimism can unleash and, conversely, the adverse effects on the body of negative states of mind.

Throughout the epic, Jason, as well as the Argonauts, vacillates between extreme states of hope and despair, in a manner that is characteristic of manic or bipolar depression. Either he leaps around joyfully, roaring like a lion, energizing his crew, or he sits in despair, head in hands, worn out by worry, ready to give up. While Jason's and the Argonauts' vacillations between exaltation and exhaustion are always direct reactions to external events (loss of comrades, grief, seemingly hopeless situations, being trapped in hostile lands), their attitudinal changes exemplify a more general cognitive and spiritual outlook toward human existence. When we find ourselves confronted with loss, or in hostile territory, or facing the other vicissitudes of life, Apollonius suggests, it is above all our state of mind that determines our potential to succeed or to perish. Hopelessness is a corrosive and highly infectious poison, while its opposites quite literally allow us to accomplish superhuman, seemingly impossible feats. In Apollonius, then, exhaustion is the result of a negative state of mind (often triggered by grief, loss, and the prospect or consequences of extreme physical challenges), but, crucially, it is a state that can be reversed through mental energizing. This view is, of course, congenial to the modern mind, being as it is an early version of the power of positive thinking.[34]

❋ ❋ ❋

In addition to energizing us, ideas can also affect us in a negative way. In *Why Do People Get Ill?*, Darian Leader and David Corfield explore unsettling psychosomatic research into the connection between mind and body, and the impact of psychological factors on what we tend to think of as purely physical illnesses. They analyze a large body of statistical and empirical evidence for mind–body dynamics that work exactly in the opposite manner from the model proposed by Galen.[35] Investigating phenomena such as the placebo effect;[36] the links between personality types and the statistical likelihood of developing certain kinds of illness; the power of metaphors and labels to shape illness experience and symptoms; the impact of loss, loneliness, and unhappiness on the body's ability to fight off infectious diseases;[37] and the often significant timing of the onset of certain illnesses, they present compelling evidence for the ways in which the mind can affect the body.

Few people would deny the reality of the following mind–body exchange: vividly imagining an anxiety-inducing situation, such as having to speak in front of a large audience, or having to present someone with criticism of his or her actions, or having to tackle something of which we might be genuinely afraid—such as climbing a steep staircase without railings, flying, or catching a spider with our bare hands—produces physical reactions similar to those we would experience if we were actually in that situation. Our pulse may quicken, we might start sweating, and our breathing may become faster and shallower.

Yet the power of our thoughts and emotions over our body reaches much further than this; for example, it is a proven fact that stress and anxiety can weaken our immune system—in other words, that psychological factors can significantly affect immune function. Research has shown that our immune system is closely connected to the nervous and the endocrine system, and that we are much more susceptible to bacterial or viral illnesses when we are feeling low or overstretched.[38] Numerous experiments (based, for example, on blood samples taken from depressed and nondepressed subjects and medical students during and after exam periods) have demonstrated that in times of mental upheaval or pressure, the cytotoxicity of natural killer cells—the key agents of the immune system that identify and destroy threats—is significantly reduced.[39] Another experiment has shown that small wounds took 40 percent longer to heal in subjects tested during exam time compared with subjects tested during a vacation period.[40] If exam-time stress can so significantly affect wound healing, one can vividly imagine the effects of chronic exhaustion, depression, fear, anxiety, and stress on the body's ability to heal and to defend itself against infectious diseases.[41] These and various other examples suggest that the connection between mind and body is much more complex than Galen imagined it to be in the second century B.C.E., and perhaps closer to the model that Apollonius proposed.

2
Sin

While the symptoms of mental and physical exhaustion were considered to be among the core symptoms of melancholia until it was replaced by the concept of depression in the twentieth century, an alternative model of theorizing states of exhaustion emerged in late antiquity and blossomed in the Middle Ages: the notion of sloth, or acedia. Just like melancholia, it included various symptoms of mental and physical exhaustion among its core indicators, such as weariness, torpor, apathy, lethargy, sleepiness, irritability, cognitive impairment, and hopelessness. Yet unlike melancholia, which was treated and theorized by physicians and was explained as being caused by an imbalance of the four humors, sloth fell into the remit of the theologians. It was understood not as an organic disease but as a spiritual and moral failing.

From the fourth century C.E., sloth featured prominently in theological treatises cataloging what would later become the Seven Deadly Sins. Indeed, it was often considered to be the most severe of the cardinal vices, a fundamental spiritual failing manifest in a bad attitude toward divine grace that gave rise to the sibling sins of envy, gluttony, lust, wrath, pride, and avarice. Yet the medieval concept of sloth is not simply to be equated with our modern understanding of the term as an aversion to effort and an undue attachment to repose, pleasure, and leisure; medieval sloth entailed an all-important spiritual dimension that is now lost and was much more complex than the secular conception of laziness as a lack of willpower, drive, and discipline.

The concept of acedia, the technical term for sloth and often used in the place of its Latin cognates such as *inertia, pigritia, desidia, socordia,* and *ignavia* in the Middle Ages, denotes a condition that shares various psychological, physical, and behavioral symptoms with melancholia, depression, and even burnout but places these in a theological framework. The term "acedia" is derived from the ancient Greek word for indifference, listlessness, or apathy. Literally, it denotes a "state of noncaring" (specifically about divine matters) and has been described as "weariness of the heart." As a theological version of melancholia, acedia was originally associated with monks and the monastic lifestyle, until it was extended to laypeople in the tenth and eleventh centuries.[1]

The concept emerged in the fourth century in the Egyptian desert near Alexandria among the Desert Fathers, a cluster of monks who lived as hermits in the wilderness. It was first theorized by the monk and theologian Evagrius Ponticus (346–399).[2] Leaving behind an ecclesiastical career in both Constantinople and Jerusalem in order to escape from what he saw as the frantic and decadent nature of urban life and to find an environment more conducive to the search for spiritual salvation, Evagrius joined the hermits populating Mount Nitria and the Desert of Cells. He became an influential teacher and wrote a number of treatises. In the *Antirrhetikos,* he drew up a list of eight fundamental "bad thoughts" or "demonic temptations," which he considered to be the cause of all sinful behavior and which would constitute the basis for the Seven Deadly Sins. His list includes gluttony, fornication (or lust), avarice, hubris (or pride), sadness, wrath, boasting (or vainglory), and acedia.

Evagrius defines the last as mental and spiritual exhaustion manifest in listlessness, apathy, boredom, restlessness, dejection, irritability, and hatred of the anachoretic lifestyle. Acedia, he writes, entices monks to abandon their spiritual calling, to leave their cells, and to neglect their spiritual duties. He associates acedia with the "noonday demon" (possibly a demon called Belphegor), who attacks at midday, when the heat is at its most oppressive and the monks are particularly vulnerable. The noonday demon (currently also associated with depression, owing in no small part to Andrew Solomon),[3] Evagrius explains, not only entices the monks to sleep during the day, but also

> makes the sun appear sluggish and immobile, as if the day had fifty hours. Then he causes the monk continually to look at the windows and forces him to step out of his cell and to gaze at the sun to see how far it still is from the ninth hour, and to look around, here and there, whether any of his brethren is near. Moreover, the demon sends him hatred against the place, against life itself, and against the work of his hands, and makes him think he has lost the love among his brethren and that there is none to comfort him. If during those days anybody annoyed the monk, the demon would add this to increase the monk's hatred. He stirs the monk also to long for different places in which he can find easily what is necessary for his life and can carry on a much less toilsome and more expedient profession. . . . To these thoughts the demon adds the memory of the monk's family and of his former way of life. He presents the length of his lifetime, holding before the monk's eyes all the hardships of his ascetic life. Thus the demon employs all his wiles so that the monk may leave his cell and flee from the race-course.[4]

Evagrius's definition of acedia thus includes the exhaustion symptoms sleepiness, lethargy, irritability, and hopelessness but also impatience and agitation, which are manifest in various unproductive displacement activities. Just like neurasthenics and the burned-out, those afflicted by acedia vacillate between sluggishness and restless, states marked by too little energy or else by aimless, nonproductive activities that waste energy. (In most cases of melancholia and depression, in contrast, there tends not to be much energy available to waste in such nonproductive dissipation activities.) According to Evagrius, acedic lethargy and restlessness are caused by an external demonic agent and an internal moral disposition.[5] He believes, however, that it is within human power to resist this temptation—indeed, that defying it is the monk's spiritual duty. Appropriate defenses against this demon are a vigorously renewed diligence and earnest dedication to one's spiritual tasks: practicing endurance and patience, insistent prayer, reading and the recitation of psalms, as well as meditation on Scripture.[6] Yet the rigorous regime that Evagrius proposes as cure is, of course, among the causes that instigated the state of exhaustion in the acedic monks in the first place, and it is questionable whether the prescription of more steadfastness and fortitude yielded the required results.

The second early Christian author to write on acedia was John Cassian (360–435). Cassian lived in a monastery in Bethlehem before visiting the hermit colonies in Egypt in 386, where he met Evagrius and was influenced by his teachings. Following bitter theological controversies between different Christian parties in the region, Cassian was driven from Egypt about fifteen years later and was also expelled from Constantinople. He finally settled near Marseille in France, where he founded the Abbey of Saint Victor. Cassian was one of the first theologians to spread Eastern theological beliefs and practices in the West. He dedicates an entire chapter to acedia in *The Monastic Institutes* (ca. 425), a practical handbook for monks that draws on the wisdom and practices of the desert eremites. In this work, Cassian addresses questions such as appropriate clothing, prayer, and other practical aspects of monastic life but also discusses at length ways in which to combat the "eight temptations," which are very similar to those originally identified by Evagrius. Book 10 of *The Monastic Institutes* explores the vice of acedia, which he defines as "weariness or distress of heart":

Acedia is akin to dejection, and is especially trying to solitaries, and a dangerous and frequent foe to dwellers in the desert; and especially disturbing to a monk about the sixth hour, like some fever which seizes him at stated times, bringing the burning heat of its attacks on the sick man at usual and regular hours. Lastly, there are some of the elders who declare that this is the "midday demon" spoken of in the ninetieth Psalm.[7]

Like Evagrius, Cassian argues that those in the grips of acedia feel disgust with the cell and contempt for their brothers. He describes a concatenation of sins in that one follows from the other: they long to be elsewhere and are unable to read, to concentrate, to pray, or to undertake any productive activity. It makes the monk "lazy and sluggish about all manner of work which has to be done within the enclosure of his dormitory." Moreover, the state of mental lethargy and unproductive hyperactivity is followed by the symptoms of extreme bodily exhaustion and starvation, accompanied by mental confusion:

> Then the fifth or sixth hour brings him such bodily weariness and longing for food that he seems to himself worn out and wearied as if with a long journey, or some very heavy work, or as if he had put off taking food during a fast of two or three days. Then besides this he looks about anxiously this way and that, and sighs that none of the brethren come to see him, and often goes in and out of his cell, and frequently gazes up at the sun, as if it was too slow in setting, and so a kind of unreasonable confusion of mind takes possession of him like some foul darkness, and makes him idle and useless for every spiritual work, so that he imagines that no cure for so terrible an attack can be found in anything except visiting some of the brethren, or in the solace of sleep alone.

Here, Cassian describes the physical symptoms of acedia in terms of what we would now call post-exertion malaise, a bodily fatigue that is as intense as that experienced after prolonged fasting, hard labor, or extended walking and that results in a craving for sustenance. Like Evagrius, he also describes the symptoms of hopelessness, restlessness, an inability to concentrate, a search for human company, and a desire for sleep. Ultimately, the monk thus harassed by the demon of acedia "is disturbed, until, worn out by the spirit of accidie, as by some strong battering ram, [the victim] either learns to sink into slumber, or, driven out from the confinement of its cell, accustoms itself to seek for consolation under these attacks in visiting some brother, only to be afterwards weakened the more by this remedy which it seeks for the present." Thus ensues a vicious circle: monks become ever more unable to meditate and contemplate things of a spiritual nature, and their ill-chosen strategies for restoring their energy reserves aggravate their condition further, just like a weary twenty-first-century sufferer who is unable to concentrate might constantly check e-mail or social media. And so "the solider of Christ becomes a runaway from His service, and a deserter, and 'entangles himself in secular business,' without at all pleasing Him to whom he engaged himself."[8]

Although Cassian describes in detail the physical, mental, and behavioral symptoms of acedia, he ultimately sees it as a moral and spiritual problem, one that pertains to the soul: "All the inconveniences of this disease are admirably expressed by David in a single verse, where he says, 'My soul slept from weariness,' that is, from accidie. Quite rightly does he say, not that his body, but that his soul slept. For in truth the soul which is wounded by the shaft of this passion does sleep, as regards all contemplation of the virtues and insight of the spiritual senses."[9]

Rather than conceiving of the various symptoms of exhaustion as having a physical cause, both Evagrius and Cassian think of it as a spiritual failing caused by a lack of willpower or a moral defect. The behavioral effects of the weariness of the soul are idleness or restless overactivity: either acedic monks remain lethargically in their cells without making any spiritual progress, or they wander about aimlessly, in search of idle chatter and refreshments.[10] Interestingly, Cassian also considers acedia as infectious in nature, a danger to the community that has to be contained like a virus. He quotes Paul, who deploys vivid medical imagery to illustrate his warning: "And so he bids them withdraw from those who will not make time for work, and to cut them off like limbs tainted with the festering sores of leisure: lest the malady of idleness, like some deadly contagion, might infect even the healthy portion of their limbs, by the gradual advance of infection."[11] Paul is gravely concerned by those who do not work: "For we have heard that some among you walk disorderly, working not at all, but curiously meddling."[12] Those who do not work, the Apostle sternly proclaims, shall not eat. Work is also Cassian's antidote to acedia: he believes that manual labor is the panacea that is able to prevent the disease of acedia from wreaking havoc in the monastic communities. The medical metaphors that he frequently employs when commenting on acedia are particularly striking in the following quotation, which presents idleness as the root cause of acedia: "The cause of all these ulcers, which spring from the root of idleness, he heals like some well-skilled physician by a single salutary charge to work; as he knows that all the other bad symptoms, which spring as it were from the same clump, will at once disappear when the cause of the chief malady has been removed."[13]

Cassian reports that the desert communities in Egypt never allowed monks, and especially not the younger ones, to be idle, "estimating the purpose of their hearts and their growth in patience and humility by their diligence in work." He even relates the example of an abbot named Paul, who lived in a lush paradisiacal garden that yielded everything he needed without any effort being required on his part. Yet to keep busy, and to stave off despair, weariness, and boredom, the monk assiduously collected the leaves of the palm trees growing on his plot and stored them in his cave, until it would be filled with foliage. Then he would burn them all and start his task all over again. He performed this chore simply for the sake of "purifying his heart, and strengthening his thoughts, and persisting in his cell, and gaining a victory over accidie and driving it away."[14]

The historian Siegfried Wenzel points out that regulated and fairly distributed manual labor is more important in a monastic context than in a desert cell, as monastic life depends on the organized participation of all its members. In a tight-knit community such as a monastery, those who refuse to perform their assigned role pose a threat to social cohesion.[15] It is interesting that Evagrius's cure for acedia differs so drastically from Cassian's: Evagrius first described acedia in the context of anchorites, where the social component was not yet so important, and proposes an intensification of prayer and meditation as acedia's antidotes. There might well, then, be a practical dimension to Cassian's proposal, which posits work as the ultimate cure for acedia and which shows a shift of emphasis to the social consequences of spiritual failure—that is, a concern with combating the risk of the failure of the group at large. Wenzel's argument can be extended further, to society as a whole: the more complex social structures become, the more those who do not contribute their share endanger the smooth functioning of the system. It is worth remembering that the establishment of the canon of the Seven Deadly Sins was generally driven not just by abstract theological reasoning but also by pragmatic social considerations—sloth, like wrath, avarice, gluttony, lust, pride, and jealousy, can breed resentment and prove to be very harmful to the social fabric. Similarly, the overworked, overstretched, and exhausted of our age pose an economic and social risk, too: sick leave owing to stress, depression, and burnout costs billions in lost earnings each year, and the strain these conditions put on public-health services continues to rise dramatically.

Drawing on both Evagrius's and Cassian's works, Pope Gregory the Great (540–604) finally compiled a list of seven cardinal vices that were to become the Seven Deadly Sins in the form we know them today. Gregory folded sorrow (*tristitia*) into acedia and vainglory into pride, and he also added envy to Evagrius's earlier list of "demonic temptations." Sloth (*socordia*) and acedia were often treated as synonymous, until *socordia* replaced acedia altogether.[16] As in the case of melancholia, depression, and neurasthenia, the meaning of the term "acedia" did not remain stable. During the centuries from the early Middle Ages to the beginning of the early modern period, the precise meaning of the word fluctuated considerably, as writers placed different emphases on distinctive aspects of the condition. Eleventh-century theologians, for example, concentrated mainly on the physical phenomena of idleness and somnolence, as well as on drowsiness and the temptation to close one's eyes, while twelfth-century writers paid more attention to the spiritual dimension of acedia, such as mental slackness, weariness, tepidity, and dejection. Concentrating on the inner life, they defined acedia primarily as a state of mind, a faulty attitude caused by a lack of faith.[17] In that period, the spiritually tepid were frequently compared to a pot of lukewarm milk on which flies settle readily.[18]

✻ ✻ ✻

In *On the Sacraments of the Christian Faith*, the mystic scholar
Hugh of Saint Victor (1096–1141) seeks to establish the difference
between vice and sin:

> [V]ices are corruptions of the soul, out of which, if they are
> not checked by reason, sins, that is, acts of injustice arise.
> Now when consent is offered to the temptation of vice, there
> is an act of injustice which is called a sin. So vice is the weak-
> ness of spiritual corruption, but sin arising from corruption
> through consent is an act of iniquity. And so vice without
> consent is weakness, to which in so far as there is weakness
> mercy is due, but in so far as it is checked from an act of iniq-
> uity a reward and a crown are due.[19]

This distinction is of considerable importance in the history of
exhaustion: while vice is a given predilection, a psychological or
characterological weakness, for which one cannot be held responsible, sin is a behavior and can therefore be influenced and controlled. According to Hugh of Saint Victor's logic, it is in our gift
not to act on our weakness, to control it through reason and willpower, and thus to take responsibility for our behavior and actions.
It is our duty to accept divine grace and to allow God, much like a
physician, to dress our spiritual wounds.[20] A predilection toward
sluggishness and torpor, according to this argument, would therefore be a vice and thus a spiritual weakness that can be forgiven,
while consenting to this predilection and succumbing to exhaustion would be considered a sin.

Hugh of Saint Victor's definition of dejection is of interest, too:
"Despair is sadness born from confusion of the mind, or weariness
and immoderate bitterness of the spirit by which spiritual enjoyment is extinguished, and by a kind of beginning of desperation
the mind is overthrown within itself."[21] The idea that confused reasoning and a weariness of the spirit can lead to a mind being "overthrown within itself" anticipates psychoanalytical models, according to which a sadistic superego might lash into the ego. It also

evokes the cognitive behavioral notion of endlessly looping negative thoughts, a self-destructive kettle-logic that uses up all one's energy and from which there seems to be no escape. A follower of Hugh of Saint Victor defines *tristitia seu acedia* (sorrow or acedia) as "an anguish of the mind that is perturbed by the frustration of its desire through something contrary, or, the weariness [*taedium*] to perform a good deed well."[22] Again, this definition evokes either conflicting internal desires that wear out the sufferer or external impediments that prevent a desire from being fulfilled.

The Italian theologian Saint Thomas Aquinas (1225–1274) defines acedia further in his famous *Summa Theologiae* (1265–1274), in which he draws up the core Christian taxonomy of sins, distinguishing between the cardinal and the venial sins, and arranging them hierarchically. In Aquinas's scholastic system, every cardinal sin is opposed to a cardinal virtue. He defines acedia as a "sorrow" that is opposed to spiritual joy and charity. According to Aquinas, charity is our relationship with God. Acedia is a "sadness about spiritual good." In other words, acedia is a form of spiritual apathy that is, if consented to, manifest in the rejection of the effort required to commit oneself to God and to all that is good. Faith requires ongoing work and effort, a constantly renewed commitment. Yet Aquinas attributes this shirking a union with God not primarily to laziness or sadness as such but to perverted forms of sadness—that is, uncontrolled sadness or sadness directed at the wrong "object" and, above all, good things. This is why Aquinas considers acedia a cardinal spiritual failing. Physical weariness, sluggishness, and torpor are not the actual crime but the effects of a failing that is spiritual in nature: acedia, according to Aquinas, is ultimately caused by human pride that is manifest in a perverted loathing of good things. Moreover, Aquinas defines acedia by proposing a behavioral model with a psychological cause, and one that is based on specific conceptions of agency:

Apathy [*acedia*] is *a sort of depression* which stops us doing anything, a weariness with work, *a torpor of spirit which delays getting down to anything good.* Spiritual goods are real goods, and taking no joy in them is bad in itself; and it is bad in its effects if it so depresses a man as to keep him back from good works. Apathy [*acedia*] then is doubly wrong. Sadness as such merits neither praise nor blame; what we praise is a controlled sadness at evil, what we blame is sadness that is either uncontrolled or is sad about good.[23]

The mental sadness or apathy about good things prevents the acting out of good things, an acting out that in return would reward us with joy, which is the opposite of sadness. It is because of this vicious circle that Aquinas considers acedia a cardinal spiritual failing that has as its ultimate cause, like all sins, human pride. He argues that acedia is a mortal sin, "saddened by the very goodness of God in which charity rejoices. Sins that by definition exclude the love of charity are of their nature fatal. Since joy in God necessarily follows on charity, and apathy [*acedia*] is sadness about spiritual good as a facet of God's goodness, apathy [*acedia*] is of its nature fatal."[24]

Like Hugh of Saint Victor, however, Aquinas distinguishes between the existence of a natural predilection toward acedia, on the one hand, and voluntary intellectual consent to give in to that predilection, on the other: the former is not as grave a sin as the latter; one is a sin of the flesh (that is, sense-appetites, which Hugh of Saint Victor would have described as vice) while the other is a sin of the spirit (that is, perverted reasoning): "But sins are completed only when reason consents to them, and if apathy [*acedia*] arises in our sense-appetites—the flesh rebelling against the spirit—but does not get at our reason—by turning into horror and loathing of God's goodness—then the sin is incomplete and non-fatal."[25] In Aquinas's view, then, it is the spiritual dimension of acedia, the aversion to all that is good, that constitutes the truly sinful core of the condition. In secular terms, this aversion could be described as a form of loathing, ungratefulness, and contemptuousness—an actively negative attitude toward the world that is stronger than mere hopelessness.

Again like Hugh of Saint Victor, Aquinas strongly believes in volition and personal responsibility—giving in to spiritual exhaustion attests not only to a bad attitude toward divine goodness but also to a lack of willpower. Human beings are by their nature rational and are capable of sin precisely because of their powers of reasoning and their ability to choose not to follow reason. If we were not able to act reasonably, we would not be able to sin:[26]

> Ignorance is a wound in reason's response to truth, wickedness in will's response to good; weakness wounds the response of our aggressive emotions to challenge and difficulty, and disordered desire our affections' reasonable and balanced response to pleasure. All sins inflict these four wounds, blunting reason's practical sense, hardening the will against good, increasing the difficulty of acting well and inflaming desire.[27]

It is precisely this notion of agency and personal responsibility, the conviction that everyone endowed with the gift of reason can at all times choose not to give in to the temptation of acedic weariness, that renders the theological conception of exhaustion distinct from medical, psychological, and psychoanalytical models. Medieval acedia is, above all, a moral and spiritual failing, as, according to the scholastics, it is always within our power as rational beings to resist spiritual weariness that expresses itself in consenting to temptation and in disinvesting in the good, including not doing good work. In most medical models, in contrast, agency and willpower do not have the authority to influence any of the processes that are understood to be organic in nature—regardless of whether they are thought to be caused by humors, nerves, viruses, infections, or immune deficiencies. Sigmund Freud, moreover, dealt a further blow to the notion of purely rational human agency and rationally based moral responsibility when he revealed the extent of the power that our drives, formative childhood experiences, and unconscious desires hold over us.

It is interesting that in current debates about the role of willpower and agency in dealing with certain problems—such as addiction, obesity, and even depression, burnout, and chronic fatigue syndrome—it tends to be people leaning to the right of the political spectrum who embrace views similar to Aquinas's; they, too, postulate the ultimate primacy of willpower, reason, and full personal responsibility for one's actions and consequently believe that not taking measures to improve one's own mental or physical welfare constitutes a morally reprehensible failing. The British prime minister David Cameron, for example, has recently proposed that disability benefits for people who are obese and for drug and alcohol addicts be cut if they fail to engage with programs designed to help them overcome their conditions.[28]

❊ ❊ ❊

Geoffrey Chaucer's parson, one of the narrators of *The Canterbury Tales* (1386–1395), delivers a speech that illustrates just how influential Aquinas's scholastic conception of acedia as a lack of commitment to the divine good had become: acedia, the parson tells us,

> loves no activity at all. Now this foul sin Acedia is also a very great enemy to the livelihood of the body, for it makes no provision regarding temporal necessity but idles away and sluggishly wastes all temporal goods by its carelessness. . . . Then comes the dread to begin any good works. For he who is inclined to sin thinks it is too great an enterprise to undertake works of goodness. . . . Now comes hopelessness, the despair of God's mercy that comes sometimes from too great a sorrow or from too great a fear, as one imagines he has committed such great sins that it would not avail him to repent them. . . . Then comes somnolence, being sluggish slumbering, which makes a man indolent and dull in body and soul; and this sin comes from Acedia. . . . Then comes negligence or carelessness, caring for nothing. . . . Then comes idleness, the gate of all sins. An idle man is like a place without walls; the devil may enter on every side and shoot at him with temptations while he's unprotected. . . . Then comes a kind of coldness that freezes a man's heart. . . . Then comes the sin of worldly sorrow, called *tristicia*, that slays a man, as Saint Paul says. For such sorrow contributes to the death of the soul and the body as well. A man becomes weary of his own life. Such sorrow, then, often shortens a man's life before his time comes naturally.[29]

Yet another poem, written at the beginning of the fourteenth century, engages with acedia in an even more sustained and systematic manner: *The Divine Comedy* (1308–1321) not only chronicles the gradual overcoming of Dante's spiritual and physical weariness in the course of his journey from hell to paradise but also features various representations of slothful and acedic characters. Dante's depictions of an array of sinners and their tailor-made punishments in *Inferno* and *Purgatory* reveal a thorough knowledge of the theological debates of his time on the nature of the Seven Deadly Sins. In the opening canto of *Inferno*, we learn that Dante, halfway through the journey of his life, found himself in a dark wood, alone and fearful, having strayed from the righteous path. He soon meets the Roman poet Virgil, who guides him through hell and purgatory, and finally to the gates of heaven, where Dante encounters the beautiful Beatrice, the love of his life who died young. In the final part of the poem, *Paradise*, Beatrice escorts him through the celestial realm, explaining to him the nature of truth, love, and grace. In the end, her systematically reeducated charge glimpses the divine and is able to return to life on Earth with renewed spiritual vigor and strengthened faith.

Dante is thirty-five years old when he starts his epic journey in early spring of the year 1300. He has lost his way both literally and metaphorically: he is full of doubts, his faith is weak, political chaos reigns in Florence, and he is not properly honoring the memory of Beatrice. Once again, we are presented with a potent mix of a more general sociopolitical atmosphere of exhaustion and an individual crisis of faith manifest in hopelessness and apathy. Moreover, the Dante we encounter in the opening canto of *Inferno* is not only lost spiritually but also lacking in energy, and his descent into hell is punctuated by recurrent moments of exhaustion. At the end of the third canto he collapses, "like a man whom sleep has seized." We learn that he was "full of sleep just at / the point where I abandoned the true path." He repeatedly finds it necessary to let his "tired body rest" and again and again bemoans his "exhausted force" (*virtute stanco*).[30] But as his teacher Virgil's influence grows, Dante's attitude changes: the closer he comes to paradise, and the more his sins are purged, the greater his energy levels become, as he sheds both his physical sluggishness and his spiritual apathy like an old skin.

On his journey—a cautionary reminder of the three dimensions of divine justice administered in the afterlife—Dante encounters various types of sinner and is forced to witness the punishments inflicted on them. In *Inferno* and *Purgatory*, the sinners are disciplined according to the law of *contrapasso*, a system by which sins are punished by tortures that either resemble or contrast with the sin in question. Flatterers, for example, are immersed in excrement, and the greedy are tied to the ground, their hands and feet bound, because they were too attached to earthly material goods.

In the Ante-Inferno, Dante and Virgil meet the lukewarm, those who "lived without disgrace and without praise" and who commingle with the angels who remained neutral in the battle between Lucifer and God. Disdained by everyone, they wail in misery and are forced to run on eternally behind an empty banner, "so quick / that any respite seemed unsuited to it." Among the lukewarm, Dante and Virgil spot the shade of "him / who made, through cowardice, the great refusal."[31] This legendary shirker is thought to be Pope Celestine V, who abdicated only five months after his election in July 1294, abandoning the holiest of offices. (After Celestine V, only Gregory XII and Benedict XVI would resign from their papacies.) For their refusal to act and properly commit in life, the lukewarm are tortured into endless activity in death.

In the fifth circle of hell, Dante and his guide encounter the wrathful and the sullen. These sinners meet their respective punishments in a shady, melancholic landscape, marked by malign gray slopes and a dark-purple stream that flows into a swamp, the Styx. It is in the muddy waters of the Styx that the wrathful are stuck, naked and with furious faces, angrily striking out with their hands, heads, and feet, and tearing at one another with their teeth. Below the surface of the muddy waters are the sullen, forced to swallow the slime, as Virgil explains:

> and I should also have you know for certain
> that underneath the water there are souls

who sigh and make this plain of water bubble,
as your eye, looking anywhere, can tell.
Wedged in the slime, they say: "We had been sullen [*tristi*]
in the sweet air that's gladdened by the sun;
we bore the mist of sluggishness [*accidïoso fummo*] in us;
now we are bitter in the blackened mud."
This hymn they have to gurgle in their gullets,
Because they cannot speak it in full words.[32]

Dante refers explicitly to acedia in this passage, by way of the adjective *accidïoso*. The pairing of the wrathful and the sullen is significant, since Dante habitually combines sins that are either similar or antithetical. The philologist Wolf-Günther Klostermann has suggested that the pairing can be explained by the Aristotelian notion of sullenness as wrath turned inward, repressed rather than expressed anger—Aristotle's conception being strikingly similar to Freud's understanding of melancholia as aggression that is directed against one's own ego.[33] As discussed in chapter 1, Galen, moreover, believed that melancholics were affected by black smoke caused by the burning of an excess of black bile (the melancholic humor) in the body. This smoke (possibly the *accidïoso fummo* [mist of sluggishness] to which Dante refers) was thought to rise from the lower bodily regions into the brain of the person, literally and metaphorically clouding the person's judgment, and also rendering the blood sluggish.

The core symptoms of melancholia, according to both Hippocrates and Galen, are causeless sorrow and fear. That the sorrow of the sullen in Dante's *Inferno* is causeless is indicated by the fact that they suffered in the sunshine: they had been sullen "in the sweet air that's gladdened by the sun." In effect, Dante blurs the line between the medical explanation of sullenness as a symptom of melancholia (which, since it has organic causes, would not count as a sin) and the theological one: within the theological framework, sullenness is understood as the product of a bad mentality, a failure to appreciate the divine creation. Moreover, the landscape in the fifth circle of hell, defined as it is by darkness and mud, externalizes the murky inland empire of the melancholic.[34]

In the eight circle of hell, Virgil reprimands the utterly exhausted Dante for his lack of energy. His tireless guide sternly warns him against the dangers of sloth:

> "Now you must cast aside your laziness [*ti spoltre*],"
> my master said, "for he who rests on down
> or under covers cannot come to fame;
> and he who spends his life without renown
> leaves such a vestige of himself on earth
> as smoke bequeaths to air or foam to water.
> Therefore, get up; defeat your breathlessness
> with spirit that can win all battles if
> the body's heaviness does not deter it."[35]

Spoltrire means "to cure someone of laziness" (it derives from *poltrire* [to lie late abed, to idle]). Laziness, exhaustion, and tepidity are clearly represented as a matter of the will and the spirit rather than the body here: the right attitude and spiritual resolve can overcome the limitations and weaknesses of the flesh. The spirit alone can defeat the body's torpor.

Yet in the Ante-Purgatory, Dante again experiences exhaustion (both proleptic-mental and physical in nature), when he is faced with having to climb the dauntingly high Mount Purgatory, on the top of which salvation awaits those who make the effort. Dante marshals his final reserves of energy, using his hands and feet to drag himself up to a low-level terrace. It is there that Virgil instructs him once again:

> And he to me: "This mountain's of such sort
> that climbing it is hardest at the start;
> but as we rise, the slope grows less unkind.
> Therefore, when this slope seems to you so gentle
> that climbing farther up will be as restful
> as travelling downstream by boat, you will
> be where this pathway ends, and there you can
> expect to put your weariness to rest [*quivi di riposar
>   l'affanno aspetta*].
> I say no more, and this I know as truth."[36]

But suddenly, Dante and Virgil hear someone say: "Perhaps you will/have need to sit before you reach that point!" They turn around and behold a massive boulder that they had not noticed before. Making their way toward it, they discover a group

> who lounged behind that boulder in the shade,
> as men beset by listlessness [*negghienza*] will rest.
> And one of them, who seemed to me exhausted [*lasso*],
> was sitting with his arms around his knees;
> between his knees, he kept his head bent down.
> "O my sweet lord," I said, "look carefully
> at one who shows himself more languid [*negligente*] than
> he would have been were laziness [*pigrizia*] his sister!"
> Then that shade turned toward us attentively,
> lifting his eyes, but just above his thigh,
> and said: "Climb, then, if you're so vigorous!"[37]

At this point, Dante recognizes his friend Belacqua, who appears to have been a Florentine musical-instrument maker renowned for his legendary laziness during Dante's lifetime. Dante is struck by the slowness of his friend's movements, the brevity of his speech, and the fact that he lifts his eyes just high enough to be able to see his visitors. Dante asks Belacqua why he sits there and whether he has fallen back into his old lazy habits. Belacqua responds:

> Oh brother, what's the use of climbing?
> God's angel, he who guards the gate, would not
> let me pass through to meet my punishment.
> Outside that gate the skies must circle round
> as many times as they did when I lived—
> since I delayed good sighs until the end—
> unless, before then, I am helped by prayer
> that rises from a heart that lives in grace;
> what use are other prayers—ignored by Heaven?[38]

Here, then, Belacqua announces that he lacks the hope and faith necessary to undertake the arduous process of repenting his sins, which, ironically, are hesitancy and sloth. He cannot muster the energy to climb Mount Purgatory, shunning the effort that would be required to achieve redemption. Belacqua's predicament illustrates one of the primary paradoxes of the acedic condition, and also of recent debates of the "active patient" experiencing chronic fatigue and/or depression:[39] to be able to free oneself from acedia, one needs to have the willpower, the optimism, and the energy to take the necessary first steps. However, the condition is of course manifest precisely in a weakening of the will and a lack of energy.

As Dante and his guide progress from the third to the fourth terrace of Mount Purgatory, Virgil lectures his charge on love. He explains that all the Seven Deadly Sins result from one of three sinful forms of love:

- Love that chooses an evil object, such as wishing evil on one's fellow human beings (as in pride, envy, and wrath)
- Love that chooses a good object (God), but the strength of which may be defective (sloth)
- Love that does not choose God or the supreme Good as its chief object but material goods that are desired to excess, such as money, food, drink, and sex (as in avarice, gluttony, and lust)

In purgatory, the human will is purified of all these defective kinds of love: one by one, those who climb the seven terraces of the mountain are purged of their antisocial desires, spiritual apathy, and material obsessions.[40]

According to Dante, then, the slothful are guilty of a love of the good that is lacking in vigor or energy. They do not feel aversion to the divine good, as Aquinas proposed; rather, their commitment to it is simply too lukewarm and tepid. It is striking that Dante grows drowsy once again during Virgil's lecture, betraying his own tendency to exhaustion, which clearly is his own cardinal spiritual failing. When he recovers his energy, he beholds the slothful compelled to run around without respite, their punishment being endless activity, to counter the lack of activity that characterized their earthly life. The sinners who rush past Dante and his guide are wild and frenzied, noisy and chaotic, forever deprived of the rest they cherished too much in the past:

> Just as—of old—Ismenus and Asopus,
> at night, along their banks, saw crowds and clamor
> whenever Thebans had to summon Bacchus,
> such was the arching crowd that curved around
> that circle, driven on, as I made out,
> by righteous will as well as by just love.
> Soon all that mighty throng drew near us, for
> they ran and ran[.][41]

Two of the penitent slothful shout out examples of biblical and historical figures whose actions illustrate zeal—one of the virtues opposed to sloth. Others urge haste, crying:

> Quick, quick,
> Lest time be lost through insufficient love;
> where urge for good is keen, grace finds new green.[42]

The crowd of repentant idlers, in whom "eager fervor now / may compensate for [the] sloth and negligence [*negligenza e indugio*]" they exhibited in "doing good half-heartedly," are so anxious to advance that they cannot even stop to converse with Dante.[43] Two shadows at the back of the crowd denounce famous examples of sloth from the Bible and from Virgil's *Aeneid*. The first reference is to the Israelites during their exodus from Egypt. Ungrateful and unappreciative of the divine intervention that saved them, many perished before reaching the promised land. The second example is the Trojans who settled halfway in Sicily rather than following Aeneas all the way on his voyage to Italy.[44]

After having listened to these cautionary tales, Dante falls asleep once again. When he wakes, he finds an angel crouching next to him and administering beatitude. The beatitude for the fourth terrace is *Beati qui lugent* ("Blessed are those who mourn, for they will be comforted" [Matthew 5:4]), which once again blurs the boundary between melancholia (associated with sadness) and acedia. The angel removes the fourth *P* (which signifies *peccatum* [sin]) from Dante's forehead, and he is thereafter purged of the sin of sloth.

The more *P*s Dante sheds, and the closer he comes to paradise, the lighter and more energetic his step becomes. Eventually he asks his master:

> "Tell me, what heavy
> weight has been lifted from me, so that I
> in going, notice almost no fatigue [*che nulla quasi per me*
>   *fatica, andando, si riceve*]?"
> He answered: "When the *P*'s that still remain
> upon your brow—now almost all are faint—
> have been completely, like this *P*, erased,
> your feet will be so mastered by good will
> that they not only will not feel travail
> but will delight when they are urged uphill."[45]

Physical and spiritual exhaustion in *The Divine Comedy* are eventually overcome, then, by repentance, purification from sin, and recommitting properly to God and the divine good. Dante illustrates this point by showing how the metaphorical gravity of sin literally weighs down not just the spiritual but also the physical body. Exhaustion is both a consequence of spiritual sin and a sign of weakness of the exertion-shunning flesh. Those blessed by divine grace will gladly accept the call to both physical and spiritual labor and will never again experience the exhaustion that threatens to interrupt Dante's journey. Stirred into action by his guide, Dante leaves his exhausted former friend Belacqua behind him, in the shadow of a great rock. For the truly exhausted, who have lost their faith both in God and in a better future, there can in Dante's world be no hope of salvation. Yet even Dante would never have been able to overcome his exhaustion without the help of Virgil, his spiritual guide and mentor figure, who leads him both metaphorically and literally from darkness into the light.

3
Saturn

An important contributor to the scholarly rediscovery of texts from the classical tradition that ushered in the Renaissance, the fifteenth-century Italian humanist Marsilio Ficino (1433–1499) also breathed new life into the link between melancholia, art, and genius. Like many before him, Ficino considers fear and sadness to be the core symptoms of melancholia, but he also counts weariness, lethargy, apathy, hopelessness, and pessimism among its related symptoms. Moreover, in *Three Books on Life* (1489), he proposes various cures that draw on the powers of the celestial bodies to reenergize the exhausted. He was the first to address the specific forms of mental and physical exhaustion experienced by scholars in a lengthy medical-spiritual treatise.

Ficino was both a Neo-Platonist scholar and a priest and was interested in medicine, astrology, magic, and music. He claims that he had two fathers: Diotifeci Ficino of Figline in Valdarno, who was a medical doctor, and the wealthy and powerful banker Cosimo de' Medici, who became his patron and encouraged him to found the Platonic Academy in Florence: "From the former I was born, from the latter reborn. The former commended me to Galen as both a doctor and a Platonist; the latter consecrated me to the divine Plato. And both the one and the other alike dedicated Marsilio to a doctor—Galen, doctor of the body, Plato, doctor of the soul." The most important duty of priests and doctors alike, Ficino believes, is "to see to it that men have a sound mind in a sound body. . . . But since medicine is quite often useless and often harmful without the help of the heavens—a thing which both Hippocrates and Galen admit and I have experienced—astronomy certainly pertains to this priestly charity no less than does medicine."[1]

Ficino translated Plato into Latin and wrote treatises on a wide range of subjects, including pestilence, Plotinus, and the music of the spheres. Born under the sign of Saturn, moreover, he also endeavored to revalorize the saturnine temperament in *Three Books on Life* and to free it from its traditionally negative connotations. "Saturn seems to have impressed the seal of melancholy on me from the beginning," he writes in a letter to a friend; "set, as he is, almost in the midst of my ascendant Aquarius, he is influenced by Mars, also in Aquarius, and the Moon in Capricorn. He is in square aspect to the Sun and Mercury in Scorpio, which occupy the ninth house."[2]

According to the astrological and Neo-Platonist doctrines in which Ficino believed, the planets influence numerous aspects of life on Earth—just as the moon rules the waters and governs the movement of ebb and tide, and the female menstrual cycle. In Ficino's cosmos, everything revolves around the principle of analogy: the microcosm is mirrored in the macrocosm; all material things have their equivalent in immaterial ideas; and all matter ultimately corresponds to and reverberates with other matter. Astrological doctrine suggests that the movement and positions of the celestial bodies at the time of a person's birth determine his or her character, disposition, and energy level, and even profession, talents, and significant events later in life. The positions of the planets are analyzed by their geometric aspects relative to one another and by their movements through spatial divisions of the ecliptic and the sky—that is, the signs of the zodiac and their positions in the so-called houses. It is, above all, the planet on the ascendant at the hour of one's birth, it was assumed, that imprints its own qualities on those who are born under its sign.

Saturn and Mars have traditionally been viewed as harmful planets, associated with misfortune and a host of disagreeable psychological qualities. Saturn's image was particularly gloomy: the slowest moving of the planets, and the one with the longest circuit, it was aligned with fear, coldness, and dryness. Similarly, in debates about whether the melancholic or the phlegmatic temperament is more disagreeable, melancholia usually won the day.[3] Yet in *Three Books on Life*, Ficino not only presents the first medical treatise dedicated specifically to the mental and physical health of the scholar but also seeks to revalorize the melancholic temperament and its related characteristics. Driven partly by personal motives, Ficino presents the saturnine disposition as one that is, or can be if fostered and nourished in the correct manner, closely connected with scholarship and genius.

Emphasizing Saturn's benign qualities—above all, perseverance, patience, steadfastness, and concentration—Ficino presents a peculiar mixture of humoral, Neo-Platonic, alchemical, and magical cures for those born under the planet's sign. His therapeutics are designed primarily to revitalize and reenergize those worn down by the negative and exhausting side effects of the saturnine disposition, such as fatigue, torpor, sluggishness, and dullness, as well as fear, sadness, madness, and frenzy. Building on the authority of Aristotle or, rather, the Pseudo-Aristotle of *Problemata* 30.1, who lavishes extended praise on melancholia and aligns it with genius and art, Ficino, too, argues that a melancholic nature is "a unique and divine gift."[4] His *Three Books on Life* were highly influential during his lifetime and ushered in what would become a veritable melancholia fashion in Europe, which was evidenced, for example, by the immense popularity of Robert Burton's *Anatomy of Melancholy* (1621) and which culminated two centuries later in the Romantic celebration of hypersensitivity, world-weariness, and artistic genius.

As the title suggests, the *Three Books* consist of three separate parts. Book 1, *On a Healthy Life* or *On Caring for the Health of Learned People*, is primarily medical in outlook, drawing on Galen's humoral theory. Book 2, *On a Long Life*, deals with the health concerns of older people and contains practical suggestions for living a long and energy-abundant life. The final book, *On Obtaining a Life Both Healthy and Long from Heaven*, is dedicated to astrological magic and how it can be deployed to reinvigorate worn-out bodies and minds. Synthesizing medical, astrological, and philosophical discourses, it is without doubt the book that is most challenging for the modern reader, owing not just to the now discredited assumptions of Ptolemaic astronomy but also to Ficino's belief in Neo-Platonic concepts, such as the existence of a world-soul, various "supramundane" or "supracelestial" gods, the intelligence of the spheres, star-souls, and a host of demons of varying moral allegiances. Ficino believes that there are three worlds: the terrestrial, the celestial, and the angelic. He conceives of the heavenly bodies as intermediaries, copies of pure Platonic ideas, whose task it is to intercede between the material and the immaterial worlds.[5]

In Book 1, *On a Healthy Life*, Ficino warns scholars not to neglect body and spirit. The spirit, in particular, is the instrument

> with which they are able in a way to measure and grasp the whole world. [It] is defined by doctors as a vapor of blood— pure, subtle, hot, and clear. After being generated by the heat of the heart out of the more subtle blood, it flies to the brain; and there the soul uses it continually for the exercise of the interior as well as the exterior senses. This is why the blood subserves the spirit; the spirit, the senses; and finally, the senses, reason.[6]

The idea that spirit is a "vapor of blood . . . generated by the heat of the heart" is a surprisingly materialistic definition of spirit for a Neo-Platonist and aptly illustrates Ficino's often conflicting intellectual allegiances. He proposes three causes of melancholia in the learned: the first being celestial; the second, natural; and the third, human. The celestial causes can be explained by the fact that

> both Mercury, who invites us to investigate doctrines, and Saturn, who makes us persevere in investigating doctrines and retain them when discovered, are said by astronomers to be somewhat cold and dry . . . , just like the melancholic nature, according to physicians. And this same nature Mercury and Saturn impart from birth to their followers, learned people, and preserve and augment it day by day.[7]

The second (and natural) cause of melancholia lies in the fact that the soul of those engaged in the sciences, especially the difficult ones, "must draw in upon itself from external things to internal as from the circumference to the center." Furthermore, the scholarly soul must stay immovably at the center, and to be fixed in the center, Ficino believes, is above all the "property of the Earth itself, to which black bile is analogous."[8] Therefore, he argues,

> black bile continually incites the soul both to collect itself together into one and to dwell on itself and to contemplate itself. And being analogous to the world's center, it forces the investigation to the center of individual subjects, and it carries one to the contemplation of whatever is highest, since, indeed, it is most congruent with Saturn, the highest of planets. Contemplation itself, in its turn, by a continual recollection and compression, as it were, brings on a nature similar to black bile.[9]

The third (and human) cause of melancholia in scholars identified by Ficino is once again based on a materialistic conception of the relationship between mind and body: frequent agitation, he argues, "greatly dries up the brain," exhausts all reserves of bodily moisture, and, as a consequence, extinguishes all heat. The brain becomes dry and cold, and, as a result of the relentless activity of intellectual inquiry, the spirit, too, is gradually depleted. The spent spiritual substance has to be replenished from the subtle and clear parts of the blood, which is thus also exhausted. The blood that remains is consequently rendered "dense, dry and black," resembling black bile. Furthermore, the scholar's dependence on the brain and the heart means that less blood and energy can flow to the stomach and the liver. Therefore, foods, especially fatty ones, are not properly digested. Finally, a lack of physical exercise, common among sedentary scholars, means that "thick, dense, clinging, dusky vapors" are not sufficiently purged.

It is Ficino's second point about the link between melancholia and the activity of self-contemplation that constitutes his most interesting and original contribution to the corpus of exhaustion theories. Unlike Galen, who believed that the spirit was a slave to the mixtures of the body, and unlike the medieval theologians, who understood acedic exhaustion as the result of a moral and spiritual failing, Ficino proposes that exhaustion can be the result of specific mental activities. Black bile, he writes, "continually incites the soul both to collect itself together into one and to dwell on itself and to contemplate itself." This statement reveals most clearly the way in which he seeks to redefine the melancholic temperament as positive: Ficino aligns it not only with scholarship and the ability to contemplate abstract philosophical questions but also with the quality of self-reflexivity as such.

The early modern period is often seen as being characterized above all by the birth of the self-reflexive, self-aware subject, the individual who questions established values and authorities, and who reflects on his or her own status as a thinking and evaluating being. William Shakespeare's *Hamlet* (1603) illustrates this changing paradigm: Hamlet can be interpreted as a representation of the acedic and melancholic type, and his story as a cautionary tale about the adverse effects of introspection.[10] Walter Benjamin, for example, writes: "The indecisiveness of the prince, in particular, is nothing other than saturnine *acedia*. Saturn causes people to be 'apathetic, indecisive, slow.' The fall of the tyrant is caused by indolence of the heart."[11] G. F. Hegel presents a similar interpretation: Hamlet's "noble soul is not made for this kind of energetic activity; and, full of disgust with the world and life . . . he eventually perishes owing to his own hesitation and a complication of external circumstances."[12]

Incapable of blindly following the old ways (that is, simply to avenge the murder of his father by killing Claudius, his uncle), Hamlet is also unable to break with the avenger's role. He is paralyzed by a form of self-reflexivity that has become an instrument of self-torture rather than enlightenment. His critical self-awareness has turned into a curse; the ability to think through a problem and to look at it from various angles results in inaction and self-loathing. Trapped in a state of pathological indecisiveness as a result of a perverted form of self-analysis that is both exhaustive and exhausting, he not only fails to solve his original problem but provokes further catastrophes and bloodshed.

The burden of contemplative self-reflexivity, and the way in which it literally weighs down the new scientifically orientated subject, are also illustrated by Albrecht Dürer's famous engraving *Melencolia I* (1514). It shows a despondent female figure who, with her head in her hand, sits surrounded by the scattered paraphernalia of science and art, staring gloomily into the distance. She listlessly holds a geometrical tool in her lap but is too weary to use it. An hourglass in the background signals that she is wasting time and that it is running out; a set of empty scales indicates that she may have lost her sense of balance; a scattering of tools suggest that she has probably worked too hard and on too many projects simultaneously; and an emaciated, sleeping dog and a limp, depressed-looking putto with a bowed head further reinforce the all-pervasive sense of exhaustion. Although the tools of critical reasoning and the keys to facilitate access to various spheres of knowledge are within touching distance, the woman is, like Hamlet, simply too weary to act, weighed down by the boundless possibilities and responsibilities that come with her newly gained status as a self-reflexive subject.

In *The Weariness of the Self: Diagnosing the History of Depression in the Contemporary Age* (1998), the French sociologist Alain Ehrenberg describes a similar struggle with the burden of autonomy and the responsibility for constant self-improvement and self-realization, a "terrible," new kind of freedom that is perceived as an affliction rather than an opportunity, and that he sees as being responsible for the rapid spread of depression-related illnesses in the post–Second World War period. Yet Ficino's, Shakespeare's, and Dürer's examples reveal that self-reflexivity and an awareness of the range of possible choices a contemplative, self-aware subject faces were considered a profoundly exhausting burden many centuries earlier. Indeed, the birth of the modern subject in the fifteenth century might be seen as entailing a sense that exhaustion is a necessary correlative of self-consciousness as such.

✳ ✳ ✳

Ficino also distinguishes between natural and pathological melancholia. Following Galen's argument on melancholic vapors and adustion, he states that when an excess of melancholic humor is burned, its fumes cloud our judgment and render us excitable and frenzied. However, when it is extinguished and only a "foul black soot remains, it makes people stolid and stupid." This pathological form of melancholia, he hastens to emphasize, is not at all conducive to genius and scholarship. By contrast, the natural—that is, the temperamental—form of melancholia can lead to refined judgment, perseverance, and wisdom. But, Ficino warns, this is not automatically the case:

> If [black bile] is alone, it beclouds the spirit with a mass that is black and dense, terrifies the soul, and dulls the intelligence. Moreover, if it is mixed simply with phlegm, when "cold blood" stands in the way "around the heart" it brings on sluggishness and torpor by its heavy frigidity; and as is the nature of any very dense material, when melancholy of this kind gets cold, it gets cold in the extreme. When we are in this state, we hope for nothing, we fear everything, and "it is weariness to look at the dome of the sky." . . . When [black bile] is too abundant, whether alone or joined with phlegm, it makes the spirits heavier and colder, afflicts the mind continually with weariness, dulls the sharpness of the intellect, and keeps the blood from leaping "around the Arcadian's heart."[13]

Black bile mixed with phlegm, then, can induce sluggishness, lethargy, and hopelessness. Excessive amounts of black bile can lead to both mental and physical fatigue and cognitive impairments, as well as slowing the movement of the blood. Yet Ficino concludes that black bile as such is not harmful, provided that it is rarefied and mixed with other humors. Combined with appropriate amounts of phlegm, yellow bile, and blood, this humor, too, can unfold its beneficent characteristics. Like Hippocrates and Galen before him, Ficino argues that the right mixture of humors is the prerequisite for both physical and mental health. Black bile differs from the other humors principally in its tendency toward extreme states: "For black bile is like iron; when it starts to get cold, it gets cold in the extreme; and on the contrary, once it tends towards hot, it gets hot in the extreme." It thus needs to be tempered by the more moderate humors. Melancholia, too, is of course a state of extremes: either its sufferers are agitated, frenzied, mad, and furious or they are subdued, weary, fearful, and hopeless. Therefore, those born under the sign of Saturn, and who are battling with an excess of black bile, need above all to learn to explore the states of mind located on the spectrum between the polar extremes.

Ficino also singles out specific behaviors that can adversely affect a scholar's natural proclivity to melancholic exhaustion and deplete his energies: among these, he counts sexual intercourse, gluttony, and sleeping in the morning. Just like the eighteenth- and nineteenth-century campaigners against masturbation, Ficino strongly believes that the loss of seminal fluid drains the spirits, weakens the brain, and ruins the stomach and the heart. Overindulging in wine and food, too, is harmful, as excessive consumption directs all human energy to the stomach and to the task of digestion. Finally, Ficino identifies staying awake during the night and sleeping after sunrise as crimes against the cosmic rhythm: the man who sleeps during the day "no doubt fights both with the order of the universe and especially with himself, while he is disturbed and distracted by contrary motions at the same time." Scholars, in particular, need to rest regularly, to give their minds the opportunity to recuperate and relax, since "fatigue of the body is bad, that of the mind is worse, and the worst is fatigue of both at the same time, distracting the person by opposite but simultaneous motions and ruining life."[14]

The main component of Ficino's therapeutic regime designed to battle melancholic exhaustion is dietetics. He compiles long lists of forbidden foods and strongly promotes the beneficial qualities of others, especially cinnamon, saffron, and sandal. He is also fond of dairy products, pine nuts, melon and cucumber seeds, light wine, gold and silver infusions, salads, and raisins. Furthermore, he praises the healing powers of sweet lyres and song and recommends "the frequent viewing of shining water and of green or red color, the haunting of gardens and groves and pleasant walks along rivers and through lovely meadows; and I also strongly approve of horseback riding, driving, and smooth sailing, but above all, of variety, easy occupations, diversified unburdensome business, and the constant company of agreeable people."[15]

He provides recipes for various energizing syrups, pills, and electuaries. One of his pills, which he calls the golden or magical one, is designed to draw out phlegm, choler, and black bile; to strengthen the body; and to sharpen and illuminate the spirits, so that they "may rejoice in their expansion and light":

> Take, therefore, twelve grains of gold, especially its leaves if they are pure; one-half dram apiece of frankincense, myrrh, saffron, aloe-wood, cinnamon, citron-peel, Melissa, raw carlet silk, white ben and red; one dram apiece of purple roses, of red sandal, or red coral, and of the three sorts of myrobalans (emblic, chebule, and Indic), with an amount of properly washed aloe equal to the weight of all the rest. Make pills with pure wine of the best possible quality.[16]

The recommendation of specific dietary regimes is a staple in the corpus of exhaustion theories: most therapeutic suggestions proposed by figures as diverse as Galen, George Cheyne, Richard von Krafft-Ebing, Silas Weir Mitchell, and various practitioners and popular writers interested in chronic fatigue syndrome revolve around cutting out specific food groups and promoting the inclusion of others.

In Book 3, *On Obtaining a Life Both Healthy and Long from Heaven*, Ficino's cures become even more esoteric and drift from the terrain of humoral medicine into that of astrological magic. Here, he seeks to draw on the natural powers of the celestial bodies and to enlist the services of various demons to reinvigorate the exhausted bodies and minds of his readers. The therapeutics suggested in the final part of his study are based on the principle of cosmic sympathy, an all-encompassing macro-microcosm analogy.[17] Ficino believes that various materials, such as stones, metals, and talismans, as well as certain herbs and spices, contain the quintessence of the "world soul" and can thus enable us to enter into a closer relationship with the world of ideas. For example, "orphic dancing"—that is, movements and music that echo the movements of the spheres—can be invigorating and calming. Song imitating the celestials "wonderfully arouses our spirit upwards to the celestial influence and the celestial influence downwards to our spirit."[18]

The key common property of the human species, Ficino proposes, is solar. He infers this to be the case "from the stature of man, erect and beautiful, from his subtle humors and the clearness of his spirit, from the perspicuity of his imagination and his pursuit of truth and honor." To replenish his energy, man should therefore surround himself above all with things solar, which are

> all those gems and flowers which are called heliotrope because they turn towards the Sun, likewise gold, orpiment and golden colors, chrysolite, carbuncle, myrrh, frankincense, musk, amber, balsam, yellow honey, sweet calamus, saffron, spikenard, cinnamon, aloe-wood and the rest of the spices; the ram, the hawk, the cock, the swan, the lion, the scarab beetle, the crocodile, and people who are blond, curly-haired, prone to baldness, and magnanimous. The above-mentioned things can be adapted partly to foods, partly to ointments and fumigations, partly to usages and habits. You should frequently perceive and think about these things and love them above all; you should also get a lot of light.[19]

Saturn, in contrast, does not represent the common quality and lot of the human race, but only that of individuals "set apart from others, divine or brutish, blessed or bowed down with the extreme of misery." Those born under the planet's sign should "beg grace from that star rather than from another, and to await from any given star not just any gift and what belongs to other stars, but a gift proper to that one." For the purpose of reenergizing the children of Saturn, Ficino thus recommends materials that are "somewhat earthy, dusky and leaden; we use smoky jasper, lodestone, cameo, and chalcedony; gold and golden marcasite are partly useful for this." He defends Saturn against the charge of being harmful by nature and instead suggests that the planet's unique gifts should be used "just as doctors sometimes use poisons: . . . The force of Saturn, therefore, cautiously taken, will sometimes profit, just as doctors say those things do which are astringent and constrictive, even those things which stupefy, as opium and mandrake." According to the macro-microcosm analogy, Saturn both resembles and shapes the intellectual because he is the head of the widest sphere and travels a lengthy circuit: "He is the highest of planets; hence they call that man fortunate whom Saturn fortunately favors."[20]

Essentially, *Three Books on Life* propagates the combination of the powers of medicine, religion, and astrology to replenish human energies and thus to counter an exhaustion seen to threaten human life as such. Astrological doctrine does of course suggest a largely deterministic worldview, in that our fate is assumed to be predetermined or at least substantially shaped by stellar constellations on which we have no influence. However, Ficino is quick to deny this charge: he repeatedly asserts the importance of free will, agency, and the responsibility of individuals to improve and enhance their fate. The gifts from the celestial bodies come into our bodies through our rightly prepared spirit: we need to understand who we are and what are the forces that shape us, and we can reach our full potential only when we, "by prayer, by study, by manner of life, and by conduct imitate the beneficence, action, and order of the celestials." To live well and prosper, it is essential to know one's "natural bent" and one's beneficial personal star.[21] Living in harmony with one's celestial patron enables us fully to tap into our energy reserves, while battling against the order of the universe will result in complete exhaustion: the heavens will feel like our personal enemy, drain our resources, and thwart our efforts, and all our labors will be in vain.

❊ ❊ ❊

In *The Rings of Saturn* (1995), the German writer W. G. Sebald (1944–2001) revives the age-old connection between astrology and mood. Sebald's essayistic and partly fictional, partly autobiographical text, in which an existentially depressed and increasingly world-weary narrator wanders through a ruin-strewn East Anglia, is based on his "pilgrimage" through Suffolk in 1992, which culminated in a nervous breakdown exactly one year later. Convalescing in the hospital, while still suffering from various, possibly psycho-somatic, ailments, including severe mental, spiritual, and physical exhaustion manifest in complete paralysis, Sebald's narrator recollects the details of his journey. It took place in August—a time of year traditionally thought to be under the influence of the dark forces of Saturn. During his wanderings, he contemplates the material traces of human history, a history that, in his view, is above all characterized by calamities and cruelty. The narrator's gaze is that of a severe melancholic, unfailingly drawn to that which is dead, dying, decaying, or vanishing. He finds evidence of human callousness and nature's indifference to our plight in the most innocent-looking flotsam and jetsam, and every object he contemplates inevitably sets in motion a process of association that builds up to yet another case in point proving the cruelty, frailty, and pointlessness of human existence and the transient nature of all our passions and efforts.

Even the sight of a seemingly innocuous dish of fish and chips, served in an empty seaside guesthouse, appears to him "dreadful." Sebald's description of the dish is reminiscent of that of a war zone or of a site where a massacre has taken place: "The tartare sauce that I had had to squeeze out of a plastic sachet was turned grey [*gräulich*] by the sooty breadcrumbs, and the fish itself, or what feigned to be fish, lay a sorry wreck among the grass-green peas and the remains of soggy chips that gleamed with fat."[22] This plate of food, like everything else he encounters on his wanderings, is viewed through a glass darkly and illustrates the ways in which someone whose judgment and perceptive apparatus are clouded by melancholia might perceive and interpret phenomena: Sebald here conjures up imagery of rust, destruction, decay, and ruins. The German word *gräulich* denotes both grayness and horror. Moreover, the dish reminds Sebald of the terrible misfortunes that herrings, the "restless wanderer[s] of the seas," suffer on a daily basis at the hands of an uncaring fishing industry and leads him to question whether the unremitting, grand-scale fish genocides that are taking place in our oceans are ethically justifiable.[23] We simply don't know anything about the inner life of the herring, Sebald muses, and therefore cannot know whether they are able to feel fear and pain like we do.

The long sentences of a seventeenth-century medical writer that meander cumbersomely across the pages remind him of "sentences that resemble processions or a funeral cortège in their sheer ceremonial lavishness." Sebald describes the decaying seaside town of Lowestoft, one of the many victims of Margaret Thatcher's neoliberal economic policies, in characteristically gloomy terms:

> The damage spread slowly at first, smouldering underground, and then caught like wildfire. The wharves and factories closed down one after the other. . . . Nowadays, in some of the streets almost every other house is up for sale; factory owners, shopkeepers and private individuals are sliding ever deeper into debt; week in, week out, some bankrupt or unemployed person hangs himself; nearly a quarter of the population is now practically illiterate; and there is no sign of an end to the encroaching misery. Although I knew all of this, I was unprepared for the feeling of wretchedness that instantly seized hold of me in Lowestoft.[24]

In the course of his pilgrimage, Sebald is drawn not only to ruins of all kinds, to decaying manor houses and disaster zones, but also to English eccentrics, many of whom are collectors of strange objects and have curious obsessions to which they dedicate all their time. To the narrator, their peculiar projects and collectibles emphasize further the absurdity of human existence and the arbitrary and futile nature of our efforts and desires. Sights that would evoke neutral or even positive associations in non-melancholic observers consistently remind him of monstrosities, acts of barbarism, and the inevitability of death: a couple making love on a beach, for example, which he observes from afar, makes him think of the last shudders of a hanged man and a beastly sea monster, the last of its kind: "Misshapen, like some great mollusk washed ashore, they lay there, to all appearances a single being, a many-limbed, two-headed monster that had drifted in from far out at sea, the last of a prodigious species, its life ebbing from it with each breath expired through its nostrils."[25]

The title of Sebald's text suggests a causal link between Saturn and his narrator's unremittingly disconsolate thoughts on the history of human cruelty, which render him increasingly hopeless and weary and drain him ever more insistently of the will to live, and references to the planet's gloomy powers are woven into the fabric of numerous reflections. Saturn is mentioned, for example, in a passage on the night in Thomas Browne's writings that chimes with the narrator's own sad song: "The shadow of night is drawn like a black veil across the earth, and since almost all creatures, from one meridian to the next, lie down after the sun has set, so, he continues, one might, in following the setting sun, see on our globe nothing but prone bodies, row upon row, as if levelled by the scythe of Saturn—an endless graveyard for a humanity struck by falling sickness."[26]

Saturn here is associated with prostration, graveyards, and the Grim Reaper. Sebald's narrator is drawn again and again to "chronicle[s] of disaster," including historical volumes that detail the horrors of the First World War, such as sinking battleships, plane crashes, the perishing masses in the swamps of Galicia, bombed cities, corpses rotting in the trenches, burst zeppelins, and many other "scenes of destruction, mutilation, desecration, starvation, conflagration, and freezing cold." One of the many calamities that preoccupy him and on which he reflects in some detail is the story of a devastating drought in China between 1876 and 1879, which claimed the lives of millions who died of exhaustion and hunger:

> A Baptist preacher named Timothy Richard, for example, noted that one effect of the catastrophe, which grew more apparent week by week, was that all movement was slowing down. Singly, in groups and in straggling lines, people tottered across the country, and the merest breath of air might suffice to topple them and leave them lying by the wayside forever. Simply raising a hand, closing an eyelid, or exhaling one's last breath might take, it sometimes seemed, half a century. And as time dissolved, so too did all other relations.[27]

Here, it is the description of the physical and behavioral symptoms of exhaustion—the slowing of movement, the astonishing effort that even such small gestures as raising a hand or lowering an eyelid require, and the gradual loss of strength—that must have chimed with the narrator's own experiences. They provide an apt image of his own melancholic exhaustion, which is represented as a form of existential hopelessness that is philosophical and historical in origin. The narrator is saddened so severely by the horrors of history that he loses all hope in the future of humanity.

It is, above all, the memory of the Holocaust that haunts Sebald's text. Sebald left Germany to work at the University of Manchester from 1966 to 1969 and, after a year in St. Gallen in Switzerland, accepted a teaching position at Norwich University in 1970, never to return permanently to Germany. Although he does not explicitly mention the Third Reich in *The Rings of Saturn* and instead focuses on tales of dreadfulness, suffering, and cruelty from other historical periods, it becomes ever more obvious that it is the unbearable memory of recent German history and the horrific cruelties carried out by his countrymen that weigh on the narrator and deprive him ever more of his energy, his faith in humanity, and, ultimately, his will to live. Human existence appears to him as nothing but a grand theater of cruelty and absurdity, and, fittingly, his body expresses his philosophical misgivings by succumbing to complete paralysis at the end of his journey into the heart of saturnine darkness.

✳ ✳ ✳

The Danish director Lars von Trier, too, pays homage to the ancient tradition that links melancholia and Saturn in his film *Melancholia* (2011), in which two sisters prepare for an apocalyptic clash between Earth and the rogue planet Melancholia, which has entered Earth's orbit. The sisters Justine (Kirsten Dunst) and Clare (Charlotte Gainsbourg) are both of a melancholic disposition, Justine being prone to existential weariness and extreme physical and mental exhaustion, while Clare is firmly in the grip of fear. Trier assigns one of the age-old core symptoms of melancholia, sadness and fear, to each sister, thus acknowledging the different guises in which melancholia can manifest itself. Part 1 of the film is dedicated to Justine's story. A beautiful advertising executive, Justine succumbs to a severe form of depression on her wedding night and, unable to keep her true feelings hidden and to participate in the lavish celebration organized in her honor on her sister's luxurious estate, loses both her husband and her job.

Although, on the surface, Justine's sadness seems "causeless," the onset of her depression appearing to be triggered by a celestial constellation and the foreboding sense of the arrival of the planet Melancholia, this reading does not hold. Rather than representing her as unreasonable, Trier shows that Justine is in fact a realist, someone who can see through social convention and who understands life as what it really is: a pointless and cruel game with no purpose, structured around empty and meaningless ritual. In various interviews, Trier emphasized that the key idea for the film came to him in a therapy session, when his analyst told him that depressives tend to be more level-headed in the face of impending disaster, since they expect the worst and, when the worst happens, are consequently less surprised.[28] Justine is very much based on Trier's own experience of depression, and *Melancholia*, together with *Antichrist* (2009) and *Nymphomaniac* (2013), forms a part of what he describes as his "depression trilogy." *Antichrist* is dedicated to the exploration of excessive grief, while *Nymphomaniac* analyzes the anatomy of addiction.

Trier carefully establishes various triggers for Justine's mental and physical breakdown, these being psychological, sociopolitical, and philosophical. Justine's connection with her new husband seems lifeless from the start—although he appears to be in love with her, he is not her intellectual match. Unable to articulate his feelings and reverting to clichés in his short and embarrassing wedding-supper speech, he fails both to read and to halt his bride's dramatic change of mood. Justine's parents, too, let her down in her hour of need. Her mother delivers a cynical and bitter address, in which she attacks the idea of marriage and love, and repeatedly advises Justine to get out of it all as quickly as she can. Justine's father is preoccupied with flirting and clowning, and although his daughter repeatedly begs him to stay because she urgently needs to speak to him, he leaves his room at night, having been unable to resist the offer of a ride home. Justine's unappetizing boss spends the evening trying to bully her into supplying a tagline for an advertising campaign, until she explodes and tells him what she really thinks of him and of the marketing business in general.

Even Clare is unsympathetic to Justine's breakdown. She is bitterly disappointed by her sister's lack of gratitude for the wedding party she has organized and cannot understand why Justine is unable at least to keep up the masquerade until everyone has left. At one point during the wedding party, Justine withdraws into a study and begins to tear down the art books that are on display there. She replaces the abstract Kazimir Malevich prints with images that externalize her state of mind, including Pieter Brueghel's *Hunters in the Snow* and John Everett Millais's painting of the drowned Ophelia. It becomes obvious that she longs for death—for snow, stillness, the end of everything. Her death wish is, of course, ultimately granted when the cataclysmic planetary collision takes place. The overture to Richard Wagner's opera *Tristan and Isolde*, which opens and closes the film, as well as the highly aestheticized cinematography and stylized images of the catastrophe further emphasize the powerful pull of the death drive: the end, to Justine, is a thing of absolute, sublime beauty, the glorious fulfillment of her greatest desire.

Justine's mental and physical decline after the wedding night is rapid—she is so exhausted that she cannot wash herself and is barely able to leave her room. She describes her condition to her sister as akin to wading through a field of gray yarn, which is slowing her movements and pulling her to the ground. She drags herself around the house like a zombie and breaks into tears during a meal because, to her, all food tastes like ashes. The film opens with a close-up of her postwedding face—an image epitomizing absolute exhaustion: her hair is limp and unwashed; her eyes are droopy and clouded, and she can barely manage to keep them open; her complexion is ashen; and her ice-blue lips are drained of all blood.

When eventually catastrophe does strike, however, Justine is the only one who is able to cope. Clare's rich, rational husband, John (Kiefer Sutherland), turns out to be a coward who kills himself when he realizes that Melancholia has not passed Earth, as he believed it would, but is indeed on collision course with it. Clare, having been obsessed with the planetary clash for months, becomes increasingly unhinged and hysterical, and, on the day the world literally ends, Justine is the one who takes control and who appeases Clare's little boy. She builds a magic tepee—a soothing illusion that provides solace for both Clare and her son and that represents the power of art and make-believe to furnish us at least with some temporary (if illusory) protection from the horror that is reality.

Like Ficino and Sebald, Trier ultimately valorizes melancholia. The existentially depressed melancholic, although paralyzed by her condition under normal circumstances, is the only figure in this film who recognizes, and is able to cope with, the truth. All the other characters are either deluded or bitter, nihilistic, or facetious. And, of course, it is the melancholic who is associated not only with insight and knowledge but also with art and the capacity to use her imagination and creativity to provide consolation to others. The most radical message of Trier's film is that the melancholic is *right*: her worldview, her pessimism, her uncompromising perception of the sad and naked truth of human existence as determined by hypocrisy, greed, cruelty, and futility are represented as the truth in the end.

The idea that melancholic or depressed people may have a more truthful or realistic view of the world around them than the nondepressed, manifest above all in their bleakly pessimistic and self-critical outlook, is embraced even by psychoanalysts and psychologists. Sigmund Freud, for example, believed that melancholics have a "keener eye for the truth than others who are not melancholic."[29] The psychologist Shelley E. Taylor writes that normal human thought and perception

> is marked not by accuracy but positive self-enhancing illusions about the self, the world, and the future. Moreover, these illusions appear actually to be adaptive, promoting rather than undermining mental health. . . . The mildly depressed appear to have more accurate views of themselves, the world, and the future than do normal people . . . [they] clearly lack

the illusions that in normal people promote mental health and buffer them against setbacks.[30]

According to Taylor and Trier, then, it is the nondepressed who are deluded about the nature of reality. The melancholics and the depressed have simply taken off their rosy glasses and put down the shield of soothing illusions, daring to stare unprotected into the abyss of human existence. In Sebald's case, it is the confrontation with the sheer horror of the truth about human nature and human history that plunges him into a vortex of existential exhaustion. Ficino, too, acknowledges the emotional, spiritual, and cognitive burden that comes in the wake of self-reflexivity and as a consequence of the new avenues of rational and critical enquiry open to the early modern subject. However, his account is essentially optimistic: as long as we know ourselves, our strengths, our weaknesses, and of course our beneficial stars, and do not fight against our astrologically predetermined nature but instead embrace it, we can learn to explore our full potential and live rich and energy-abundant lives.

4

Sexuality

The link between exhaustion and sin, established in late antiquity and the Middle Ages by the theologians who wrote on acedia and sloth, was revived four hundred years later in eighteenth- and nineteenth-century discourses on sexuality. The eighteenth century saw a surge in anxieties related to what were taken to be sinful sexual practices, particularly masturbation. The afterlife of the partly humoral, partly theological, and partly moralistic anti-masturbation discourse first formulated in that period extended well into the nineteenth century, during which a "science of sex" (*scientia sexualis*) emerged, as biological and psychological models replaced the predominantly Christian taxonomies of sexual sin.[1]

Premodern sexual deviance was essentially seen as a crime "against nature," with the church delineating the parameters of what was "natural" and thus acceptable and normative, and the state and the community policing its boundaries.[2] In the second half of the nineteenth century, sexual deviance was no longer understood primarily in terms of sinful and immoral behavior but increasingly categorized as either normal or pathological. However, one specific, age-old humoral belief continued to haunt these new "scientific" discourses—the idea of the harmfulness of masturbation. Masturbation, it was assumed, upset the balance of the four humors and drained the individual of precious life energy, leading to permanent exhaustion and potentially even death.

The belief in the harmfulness of masturbation in particular, and excessive sexual activity in general, can be traced back to Greek antiquity and is rooted in the humoral medical system. It was generally assumed that the loss of seminal fluids brought with it a decrease in vital elements and bodily strength. Although physicians were predominantly worried about male sexual excesses, for a long time it was also assumed that females, too, emitted a less visible, ejaculation-like liquid when engaging in sexual activities and were thus also prone to experience the adverse effects of upsetting the humoral bodily economy. Pythagoreans writing in the fifth century B.C.E., for example, asserted that with each sperm secretion a part of the soul was lost. Aristotle maintained that "the loss of [semen] from the system is just as exhausting as the loss of pure healthy blood." For most men, Aristotle wrote, "the sequel to sexual intercourse is exhaustion and weakness rather than relief" because "semen has some *dynamis* [potency] within itself."[3] Galen, and most humoral physicians who adopted his theories, also believed in the highly damaging nature of seminal expulsion. Moreover, it was generally assumed that when all vital spirits are concentrated in the genitalia, the rest of the body—in particular, the brain—is left depleted of essential life energy. (A similar argument was also often made about the stomach and the dangers of overeating.) Consequently, if someone indulges in excessive sexual activities over an extended period of time, the depletion of energy in the rest of the body becomes chronic and dangerous.[4]

The medieval Arab physician Avicenna famously maintained that the loss of one part of semen was as harmful as the loss of forty parts of blood—a quantitative claim that would be much repeated in the medical literature until the advent of sexology in the late nineteenth century.[5] Marsilio Ficino, too, cites Avicenna when he writes in his *Three Books on Life* that excessive sexual intercourse is one of the primary causes for exhaustion,

> especially if it proceeds even a little beyond one's strength;
> for indeed it suddenly drains the spirits, especially the more

subtle ones, it weakens the brain, and it ruins the stomach and the heart—no evil can be worse for one's intelligence. For why did Hippocrates judge sexual intercourse to be like epilepsy, if not because it strikes the mind, which is sacred. . . . So it was with good reason that the ancients held the Muses and Minerva to be virgins.[6]

The architects of premodern conceptions of the so-called sexual perversions were ecclesiastical scholars. The most influential of these, Saint Thomas Aquinas, not only wrote on acedia but also drew up the core Christian taxonomy of sexual sins in his *Summa Theologiae*. Aquinas defines any sexual act from which procreation cannot follow as "unnatural vice." He furthermore divides unnatural vice into different species of lechery. All sins of lechery are, first, in conflict with right reason, and, second, in conflict with the "natural pattern of sexuality for the benefit of the species." The species of lechery are self-abuse (that is, masturbation), bestiality, sodomy (sex with a person of the same sex), and deviations from the natural (genital) form of intercourse such as anal and oral sex. Aquinas then compares the different modalities of lechery and draws up a hierarchy. "The gravity of a sin corresponds rather to an object being abused, than to its proper use being omitted," he reasons, and thus the lowest rank is held by the solitary sin masturbation, while the greatest sin is that of bestiality as it crosses the species barrier.[7]

It was only at the beginning of the eighteenth century that Aquinas's hierarchy of the worst sexual sins was challenged: masturbation, formerly classified as the least harmful of the unnatural vices, suddenly became the most vilified and feared act of sexual deviance. The historian Thomas Laqueur relates the sudden rise of the masturbation pandemic at the dawn of the Enlightenment to the advent of individualism and moral self-government. He identifies the privileging of the imagination, secrecy, and privacy, as well as a valorization of excess, as some of the main reasons why masturbation graduated from a marginal vice to an emblematic disease capturing the core anxieties of the modern subject. Masturbation, he writes, "became ethically central and construed as dangerous precisely when its component parts came to be valued."[8] Print culture, the novel, and solitary reading practices were not just deemed dangerous because they could stimulate the imagination in undesired ways but also considered to be essential qualities of the cultured individual. Similarly, overindulgence was both feared and celebrated, for the rapidly changing laws of the marketplace depended on a fetishization of consumer goods and on generating an ever-increasing appetite for them.

In 1712, an anonymous pamphlet, *Onania; or, the Heinous Sin of Self-Pollution, and All Its Frightful Consequences, in Both Sexes, Considered, with Spiritual and Physical Advice to Those Who Have Already Injur'd Themselves by This Abominable Practice*, written by an English quack, was the first of a number of texts that triggered what was to become known as the masturbation pandemic in the eighteenth and nineteenth centuries. The author declares as the aim of his study the promotion of "Virtue and Christian Purity" and the discouragement of "Vice and Uncleanness," and in particular "self-pollution."[9]

Apart from the fact that masturbation stands in the way of marriage, puts a stop to procreation, and is generally "displeasing to God," the author of *Onania* asserts that it also causes weakness and exhaustion, gonorrhea, nocturnal effusions, seminal emissions, gleets, oozings, infertility, and impotence.[10] Here, we can already observe a shift from a purely religious register to an increasingly medical one. Immoral action is declared to have material, organic consequences; the evocation of frightful medical scenarios, such as the loss of precious life energy, is deployed as a new pedagogical tool. Masturbation is defined as a practice that "perverts" nature because it endangers the survival of the species and thus by implication attacks God's design. Overall, *Onania* contains a curious mixture of Christian, medical, and demographic arguments, culminating in a worldly plea: afflicted readers are urged to buy the "prolifick powder" produced by the author and promising a cure from their ailments.

In 1760, a second influential treatise on masturbation appeared, written by the Swiss physician Samuel-Auguste Tissot (1728–1797). In the preface, Tissot makes explicit the change of strategy already present in *Onania*, a shift from moral appeals to the intimidating illustration of the physical consequences of immoral behavior:

> My design was to write upon the disorders occasioned by masturbation, or self-pollution, and not upon the crime of masturbation: besides, is not the crime sufficiently proved, when it is demonstrated to be an act of suicide? Those who are acquainted with men, know very well that it is much easier to make them shun vice by the dread of a present ill, than by reasons founded upon principles, the truth of which has not been sufficiently inculcated into them.[11]

Here, Tissot openly acknowledges that the suggestion of physical ailments as a result of immoral practices is a much more effective tool for convincing human beings to shun evil than are appeals to religious and moral principles. This shift is significant not only because it illustrates a secular focus on the here and now rather than the afterlife, but also because it demonstrates how and why medical arguments were more and more regularly used as pedagogic, ideological, and political tools.

Tissot consequently produces a long list of terrifying symptoms allegedly caused by the practice of masturbation. These include, above all, loss of life energy, weakness, and exhaustion, but also convulsions, sleeplessness, paleness, pimples, consumption, diarrhea, the weakening of intellectual powers, bad digestion, vomiting, anguish, paralysis, spasms, melancholy, catalepsy, epilepsy, imbecility, loss of sensation, disorders of the urinary system, and even death. Tissot still adheres to key principles of humoral theory and argues that the loss of seminal liquor causes dangerous impoverishments in the bodily economy that adversely affect the soul, the nervous system, and the senses. He, too, repeats Avicenna's formula when he writes that the loss of one ounce of seminal liquor weakens the body more than does the loss of forty ounces of blood.

Assumptions of this kind were to prevail for many years after Tissot. Many theorists of neurasthenia, for example, established a direct link between masturbation and exhaustion.[12] In his early works, even Sigmund Freud argues that masturbation substantially weakens the organism and causes lassitude in the patient. Like his eighteenth- and nineteenth-century colleagues before him, Freud believed that the fragile energy-economy of the human body could be severely damaged by the careless waste of sexual energy (libido) that occurs during the act of masturbation.[13] Sándor Ferenczi, elaborating on Freud's brief comments on the topic, believed that masturbation puts a specific strain on the sources of neuropsychological energy because "such a willed gratification requires a greater consumption of energy than the almost unconscious act of coitus."[14] Many of Freud's successors, however, abandoned this increasingly untenable biophysical argument and suggested that the loss of energy during and after masturbation was less a physical phenomenon than the result of excessive feelings of guilt.[15]

* * *

While the treatises on masturbation by the anonymous English author and Tissot were grounded primarily in a mélange of Christian dogma and humoral theory, an alternative model with which pathologies could be assessed and explained rose to prominence in the second half of the nineteenth century: the degeneration paradigm. In 1857, in his study *Treatise on Physical, Intellectual and Moral Degeneracy in the Human Species and the Causes That Produce These Diseased Varieties*, the French physician Bénédict Augustin Morel (1809–1873) introduced the idea of degeneration as a negative, retrogressive cultural development, a form of "perverse evolution," that results in the gradual weakening of certain groups of individuals and increases from generation to generation. Degeneration, in other words, was considered a form of genetic exhaustion, with dire biopolitical consequences for the strength and vigor of the nation. Morel defines degeneration in the following terms:

> The clearest notion we can form of degeneracy is to regard it as a morbid deviation from an original type. This deviation,

even if, at the outset, it was ever so slight, contained transmissible elements of such a nature that anyone bearing in him the germs becomes more and more incapable of fulfilling his functions in the world; and mental progress, already checked in his own person, finds itself menaced also in his descendants.[16]

Harry Oosterhuis argues that Morel "translated the Christian doctrine of man's regression after original sin into a biological metaphor," and that degeneration theory "signalled a crisis in the social optimism that had characterized both liberalism and positivist science."[17] Indeed, it is possible to identify the advent and rapid proliferation of degeneration theory as the point at which the Enlightenment notion of unlimited progress turned sour, when modernity began to be construed as decadence, and when both cultural and medical theorists suddenly feared a general progressive weakening not just of individual groups but of Western civilization as a whole. Although degeneration theory was based on purportedly biological arguments, it essentially pathologized behavior and qualities that were thought of as immoral, criminal, sinful, or otherwise unwelcome.

Cesare Lombroso (1836–1909), an Italian criminal anthropologist most famous for the concept of the "born criminal," further popularized degeneration theory. Another highly influential text on the matter is the German cultural critic and physician Max Nordau's *Degeneration* (1892–1893), an international best seller in which Nordau rejects contemporary art and music as decadent products of degenerate artists and, more significantly, as driving forces of further cultural degeneration and decline. The fear of degeneration—be it physical and mental on the individual level, biopolitical on the demographic level, or sociocultural on the political and philosophical level—attests to a pessimistic, exhausted cultural climate in which the myth of progress itself appears to have run out of steam. It was not until the publication of Freud's *Three Essays on the Theory of Sexuality* in 1905 that another powerful paradigm—that of arrested psychological development—finally challenged and ultimately replaced the hegemony of degeneration theory in sexological discourse, if not elsewhere.

While earlier writers such as Jean-Jacques Rousseau and doctors such as Tissot perceived civilization as a polluting force contaminating and weakening the body and mind of the individual, later sexologists instead saw the so-called perverts as corruptor figures who weakened the social body. The "degenerates" were construed as dangers to civilization, halting progress by their regression to pre-Christian rituals such as fetishism and even bestiality. They were frequently viewed as retreating atavistically from the intellect to the senses, from reality to the imagination, and from civilization to a primitive state of being.[18] As Vernon A. Rosario observes, what "emerges from the antimasturbatory literature of the nineteenth century is the perception of 'deviant' individuals as viruses of the social corps—polluting its national strength and purity."[19] While in the eighteenth and early nineteenth centuries, moralistic messages that were clearly still grounded in the Christian notion of sin were increasingly presented with medical health warnings in order to scare masturbators into submission by suggesting that they were in danger of squandering for good their nonrenewable life energy, the late nineteenth century gave this argument a decidedly biopolitical twist by suggesting that degenerate individuals were not just endangering themselves but also weakening and indeed exhausting the health of the nation.

✳ ✳ ✳

In the eighteenth and nineteenth centuries, the Gothic emerged as a significant literary and artistic movement through which the Western imagination figured its concerns about exhaustion, decrepitude, decay, and ruination. The Gothic is also teeming with references to the entire spectrum of what Freud would later identify as polymorphous perversions. One need only think of Matthew Lewis's novel *The Monk* (1796), for example, which includes graphic scenes of rape and incest. And within the Gothic supernatural bestiary, no creature combines the themes of exhaustion and sexuality as effectively as the vampire. Literary representations of vampires frequently serve as vehicles to voice anxieties about racial others and about sexual deviance in its various manifestations:

in works such as Ludwig Tieck's *Wake Not the Dead* (1823),[20] Théophile Gautier's *The Dead in Love* (1836), and, of course, Bram Stoker's *Dracula* (1897), the vampiric protagonists are aligned with necrophilia, homosexuality, polygamy, fetishism, obsession, gynophobia, and oral sex. Moreover, often of aristocratic descent, vampires such as John Polidori's Lord Ruthven, protagonist of the story "The Vampyre" (1819), and Stoker's Count Dracula are recurrently associated with capitalist exploitation, as they quite literally suck their victims dry, parasitically draining their life energy and ruthlessly depleting their resources for their own precarious survival. Karl Marx was keenly aware of the metaphoric power of vampires when he wrote in *Capital*: "Capital is dead labor, which, vampire-like, lives only by sucking living labor, and lives the more, the more labor it sucks."[21]

As attitudes toward otherness and sexuality changed in the course of the nineteenth and twentieth centuries, so did the status of the bloodsucking creatures of the night. While most nineteenth-century vampire texts cast the undead as seductive but ultimately monstrous threats to the social order that are generally destroyed in the end by the forces of good, twentieth-century, and especially postwar, representations of vampires focus instead on the loneliness of the social outcast, on the attractions of narcissism, and on attitudes toward minorities, or else they glamorize the otherness of the vampire. Teenagers, in particular, are prone to identify with the pale, brooding, and misunderstood outsiders, whose difference is now frequently recast not just as acceptable but as superior: Ann Rice's *Vampire Chronicles*, Stephenie Meyer's *Twilight* saga, and Kevin Williamson and Julie Plec's television series *The Vampire Diaries* are clear cases in point.

In nineteenth-century vampire texts, the supernatural frequently functions as a guise to discuss then-taboo sexual practices.[22] John Sheridan Le Fanu's *Carmilla* (1872) is a highly representative example of this tendency: allegorically deploying the figure of a female vampire, it is a cautionary tale against the assumed physical and moral dangers of lesbian love. Motherless Laura, a classic Gothic victim, lives with her aging father in an isolated castle in Styria, where she falls under the spell of the beautiful and mysterious houseguest Carmilla. Blatantly abusing the father's hospitality, and capitalizing on Laura's loneliness and naivety, Carmilla talks the talk of lovers and woos her victim with romantic phrases and gestures, while feeding on peasant girls in the vicinity and gradually depleting Laura of her own life force. Psychologically and physically seductive, Carmilla is a highly skilled deceiver, and it takes the father a long time, as well as outside help, before he understands why his beloved daughter is literally wasting away at such alarming speed.

The literary critic Richard Dyer argues that the frequent association of homosexuality with vampires is due, first, to the fact that the public face of homosexuality and decadent sexuality in general was frequently associated with aristocrats such as the Marquis de Sade, Lord Byron, and Oscar Wilde. Vampires, too, are traditionally of aristocratic origin. Second, a Freudian reading of monsters in general suggests that they represent the threatening forms that repressed sexual desires can take. Third, the importance of sucking and biting, and the fact that most acts of vampirism take place in private spaces such as bedrooms and at night, speak for themselves. Fourth, and most important, both vampirism and homosexuality are also aligned with secrecy, mystery, and clandestine identities, which are decodable only by the initiated. "[T]he vocabulary of queer spotting," Dyer writes, "has been the languid, worn, sad, refined paleness of vampire image." He suggests that this is owing once again to the idea of the decadence of the aristocracy, who do not work and who live their lives indoors or in the shade.[23]

A much more plausible origin for the association of languor, paleness, apathy, and exhaustion with homosexuality and vampirism, however, is the link between masturbation and other nonprocreative sexual practices and the waste of precious life energy discussed earlier. As a direct result of the humoral doctrines that dominated medical practice for centuries, the belief in the damaging physical consequences of excessive sexual activities in general, as well as of sexual activities seen as perverse, was still widely accepted in the nineteenth century. It was based on the idea that nonrenewable life energy was wasted in such acts, while it also served as a medically supported moral tool to vilify and pathologize

them. Weakness, paleness, and languor were thus frequently interpreted as signs for sexually improper activities.

Le Fanu's *Carmilla* abounds in references to the female vampire's languor: Laura repeatedly notices "something of languor and
exhaustion" in her friend's pretty countenance; she observes that
Carmilla's movements are "languid—*very* languid," and that she has
"languid and burning eyes." When the two of them go for even the
shortest of walks, Carmilla seems "almost immediately exhausted"
and has to return to the castle. When a doctor is summoned to
investigate Carmilla's mysterious chronic exhaustion, she tries to
deflect his and Laura's concern: "There is nothing ever wrong with
me, but a little weakness. People say I am languid; I am incapable of
exertion; I can scarcely walk as far as a child of three years old; and
every now and then the little strength I have falters and I become
as you have seen me. But after all I am very easily set up again; in a
moment I am perfectly myself. See how I have recovered."[24]

Of course, as the reader soon discovers, Carmilla's method
of restoring her energy is far from wholesome, and thus it is
no surprise that Laura, too, should soon suffer from weakness
and exhaustion:

> For some nights I slept profoundly; but still every morning
> I felt the same lassitude, and a languor weighed upon me all
> day. I felt myself a changed girl. A strange melancholy was
> stealing over me, a melancholy that I would not have inter-
> rupted. Dim thoughts of death began to open, and an idea
> that I was slowly sinking took gentle, and, somehow, not
> unwelcome, possession of me. If it was sad, the tone of mind
> which this induced was also sweet. Whatever it might be, my
> soul acquiesced in it.

Carmilla is clearly excited by the fact that her victim is slowly fading away and succumbing to morbid longings as a result of her
indecent nocturnal undertakings, her "strange paroxysms of languid adoration" becoming ever more frequent. She attends to Laura
"with increasing ardour the more [her] strength and spirit waned,"
which suggests that she not only thrives while Laura withers

away but also derives some sadistic-necrophiliac sexual pleasure from the parasitical energy transfer.[25]

Le Fanu's equation of vampirism with lesbianism is far from subtle: he likens it to a highly infectious epidemic, thus suggesting the dangers of moral and sexual corruption. Moreover, Carmilla frequently talks of love, and Laura is not entirely unaware of (or immune to) the nonplatonic nature of her houseguest's attention, which she experiences as simultaneously fascinating and repulsive. Vampires traditionally have to be invited in—they seduce rather than use violence—which renders their victims at least partly responsible for what happens to them. Moreover, the vampiric act itself and the sensations it triggers are clearly related to orgasmic sexual activities in Le Fanu's novella. Laura reports that

> certain vague and strange visited me in my sleep. The prevailing one was of that pleasant, peculiar cold thrill which we feel in bathing, when we move against the current of a river. This was soon accompanied by dreams . . . they left an awful impression, and a sense of exhaustion, as if I had passed through a long period of great mental exertion and danger. . . . Sometimes there came a sensation as if a hand was drawn softly along my cheek and neck. Sometimes it was as if warm lips kissed me, and longer and more lovingly as they reached my throat, but there the caress fixed itself. My heart beat faster, my breathing rose and fell rapidly and full drawn; a sobbing, that rose into a sense of strangulation, supervened, and turned into a dreadful convulsion, in which my senses left me and I became unconscious.[26]

These nocturnal happenings soon leave their mark on Laura's appearance: "I had grown pale, my eyes were dilated and darkened underneath, and the languor which I had long felt began to display itself in my countenance."[27] Increasingly alarmed by these changes, Laura's father calls in a doctor and, by coincidence, also hears the story of another man who recently lost his beloved niece to Carmilla the vampire. With the aid of someone initiated into the mysteries of the bloodsucking predators and adept at vampire slaying, the men eventually decapitate Carmilla and thus vanquish for good the threat that subversive lesbian activities pose to the patriarchal order. As in the case of the early sexological literature on the dangers of masturbation, then, Le Fanu effectively deploys exhaustion imagery to suggest grave physical and moral damage in his cautionary tale against the highly contagious menace of lesbianism.

In most Western cultures, the link that was thought to exist between sexuality and exhaustion is now largely a thing of the past, since both humoral theories and overly moralistic and judgmental attitudes toward sexual difference no longer dominate the cultural imagination. Similarly, our ongoing fascination with vampires does not revolve around taboo forms of sexual desire that are represented as both fascinating and monstrous, as was the case in the nineteenth century, but is based a celebration of difference that is recast as a positive and highly desirable form of exceptionality (and one that, unsurprisingly, appeals particularly to teenagers). Yet what remains culturally relevant even today is the basic assumption that underpins the link between exhaustion and sexuality—the belief that exhaustion may be caused by specific behavior and actions, which are, to a certain extend at least, deliberate choices and thus fall into the remit of the moral responsibility of the individual.

5
Nerves

If we had to describe the characteristic features of a "nervous" type, we might think of an easily excitable, an anxious, or a very sensitive person—someone like the ailing lord of the manor in Edgar Allan Poe's famous tale "The Fall of the House of Usher" (1839), for example. Roderick Usher—a product of cross-generational inbreeding and a thinly veiled parody of the high-strung Romantic artist—constantly vacillates between states of feverish agitation and melancholic listlessness. We learn that he "suffered much from a morbid acuteness of the senses; the most insipid food was alone endurable; he could wear only garments of certain texture; the odors of all flowers were oppressive; his eyes were tortured by even a faint light; and there were but peculiar sounds, and these from stringed instruments, which did not inspire him with horror."[1]

Usher's nerves are exceptionally responsive to external stimuli, but he is also tortured by anxieties generated by his overactive, morbid imagination (and Poe leaves open the question whether the cause of these anxieties is real or imagined). We might also think of Woody Allen as another example of a typically nervous character—a neurotic intellectualizer plagued by a catastrophic imagination, who cannot stop articulating his endless stream of worries about his body, his relationships, and his state of mind. Or we might think of an extremely shy and timid person, who feels uncomfortable in social situations and blushes and stutters when addressed, or someone who jumps every time a door closes or a phone rings. The word "nervous," in brief, still essentially makes us think of character qualities.

Yet this connection between personality traits and bodily fibers is a residue from a bygone age in which the concept of "nerves" was embedded in a framework of beliefs that assumed a direct link between human energy, behavior, and the constitution of the nervous system. In the eighteenth and the nineteenth centuries, nerves resided at the heart of all medical theories of exhaustion: exhaustion during that period was essentially conceived as "nervous exhaustion," as a condition triggered by a lack of "nerve force." Nowadays, we no longer believe that nerves influence character, nor do we believe that they regulate our energy supply. We think of nerves as fibrous, cord-like structures whose main task is the transmission of impulses from the central nervous system to peripheral organs and vice versa. We divide them into sensory nerves, motor nerves, and autonomic nerves, which control the involuntary or partially voluntary activities of our bodies, such as the rhythm of our breath and the beating of our hearts. We know that electrochemical impulses can travel through the nerves at a speed of up to 200 miles per hour and that nervous damage is difficult to repair. Generally, most medical practitioners tend to differentiate rigorously between neurological (that is, physical) and psychological ailments.

Yet nerves have attracted much speculation about their shape, structure, and functions in the past. Galen considered nerves to be hollow tubes through which life energy (the "animal spirits") was distributed in the body. The animal spirits, Galen conjectured, were invisible and weightless, transmitting sensory impressions to the brain and motor impulses to the muscles. In the seventeenth century, the French philosopher René Descartes proposed that the animal spirits were of a liquid nature. It was only in the eighteenth century that Galen's basic assumptions were questioned and the modern conception of nerves as fibrous rather than hollow emerged.

Eighteenth-century medical thinking on nerves revolved primarily around new insights into the reflex functions of the nervous system and speculations about the role of electricity in the activities of nerves. Luigi Galvani's experiments, for example, showed that animals such as frogs and sheep possessed intrinsic "animal electricity," which controlled their motor activities. In the wake of these new theories, however, nerves were increasingly associated with irritability, fragility, and hypersensitivity. This was also reflected in a change of the meaning of the word "nervous": "nervous" originally meant "tough," "sinewy," and "vigorous" but gradually came to denote a heightened receptiveness. Nerves were imagined as quivering and vulnerable bodily filaments, comparable to taut violin strings perpetually in danger of snapping and in need of constant safeguarding from being overstrained. Moreover, "nerve force" (a form of life energy and essentially a slightly modernized version of the animal spirits) was imagined as strictly limited in supply and vulnerable to harmful depletion.

Among the first studies of specifically "nervous" diseases is George Cheyne's *The English Malady: or, A Treatise of Nervous Diseases of All Kinds, as Spleen, Vapours, Lowness of Spirits, Hypochondriacal, and Hysterical Distempers, etc.* (1733). Cheyne (1671–1743), a Scottish physician, proposed nervous weakness as the primary cause of various ailments we would now describe as psychosomatic, which hamper the body's and the mind's vivacity. These ailments include "Lowness of Spirits, lethargick Dullness, Melancholy and Moping," as well as hypochondria and hysteria. Cheyne, who still subscribed to many of the principles of ancient humoral theory, imagines the body as a machine made of "an infinite Number and Variety of different Channels and Pipes, filled with various and different Liquors and Fluids, perpetually running, glideing, or creeping forward, or returning backward, in a constant *Circle*, and fending out little Branches and Outlets, to moisten, nourish, and repair the Expense of Living."[2]

Nerves, in Cheyne's view, are solid and fibrous and help to circulate and break down the vital juices that are necessary to keep the body alive. Nervous weakness and various mood disorders can occur when the fluids are unable to circulate freely in the body, which causes "Laxity or want of due Tone, Elasticity and Force in the *Fibres* in general, or the *Nerves* in particular." Weak nerves, then, create a vicious circle: a "due Degree of Strength, Power and Springyness" is required in the nerve fibers to make the juices circulate smoothly to begin with, but when the juices do not flow freely the fibers are further weakened owing to lack of nourishment and lubrication. The body then falls prey to "vicious and morbid Juices." "All Nervous Distempers whatsoever," Cheyne concludes, "seems to me to be but one continued Disorder . . . arising from a Relaxation or Weakness, and the Want of a sufficient Force and Elasticity in the Solids in general, and the *Nerves* in particular." When the nervous system is weakened, an "Interruption of their Vibration or proper Action" occurs, "whereby the Soul is disabled to communicate its *Energy* or Principle of Motion to the Muscular Fibres," which leads to various states of mental and physical exhaustion.[3]

Cheyne argues that weak nerves can be inherited or acquired, the latter primarily through bad lifestyle choices. His greatest preoccupation is diet, and his tone verges on the messianic when he warns about the dangers of excessive consumption. Civilization and progress, in his view, are a mixed blessing: in their wake followed refinement, education, and enhanced sensitivity, on the one hand, but also the dangers of overindulgence and nervous weakness, on the other. Cheyne relates the epidemic rise of nervous weakness that he observed in the early decades of the eighteenth century to the fast-growing wealth of the seafaring English nation and the adverse consequences of immoderation, laziness, and luxury lifestyles. He urges his readers to follow a diet of milk, seeds, and vegetables; to avoid heavy wines, liqueurs, chocolate, spices, red meat, and snuff; and to take regular exercise. He also mentions city life, the moist climate and the rankness of England's soil, as well as astral and aerial influences, as further generators of nervous weakness.

Cheyne claimed that the "atrocious and frightful Symptoms" of the nervous complaints he studied were "scarce known to our Ancestors, and never r[ose] to such fatal Heights, nor afflict[ed] such Numbers in any other known Nation."[4] His assertion is characteristic of a more general tendency among theorists of exhaustion: as we have seen, many ages tend to present themselves as the most exhausted, as if exhaustion were a badge of honor and competing for the title of the most shattered were a kind of sport. A nostalgic vision of a quieter, more peaceful past and a romantic idealization of rural life often feature at the center of the many jeremiads that identify modern civilization as the major cause of exhaustion.

Cheyne, who was morbidly obese, includes his personal story in *The English Malady,* which functions both as a case study and as a cautionary tale. We learn that he gorged himself on the world's most extravagant delicacies with an insatiable appetite, growing ever fatter and ever more short of breath. Moreover, by thus destroying the "springyness" of his nervous system, he grew physically exhausted and weary of life:

> Upon my coming to *London,* I all of a sudden changed my whole Manner of Living . . . being naturally of a large *Size,* a cheerful Temper, and tolerable lively *Imagination* . . . I soon . . . grew daily in *Bulk* . . . constantly Dineing and Supping . . . my Health was in a few Years brought into great Distress, by so sudden and violent a Change. I grew excessively *fat, short-breath'd, Lethargic* and *Listless.*[5]

The epicurean Cheyne's mood and weight were to yo-yo dramatically for years to come, until he finally banished "animal foods" and "fermented liqueurs" from his menu for good; settled for a moderate diet of milk, seeds, and vegetables; and undertook regular daily outings on horseback. Like Galen's and Marsilio Ficino's before him, Cheyne's therapeutic regime centers above all on the connection between diet, lifestyle, and exhaustion, and surprisingly many of his suggested cures still sound convincing.

A few decades after the publication of *The English Malady,* another Scottish physician, John Brown (1735–1788), introduced the distinction between "sthenic" nervous diseases (defined by an excess level of energy) and "asthenic" nervous diseases (defined by a lack of energy). So great was his influence that an entire system of medical thinking was named "Brunonian" in his honor. Recommended cures for nervous patients treated by Brown depended on whether they were thought to lack nerve force owing to too much stimulation, in which case they were urged to rest, or to too little stimulation, in which case they were prescribed tonics and stimulants (Brown recommended mainly alcohol).

The repercussions of Brown's theory were felt for a long time, and, among many other popular therapies such as hydrotherapy and electrotherapy, shaped Silas Weir Mitchell's conception of the infamous "rest cure."[6] Brunonian thinking was also responsible for the precursors of what we would now call occupational therapies: some nineteenth-century doctors in America, for example, sent listless male patients thought to suffer from understimulation to the Dakotas for rough-riding exercise cures.[7] It was assumed that their sluggish life energies could be reawakened if only they were exposed to stimulating sights, sounds, tastes, and experiences. It was, however, predominantly the asthenic diseases caused by a surplus of stimulation that captured the imagination of the nineteenth century and most worried its medical men.

※ ※ ※

In the 1840s, it was discovered that electricity was the true agent of nerve action—a finding that revolutionized the field of neurology. In the 1850s, it became common to think of the brain as a kind of battery, and nerve fibers as resembling electrical wires that conducted power though the body.[8] The idea that nerve force, just like the power of a battery, was limited in quantity and could be depleted if not managed wisely also chimed with the perturbing principles of the second law of thermodynamics. This law, proposed in the middle of the nineteenth century, suggested that the amount of energy in the universe was not only limited but also steadily decreasing.

The period between 1880 and the beginning of the First World War has often been described as the "nervous age." The German historian Joachim Radkau, for example, claims that "nervousness" was not only a very common individual diagnosis but a state of affairs, a way of collectively experiencing and thinking about various cultural processes, including social, biological, and aesthetic developments.[9] Nervousness, he argues, was in the air, colored all debates, and even influenced the jittery political decisions that culminated in the war. Nerves had turned into civilization's greatest weakness and threatened the stability of both the individual body and the body politic.

It was in the context of this ongoing preoccupation with nervousness and nervous weakness that the neurasthenia diagnosis was born. Neurasthenia was a baggy and infinitely expandable diagnostic concept, an umbrella term for a range of other symptoms that were clustered around its core symptom: nervous exhaustion. As in Cheyne's theory, weak nerves were thought to be the main agents causing both mental and physical fatigue.

The term "neurasthenia" and its diagnosis were first proposed in the United States in 1869 and popularized in the early 1880s by the physician and electrotherapist George M. Beard.[10] His version of neurasthenia would remain by far the most influential until the diagnosis gradually disappeared from Western medical handbooks after the First World War. In *American Nervousness: Its Causes and Consequences*, Beard defines neurasthenia as a "deficiency or lack of nerve-force." "*Nervousness,*" he writes, "*is nervelessness.*" The long list of symptoms explored in his sprawling study includes, above all, physical and mental exhaustion, but also irritability, indigestion, insomnia, inebriety, drowsiness, hopelessness, phobias of all kinds (including "fear of everything" and "fear of fears"), hay fever, bad teeth, ticklishness, cold feet, dry hair and skin, and premature ejaculation.[11] Oscar Wilde mocks the sweeping inclusiveness of the diagnosis in a letter dating from 1900 (the year of his death, following his imprisonment for homosexuality): "I am now *neurasthenic*. My doctor says I have all the symptoms. It is comforting to have them *all*, it makes one a perfect type."[12]

Yet Beard clearly hit a nerve with his diagnosis: soon it was highly fashionable to be neurasthenic in America and western Europe. The popularity of Beard's diagnosis has partly been explained by the fact that he drew together into a single medical condition a whole range of more or less trivial symptoms.[13] Moreover, Beard clearly signposts neurasthenia as a physical rather than a psychological disorder, thereby freeing its sufferers from any stigma that might be attached to mental illness. Those who adopted the diagnosis could derive solace from the fact that there was a "real," organic dimension to their sufferings, as opposed to "just" a mental one, as, for example, in the case of hysteria.

Like Cheyne before him, Beard explicitly declares neurasthenia a disease of civilization, triggered by various characteristics of the modern age, including "steam-power, the periodical press, the telegraph, the sciences, and the mental activity of women."[14] The causes of neurasthenia were firmly attributed to the outside world, to technological and social changes that drained the limited energy reserves of modern men and women. The modern environment, particularly the urban environment, was thought to generate too many stimuli, such that the senses were incessantly assaulted by noise, sights, speed, and information. Beard feared that the sensitive nervous systems of the modern subject would be unable to cope with this sensory overload. Interestingly, similar arguments about the dangers of permanent overstimulation caused by new communication technologies, and other adverse psychological effects of neoliberal techno-capitalism and globalization, also feature prominently in current theories regarding the origins of stress and burnout.

Furthermore, Beard associates neurasthenia with the middle and upper classes, arguing that its symptoms are the result of too much "brain work," particularly common among businessmen and captains of industry.[15] The "brain-working, indoor-living classes" are repeatedly contrasted in his study with the "lower orders"—muscle workers, day laborers, and peasants, as well as with "savages and barbarians of all times and ages." Beard defines "a fine organization" as the key characteristic of a person with a nervous disposition:

The fine organization is distinguished from the coarse by fine, soft hair, delicate skin, nicely chiselled features, small bones, tapering extremities, and frequently by a muscular system comparatively small and feeble. It is frequently associated with superior intellect, and with a strong and active emotional nature. . . . It is the organization of the civilized, refined and educated, rather than of the barbarous and low-born and untrained—of women more than of men. It is developed, fostered, and perpetuated with the progress of civilization, with the advance of culture and refinement, and the corresponding preponderance of labor of the brain over that of the muscles. As would logically be expected, it is oftener met with in cities than in the country, is more marked and more frequent at the desk, the pulpit, and the counting room than in the shop or on the farm.[16]

As is clear from this extract, Beard associates so many positive and flattering qualities with the neurasthenic disposition that in effect he turns it into a distinction rather than a disease. In his account, neurasthenia is construed as a marker of evolutionary refinement and social and intellectual status, a condition signaling sensitivity, industriousness, and sophistication. It is not surprising, then, that neurasthenia became so fashionable and that so many embraced the diagnosis with enthusiasm. Moreover, Beard also furnishes his diagnostic invention with a patriotic dimension, as neurasthenia is to be found not simply among the "highest social orders" but only among the most highly developed and civilized nations, and in particular, of course, in America, which he frequently compares favorably with England, Germany, and France.

To render his diagnosis even more palatable to the general readership at which his study was aimed, Beard repeatedly uses metaphors from the fields of economics, engineering, and physics to illustrate the workings of neurasthenia. For example, in the chapter "Nervous Bankruptcy," he uses an extended "wise management of limited funds" simile. We learn that there are those among us who are

very poor in nerve force; their inheritance is small, and they have been able to increase it but slightly, if at all; and if from overtoil, or sorrow, or injury, they overdraw their little surplus, they may find that it will require months or perhaps years to make up the deficiency, if, indeed, they ever accomplish the task. The man with a small income is really rich, as long as there is no overdraft on the account; so the nervous man may be really well and in fair working order as long as he does not draw on his limited store of nerve-force. But a slight mental disturbance, unwonted toil or exposure, anything out of and beyond his usual routine, even a sleepless night, may sweep away that narrow margin, and leave him in nervous bankruptcy, from which he finds it as hard to rise as from financial bankruptcy.[17]

These similes are telling—they not only connect the diagnosis with distinctly modern social and technological developments but also frame it in popular imagery that reflects the dominant economic values of the time. Like capital, nerve force can be squandered and wasted by ill-judged expenditure and overinvestment in potentially ruinous activities. One's limited energy supply needs to be managed as prudently as one's financial assets: bodily economies, Beard suggests, adhere to the same rules as apply to household or national budgets. Yet, as Janet Oppenheim points out, there is one crucial limitation to the explanatory potency of Beard's financial metaphors: bodily economies, in contrast to national ones, cannot accommodate profits. Unlike wealth and capital, nerve force is not suited to include aspirations of expansion and growth.[18] In other words, one can neither reinvest nerve force nor stockpile it for the future.

After the publication of Charles Darwin's *On the Origin of Species* in 1859, medical and cultural debates began to draw on evolutionary biological models and became increasingly preoccupied with the idea of "degeneration." Particularly in France and Germany, fears about degeneration as a form of perverse, backward evolution, and as a process that entails the gradual exhaustion and weakening of a nation's genetic capital, created a climate of cultural pessimism. Works such as Richard von Krafft-Ebing's famous sexological compendium *Psychopathia Sexualis* (1886) and Max Nordau's *Degeneration* (1892), a polemical attack on various aspects of modern culture, warned of the grave dangers of deficiencies that could be passed on to, and intensified in, the next generation. Nervous weakness, "perverse" sexual desires, alcoholism, criminal inclinations, effeminacy, and feeble-mindedness, for example, were all thought of as qualities that could be inherited. Many Continental theorists who embraced the idea of hereditary diseases painted gloomy pictures of the future, fearing an ever-increasing contamination of their nations' gene pool and work-force. In Beard's account, however, the figure of the neurasthenic is not a representative of decadence, decline, and degeneration but instead is cast as its opposite: his neurasthenic is the very pinnacle of evolutionary refinement. Beard thus turns the idea that nervous weakness is a bad thing on its head—his account is essentially optimistic and affirmative.

Beard's writings on neurasthenia show once again the ways in which ideological and cultural factors shape the theorization of medical symptoms more generally, and of theories of exhaustion more specifically. In an age dominated by the values of productivity, activity, and efficiency, the exhausted were considered a major problem. However, Beard gives these anxieties a positive spin: since he believed that exhaustion was caused by the very processes that characterized the modern age—recent technological inventions, the faster pace of life, a shift from physical to intellectual labor—being exhausted could be seen as a positive quality. As a wound inflicted by modernity, exhaustion could be borne as proudly as a battle scar. In our age, too, burnout is not as stigmatized a condition as depression, for example, but almost viewed as a distinction, as it implies that one has simply worked too hard and invested everything, and more, in one's job. It is thought to affect, above all, hard-working, ambitious, successful, caring, and conscientious types. Furthermore, it is the twenty-first-century workscape itself (with its unique set of sociopsychological stressors) that is held responsible for the spread of the condition, and not so much the individual who experiences it.

✻ ✻ ✻

Given that a range of positive characteristics manifest in dubious claims about the social, intellectual, and racial superiority of the neurasthenic individual were integral to Beard's diagnosis, it is not surprising that neurasthenia quickly became not just a disease of

civilization but a *maladie à la mode* (melancholia, too, was a similarly fashionable disease at certain points in history, such as in the
age of Romanticism).[19] Neurasthenia traversed the Atlantic and
soon passed from medical into popular and literary debates. In
addition to Oscar Wilde, Franz Kafka, Marcel Proust, Henry James,
and Virginia Woolf, to name just a few, were among the many mod-
ernist authors diagnosed with neurasthenia. In 1913, when Kafka
was torn apart by his inability to decide whether to marry his fian-
cée, Felice Bauer, he named neurasthenia as one of his many ailments. In his diary entry from May 4, he arranges his complaints
into the following hierarchy: "1. Digestion. 2. Neurasthenia. 3. Rash.
4. Inner insecurity."[20] Just like John Cassian in the case of acedia, he
hoped that he could cure his neurasthenia with work.

The German writer Heinrich Mann (brother of the better-known
Thomas Mann), too, frequently describes himself as neurasthenic
and as nervous in his correspondence and in other nonfictional
works. Neurasthenic characters feature repeatedly in his oeuvre. In
his satirical novella *Dr. Bieber's Temptation* (1898), for example, a
character called Herr Sägemüller, who is in a sanatorium for nervous patients and has embraced his neurasthenia diagnosis with
an eagerness that borders on religious fervor, explains his condition in the following terms:

> As you probably know very well, my dear Fräulein, in the
> past intellectual activities took place in monasteries. While
> intellectuals have never been on good terms with the bru-
> tality and coarseness of reality, we can no longer escape it
> today—it assaults us both at home and outdoors. The electri-
> cal tram . . . intervenes as insolently into my life as the phone
> wires that are whirring outside my bedroom window at night.
> Advertisements on the street corners and the howling of the
> trade people and the press, bells ringing everywhere, bikes
> and motorcars—all of these phenomena rape my senses; I am
> entirely defenseless. Another aggravating factor is that while
> the conditions of material life have become ever more com-
> plicated, our intellectual organization has become infinitely
> finer. Yet unlike in the case of the cruder scholar of the past,

there is no safe haven for the much more sensitive intellectual worker of today. This is why you find me here. The clinic
is a sanctuary where I can find relief from the preoccupation with my physical existence. As far as possible, I have sur-
rendered my will to that of the doctor, and you can barely
believe how good a so-called modern person feels when they
are finally allowed to cease desiring and wanting things.[21]

In this speech, Sägemüller concisely lists the then-prevalent
anxieties about the vulnerability of the self in the modern world
and the impact on that self of new technologies. This vulnerability
is particularly manifest in the porous boundary between inside
and outside (Sägemüller feels "raped" by the noise from the streets),
the recurrent penetration of technology into all spheres of life, and
the sense of being unable to find shelter from the vicissitudes of
modernity. Sägemüller blames external forces for his condition
and does not fail to emphasize his superior "fine organization"—a
detail that is clearly derived from Beard's account of neurasthenia. It is also interesting to compare Sägemüller's lament with the
breathless jeremiad of the psychiatrist Wilhelm Erb, who, together
with Krafft-Ebing, was the most important theorist of neurasthenia in Germany:

Owing to the excessive increase in traffic and the wire-net-
works of our telegraphs and telephones, which now span the
entire globe, our trading patterns and circumstances of life
have been transformed completely: all affairs are conducted
in haste and excitement, nights are used for travelling, days
for doing business, and even "recreational journeys" have
turned into strains on the nervous system; the worrying
repercussions of serious political, industrial, and financial
crises permeate into much wider circles of the population
than in the past; the general public now participates in public life; political, religious, and social battles, party politics,
election campaigns, and the excessive dominance of clubs
and societies overheat people's heads and force their spirits
to undertake ever new exertions while robbing them of the

time for rest, sleep, and stillness; life in big cities has become ever more refined and restless.[22]

Unlike Erb, however, Mann does not subscribe to the conception of neurasthenia that his character embraces. In the course of the novella, he mercilessly exposes Herr Sägemüller as a highly dubious and self-pitying malingerer, completely lacking in self-knowledge, who has adopted the fashionable identity of a neurasthenic to excuse his own shortcomings, to abdicate responsibility for his actions, and to be able to look down on others. Ultimately, Mann suggests that what is really sick is not the modern age as such but the very people who argue that this is the case—people like Herr Sägemüller.

Mann was not the only one to ridicule the neurasthenia fashion—many other writers and caricaturists, too, produced scathing satirical portraits of malingerers, shirkers, and hypochondriacs who readily embraced the diagnosis. Thomas Mann, for example, criticizes an entire industry based on a morbid preoccupation with illnesses—minor, major, and imagined—in *The Magic Mountain* (1924) and created a character much like Herr Sägemüller in his novella *Tristan* (1903). Other novels that present negative portraits of neurasthenics include Marcel Proust's *In Search of Lost Time* (1913–1927) and Italo Svevo's *Zeno's Conscience* (1923). An aphorism penned by the Viennese cultural commentator Karl Kraus neatly encapsulates the gist of the less sympathetic attitudes toward neurasthenics at the turn of the twentieth century: "Anesthesia: wounds without pain. Neurasthenia: pain without wounds."[23]

❋ ❋ ❋

Beard's theories were received particularly positively by the medical establishment in Germany. The most important German theorists to spread the neurasthenic gospel were Wilhelm Erb and Richard von Krafft-Ebing, the forensic psychiatrist and author of *Psychopathia Sexualis*, who also wrote the influential study *On Healthy and Sick Nerves* (1885). Krafft-Ebing repeatedly refers to Beard and reproduces many of his arguments. His version of neurasthenia differs from Beard's in various important respects, however, and is ultimately much more pessimistic in outlook. Krafft-Ebing argues that given the large number of developments that have taken place in the name of progress, one might reasonably be inclined to assume "that modern civilized man would advance ever more towards happiness and satisfaction, as Enlightenment, education, the comforts and luxuries of the refined cultural life suggest." Yet nothing could be further from the truth: a murky shadow looms over modern culture:

> People appear pale, glum, excited and unsteady in our modern civilization, particularly in the centers, in the big cities, and that they are not happy is evident among other things in the fact that the sorry philosophical *Weltanschauungen* of Schopenhauer and E. v. Hartmann have been met with so much praise.
>
> The worm that gnaws at the fruit of cultural life and that poisons the love of life and life energy of so many people is the so-called nervousness. . . . It is the sickly reaction of nerves that is to a large extent responsible for the epidemic of *Weltschmerz* and pessimism that has penetrated large strata of modern society and that is, among other highly worrying symptoms, statistically manifest and expressed in the ever growing number of suicides and mental illnesses.[24]

Krafft-Ebing fears that "modern society is heading toward inevitable moral and physical ruin." Like Beard, he uses economic metaphors to illustrate his theories and refers to "nerve capital" and "nerve labor." The idea of overspending or wasting precious and limited resources features prominently in his account, too: "The various symptoms of nervous weakness . . . are nothing but the permanent symptoms of a nerve-life that is unable to strike a balance between production and consumption of nerve-power."[25] Yet Krafft-Ebing, unlike Beard, does not celebrate nervous weakness as a sign of refinement. Rather, he views nervous exhaustion both as a symptom of moral decline and as what we would now call a biopolitical problem, as it threatens the nerve capital of the entire body politic.

Krafft-Ebing, again unlike Beard, does not believe that the increase in external sensory stimuli in cities is the reason for the loss of the population's nervous capital. Instead, he shifts the blame to those who seek out the hustle and bustle of the big cities, those "poor wretches" who are addicted to diversion and distraction.[26] He believes that the more irritable, weak, and unhealthy the nervous system becomes, the more it requires diverse and ever stronger stimuli.[27] In other words, Krafft-Ebing assumes that nervous weakness blunts the senses, rather than rendering them more refined. Like debauched libertines who have seen and done it all, restless nervous people incessantly have to search for new, ever more elaborate excitements.

Krafft-Ebing is a declinist thinker, a culturally conservative pessimist focusing on the night side of modern civilization. His study is, above all, a nostalgic, Rousseauian lament that contrasts a more inward, learned, and harmonious past with the modern, fast-paced rat race, in which idealism has been replaced by crude materialism, rampant egotism, hedonism, and degenerate forms of entertainment. Among the urban phenomena that vex him most are "shocking dramas, adultery comedies, trapeze artists, nerve-wrecking and agitating music, images that generate sensual responses and irritate the eyes, expositions, strong wines, cigars, liqueurs, clubs, gambling dens, amorous adventures, and news stories about crimes and people's misfortunes in the daily press, etc."[28]

Finally, while Beard blames the rise in neurasthenic symptoms on technological advances, overwork, and an increase in sensitivity, Krafft-Ebing believes that the key factor behind the growing nervousness of the modern age is a "neuropathic constitution"—that is, inherited qualities. These hereditary qualities, combined with the various lamentable social developments listed earlier, among which Krafft-Ebing also counts the emancipation of women, would lead, if unchecked, to the decline of the entire Western world.[29] Most late-nineteenth-century explanations of nervous exhaustion ultimately vacillate between the two poles represented by Beard and Krafft-Ebing: the spread of nervous diseases is blamed either on external environmental factors or on heredity and the somber laws of degeneration.

* * *

Nerves, nervous exhaustion, and degeneration also feature at the very center of Joris-Karl Huysmans's decadent masterpiece *Against Nature* (1884)—the model for the infamous "yellow book" so cherished by Oscar Wilde's Dorian Gray. The novel's protagonist, Duc Jean Des Esseintes, is the last scion of an ancient noble line whose male members have grown progressively more effeminate, sickly, and weak owing to two centuries of inbreeding. Des Esseintes, "a frail young man of thirty, nervous and anaemic," is the very embodiment of the degenerate fin-de-siècle aesthete, permanently plagued by ennui and spleen. His nervous system is so extraordinarily hypersensitive that every smell, taste, sound, or sight that jars with his refined tastes is experienced as excruciatingly distressing. Exhausted, world-weary, and disgusted with what he perceives as the vulgarity and stupidity of contemporary society, which he associates primarily with the rise of the moneyed middle classes, Des Esseintes decides to retreat to the outskirts of Paris. Having escaped the hustle and bustle of metropolitan life, he attempts to create a refuge "from the incessant deluge of human folly," in which good taste and eternal quietude reign.[30]

Des Esseintes has tried everything to alleviate his weariness, including studying Latin theology, socializing with the Faubourg Saint-Germain set, indulging in debauched sexual practices, and seeking solace in the arts. Yet eventually, all his passions burn themselves out. "Having lost faith in everything" and "ravaged by spleen," "he had reached such a pitch of nervous sensibility [*sensibilité de nerfs*] that the sight of a disagreeable object or person would etch itself into his brain so deeply as to require several days for its imprint to be even slightly dulled; during that period, the touch of a human form, brushed against in the street, had been one of his most excruciating torments."[31] His weak nerves propel him on a quest to abolish unpredictable "natural" stimulation from his life and to seek out controllable, artificial sources of stimulation instead. Having moved to his suburban refuge, he dedicates much energy to the interior design of his retreat. The furnishings are to correspond precisely to his mood—providing or weakening stimulation as necessary. Even the color scheme he chooses is designed to match his nervous tastes: like all "weak and nervous people" (*affaiblis et nerveux*), Des Esseintes is inevitably drawn to "that irritating, morbid colour, with its deceptive splendours, its febrile sourness: orange."[32] He decides to have his walls bound like books, in heavy, smooth Moroccan leather; wild animal skins lie scattered across the parquet; bluish panes in the casement windows filter the unbearably shrill daylight; and heavy draperies made out of the darkened, smoky gold thread work of antique stoles help to shield him further from the vicissitudes of nature.

Des Esseintes also gilds the shell of a giant lethargic tortoise and has it encrusted with rubies, which he hopes will offset the intricate pattern of his Oriental carpets when the creature crawls across them. However, the animal proves resistant to becoming a part in his ambitious interior design project and dies, just like a host of rare and exotic orchids, with which Des Esseintes is temporarily enchanted. Even his cutlery is designed to satisfy his morbid obsessions: it is silver-gilded, "so that the silver, barely visible through the faintly eroded layer of the gold, gives it a suggestion of something sweetly old-fashioned, a vague hint of something utterly weary and close to death [*tout épuisée, toute moribonde*]."[33]

Having sold his ancestral chateaux, Des Esseintes keeps only two old servants, whom he forces to wear thick felt slippers, so as not to be disturbed by the sound of their footsteps. Everything in his new house is hermetically sealed and padded; double-doors are installed, with well-oiled hinges; thick carpets muffle any sound of life; an aquarium positioned in front of a window breaks the light in such a way that it is not too tiring for his strained sensory apparatus. Des Esseintes, in short, turns "against nature" and embraces artistry, as the artificial can be both controlled and shaped according to one's tastes. He lives in a house filled with imitations: he possesses, for example, an array of scents that evoke natural ones and occasionally infuses the air with these synthetic perfumes to conjure up memories of past experiences or faraway places. Artifice, he believes, is "the distinguishing characteristic of human genius. As he was wont to remark, Nature has had her day; she has finally exhausted [*lassé*], through the nauseating uniformity of her landscapes and her skies, the sedulous patience of men of refined taste."[34]

The majority of the novel's chapters are dedicated to detailed descriptions of Des Esseintes's decadent tastes. Above all else, Des Esseintes cherishes his library, as he deems the pleasures of the imagination preferable to genuine experiences. Unsurprisingly, he is most drawn to the works of late Latin authors, the chroniclers of the fall of Rome detailing "a decayed civilization, a splintering empire."[35] He appreciates, above all, literary styles that mirror decline in their syntax, that enact decadence in the very texture of their verbal material. He also holds some contemporary prophets of ennui in high esteem, especially Charles Baudelaire, Edgar Allan Poe, and Stéphane Mallarmé. According to Des Esseintes, Baudelaire expertly exposes the morbid psychology of the soul "which has reached the autumn of its capacity to feel" and shows the moment "when the enthusiasms and convictions of youth are exhausted [*sont taris*], when nothing remains but the arid recollection of hardships endured."[36] Baudelaire probes the wounds inflicted by satiation, disillusionment, and contempt, chronicling the "morbid conditions that afflict exhausted minds and despairing souls."[37] In Poe, in contrast, Des Esseintes admires the writer's astute dissections of the torpor of the will: "Violently agitated by hereditary neuroses, maddened by convulsive moral disturbances, [Poe's] creatures lived solely on their nerves."[38] Yet it is a collection of Mallarmé's prose poems that is the most treasured item in his library. Mallarmé's is a literature that is

> enervated by old ideas and exhausted by a surfeit of syntax [*affaiblie par l'âge des idées, épuisée par les excès de la syntaxe*], which responds solely to the peculiar interests that exacerbate the sick and yet, in its decline, feels impelled to give expression to everything, and on its deathbed desperately longs to compensate for all the pleasures it has missed and to leave behind a legacy of the subtlest memories of pain.[39]

Huysmans, it is obvious, feels a deep kinship with the aesthetic projects of the writers his protagonist admires. Huysmans's own highly embellished, complicated, and often feverishly obsessive literary style, too, powerfully communicates the demise of established classical ideals and literary models, and enacts the nervous exhaustion it depicts on the level of content.

During the course of the novel, Des Esseintes mainly languishes in his armchair, dwelling in memories. But even his ruminations about the past leave him "feeling drained, exhausted, half dead" (*anéanti, brisé, presque moribond*), and his numerous physical ailments increase and become ever more worrisome.[40] They include dyspepsia, vomiting, nausea, migraines, irritable bowel syndrome, sweating, insomnia, nightmares, lack of appetite, weight loss, and auditory and olfactory hallucinations. In the end, seriously weakened and worried that he will perish, he calls in a specialist for nervous diseases, who prescribes pepsins, cod-liver oil, beef tea, burgundy, and egg yolk. Following the physician's dietary regime, Des Esseintes manages to regain his physical strength. However, the doctor does not leave it at that: to tackle the underlying psychological causes that have generated the other ailments, he insists, Des Esseintes must abandon his solitary existence and morbid dwelling and return to society. Fearing death and the reappearance of his numerous debilitating ailments, Des Esseintes resentfully consents to the doctor's orders, packs up the paraphernalia of his artificial paradise, and prepares to move back into the center of Paris. In the end, Des Esseintes collapses exhausted into a chair and succumbs to the "waters of human mediocrity" that are about to engulf him. He wishes that he were able to force himself to possess faith, to embrace Catholicism, and "to make it a protective crust, to fasten it with clamps to his soul, to place it beyond the reach of all those ideas that undermine and uproot it."[41]

A nostalgic longing for the long-lost spiritual certainties of Catholicism runs like a red thread through the entire novel. It is certainly neither a coincidence nor a surprise that its creator, Huysmans, not long after the publication of *Against Nature*, rediscovered his own faith. Yet Des Esseintes's decadent tastes not merely are caused by a loss of faith but also constitute the direct result of his nervous exhaustion: "[A]s his constitution had become unbalanced and his nerves had gained the upper hand, his tastes had altered and the objects of his admiration had changed."[42] In other words, decadence, aestheticism, and nervousness go hand in hand.

Huysmans's representation of exhaustion powerfully illustrates the ways in which it is tied up with a certain zeitgeist and how a more general cultural atmosphere can affect the energy levels of an individual. It also reinforces the link proposed by Beard and many other theorists of neurasthenia between a highly refined disposition and a propensity to suffer from exhaustion, as well as the association of exhaustion with the upper classes, artists, and "brain workers." The causes that Huysmans offers as explanations for Des Esseintes's nostalgia for the past and his spiritual disenchantment with the present are many and include the decline of the aristocracy and the rise of the bourgeoisie; the advent of positivism, scientism, and materialism; and the cultural pessimism that reigned in France after it suffered military defeat in 1870/1871 at the hands of the Prussians.

It is evident that Huysmans was well informed about then-current medical and psychiatric debates about nervous exhaustion, and he directly weaves this knowledge into his fiction. He clearly supports the argument that many French and German psychiatrists in particular propagated: that the causes of nervous diseases are, above all, hereditary: Des Esseintes is the product of incest and degeneration—the final offspring of an "exhausted bloodline." Huysmans also refers to then-common medical cures for exhaustion: Des Esseintes is prescribed pepsins, tonics, and a moderate diet and at some point tries to follow a hydrotherapy regime in his house. Like Krafft-Ebing, Huysmans suggests that the more strained and exhausted someone's nerves are, the more "decadent" their tastes will be. As many others before him, he firmly aligns the nervous temperament with artistic inclinations. Finally, it is telling that it is a medical man who is granted the last word in this novel: it is the nerve specialist who terminates Des Esseintes's aestheticist extravaganzas and his doomed experiment with solipsistic seclusion.

* * *

Although their accounts differ in many respects, both Beard and Krafft-Ebing, and the majority of their contemporaries, believed that nervous exhaustion could be explained primarily by organic factors—that is, a lack of nerve force, which was essentially a version of human energy. This lack of nerve force, they conjectured, could be brought on either by external factors that vampirically deplete limited supplies of nervous energy or by an inherited weak nervous constitution. To a certain extent, somatic narratives of this kind protected sufferers from being held responsible for their condition, an idea that the famous goodnight-kiss episode at the beginning of Proust's *In Search of Lost Time* neatly illustrates. In that scene, the narrator, Marcel, is subjected to a medical reassessment that encapsulates the way in which nervous weakness was theorized in the age of neurasthenia. The narrator's mother previously considered her son's anguished and obsessive longings for her evening embrace as morally bad but voluntary and thus curable behavior. Yet after the narrator's despair culminates in a particularly dramatic nocturnal scene on a staircase following a dinner party, his mother begins to regard him as sick and nervous, as someone whose behavior is determined by a medical condition. "[I]t's his nerves," she apologetically explains to the family servant. "And thus for the first time," the narrator writes, "my unhappiness was regarded no longer as a punishable offence but as an involuntary ailment which had been officially recognised, a nervous condition for which I was in no way responsible: I had the consolation of no longer having to mingle apprehensive scruples with the bitterness of my tears; I could weep henceforth without sin."[43]

Yet the period in which patients were able to derive solace from the neurasthenia diagnosis was short-lived. Neurasthenia's heyday occurred between 1880 and the beginning of the First World War. Thereafter, it gradually disappeared from the medical handbooks and was no longer widely used as a diagnostic category. That said, neurasthenia was dropped officially from the *Diagnostic and Statistic Manual of Mental Disorders* (*DSM*) only in 1980 and is still included in the tenth revision of the *International Classification of Diseases* (*ICD-10*). The *ICD-10* identifies mental and/or physical fatigue as its core symptoms and currently differentiates between two types of neurasthenia:

In one type, the main feature is a complaint of increased fatigue after mental effort, often associated with some decrease in occupational performance or coping efficiency in daily tasks. The mental fatiguability is typically described as an unpleasant intrusion of distracting associations or recollections, difficulty in concentrating, and generally inefficient thinking. In the other type, the emphasis is on feelings of bodily or physical weakness and exhaustion after only minimal effort, accompanied by a feeling of muscular aches and pains and inability to relax.[44]

In both types of neurasthenia, a variety of other symptoms may be present, including dizziness, tension headaches, feelings of general instability, insomnia or hypersomnia, worries about decreasing mental and bodily well-being, irritability, anhedonia, and varying minor degrees of both depression and anxiety.

The reasons for the diagnosis's gradual disappearance after the First World War are manifold. As is evident even from the *ICD-10* entry, neurasthenia is an imprecise category that overlaps with others that are now more commonly used, and it comprises too many disparate symptoms. When diagnostic tools became more refined at the beginning of the twentieth century, neurasthenia was broken down again into its constituent parts.[45] However, the most important reason for the disappearance of neurasthenia as a widely used diagnostic category was a major paradigm shift in the fields of psychiatry and psychology: the advent of psychoanalysis.[46] The somatic explanation of the many symptoms of neurasthenia was increasingly questioned, and in the early decades of the twentieth century, psychoanalytic explanations began to replace the biological models.[47] Freud sweepingly dismissed all the causes that Beard, Krafft-Ebing, and many other theorists had established as triggers for the condition and argued that neurasthenia, like all neuroses, could be explained with recourse to one phenomenon only: sexuality. In addition, from the 1930s onward, the concept of depression, which comprised some of the symptoms that were also present in neurasthenia, grew ever more popular. Depression was to become the most frequently diagnosed condition in the field of mental health in the second half of the twentieth century.

While neurasthenia is now diagnosed only very rarely in western Europe and the United States, it is still considered a valid diagnostic category in some Asian countries precisely because it does not carry the same social stigma as depression and other illnesses that are deemed to be mental rather than physical in nature. Many who experience chronic fatigue syndrome strongly argue for the purely organic origins of their illness for similar reasons.[48] In China, for example, neurasthenia (*shenjing shuairou*) is considered to be caused by a decrease in vital energy (*qi*). Neurasthenia functions essentially as a culturally sanctioned and stigma-free label for symptoms of distress that are very similar to those experienced by depressives in the West.[49] Yet in Japan, in contrast, the explanatory model for neurasthenia (*shinkeisuijaku*) verges more toward psychological causes. Japanese neurasthenia is associated with a specific personality type characterized by hypersensitivity, introversion, self-consciousness, perfectionism, and hypochondriac tendencies and is frequently treated by the Morita therapy, which combines insights from modern psychology and Zen Buddhism.[50]

The rise and fall of the neurasthenia diagnosis, and the fact that it is defined differently in different cultural contexts, illustrate once again that there is nothing "natural" or inevitable about the ways in which specific sets of symptoms are clustered together into distinctive diagnostic entities. The history of medicine shows us that disease categories change, sometimes quite dramatically, and especially at the borders between physical and mental health. Nowadays, the long list of symptoms associated with neurasthenia appears rather random and peculiar, and it is difficult to see how conditions as distinct as physical and mental exhaustion, toothaches, hay fever, phobias, and dry hair could ever have been imagined as sharing a singular physical cause. It is also extremely rare to encounter the underlying value judgments and dominant cultural attitudes that often shape medical diagnoses in such an explicit, unapologetic form as in Cheyne's, Beard's, and Krafft-Ebing's narratives; it is plainly visible that their personal attitudes to various cultural, political, and social developments substantially influenced their medical theories and their therapeutic recommendations. In Cheyne's and Beard's cases, national pride, classism, and a celebration of progress are particularly pronounced, while Krafft-Ebing's account is that of a pessimistic declinist, who feels profoundly ill at ease with many of the developments of the modern world.

* * *

Even after the golden age of the neurasthenia diagnosis in the West, and the advent of neurology proper, the idea of nerves as determiners of moods, energy levels, and behaviors continues to haunt our language, as is evident in the meaning of the word "nervous" discussed at the beginning of the chapter, and in figurative expressions such as "to get on somebody's nerves," "nervous wreck," "shattered nerves," "nerves of steel," and "bundle of nerves." Nerve imagery also still features prominently in many literary works written after the heyday of neurasthenia. T. S. Eliot, for example, uses it in his poem *The Waste Land* (1922), in which one of the many distraught narrative voices declares:

"My nerves are bad to-night. Yes, bad. Stay with me.
Speak to me. Why do you never speak? Speak.
What are you thinking of? What thinking? What?
I never know what you are thinking. Think."

The erratic anxious woman who is uttering these lines in the second part of the poem might be modeled on Eliot's first wife, Vivienne, who was struggling with an array of physical and mental problems that included bouts of fatigue, feverish agitation, migraines, and insomnia. Eliot himself suffered a nervous breakdown in the early 1920s. Unlike nervous exhaustion, a nervous breakdown entails a sudden, severe, and usually temporary decline in mental health that is often brought on by stress or trauma. It is an acute rather than a chronic condition and affects people who ordinarily cope well with life's vicissitudes.

When Eliot's mental well-being abruptly deteriorated, his doctor recommended that he take the rest cure for three months.

Eliot followed his advice and sought recovery first on the shores of Margate and then in a sanatorium in Lausanne. It was during this period that he completed his famously bleak, disjointed, and desolate poem ("On Margate Sands / I can connect / Nothing with nothing"), which was to become one of the most iconic representations of the weary and apocalyptic mood of the postwar period. Even spring, traditionally associated with renewal and rebirth, is represented as a negative force in *The Waste Land*:

> April is the cruellest month, breeding
> Lilacs out of the dead land, mixing
> Memory and desire, stirring
> Dull roots with spring rain.

Spring's crime is that it perpetuates the cycle of life, which, in the poet's view, entails nothing but suffering, sordidness, and slow decay. Everything in Eliot's bleak vision has gone to waste: he deems it preferable that the exhausted soil and the weary, ghost-like inhabitants of the ruin-strewn present should be allowed to expire peacefully, rather than having to be forced to continue with their pointless plight.

6

Capitalism

On a mild spring morning full of the promise of new life, a man in his early thirties refuses to get out of bed. It is the same story as every day. He is not physically ill, although he is plagued by a range of minor ailments, such as sties, shortness of breath, and a persistent itch on the back of his head, to which he dedicates much attention. He is wrapped in a threadbare Oriental dressing gown. His soft, chocolate-colored eyes glide wearily over the dusty objects in his derelict bedchamber; his skin is pale, and his features appear curiously slack, as though even his facial muscles lack energy. Around him, filth and cobwebs reign—his room has not been cleaned for years, and the plaster ceiling is crumbling. His man-servant repeatedly beseeches him to get up, to dress, and to shave, but his efforts are in vain.

During the course of the day, the man in the dressing gown receives a string of visitors, all of whom try to lure him out of his bed and to convince him to accompany them to a May celebration that almost all of St. Petersburg will be attending. But the man in the dressing gown firmly resists their offers and remains in bed. His lethargy is disturbed only momentarily, when he remembers some pressing worries—he has recently been told that he has to vacate his lodgings, as his landlord intends to renovate the apartment. He has also just learned that his estate in the country is no longer yielding much profit, owing to neglect and poor management—his annual allowance is about to decrease dramatically. In spite of the urgency of these problems, he is unable to rouse himself into action. He resolves to write some letters to put his affairs in order but cannot muster the energy to do so. He procrastinates and despairs. Days, then weeks, and then the seasons pass. Sometimes he gets as far as putting a few lines to paper but then becomes caught up in the vexing grammatical question of when to use "which" and when to use "that." The letters are never sent, and the man's affairs deteriorate at an alarming pace.

The man in the dressing gown is Ivan Ilyitch Oblomov, the antihero of Ivan Goncharov's (1812–1891) eponymous novel, published in 1859.[1] Although his name has become synonymous with a pathological form of laziness, Oblomov's refusal to get out of bed and to live an active life is due to more complex causes. Laziness implies a moral judgment based on the idea that the lazy person voluntarily chooses to remain inactive and that his or her condition is the result of a lack of willpower or moral fiber. But Oblomov also suffers from a complex range of psychological ailments that challenge this assessment and include depression, anxiety, nervous weakness, and world-weariness.

Oblomov is the only son of a landowning and serf-holding family. He lives at a time when Russia is still essentially feudal but is also seeing the emergence of progressive thinkers, who are proposing radical reforms of the social order and the management of labor. Oblomov never has had to work—from the moment of his birth, he was assigned a man-servant, Zahar, who put on his socks and boots for him and who was supposed to do many other things besides. Zahar, however, is as work shy as his master and also stubborn, clumsy, inefficient, and ill-tempered. Unlike Oblomov, who is at heart a gentle, pure, and loving soul, Zahar has no redeeming qualities.

On one level, Goncharov's novel may be read as social critique, a cautionary tale that reveals the unhealthy consequences of traditional master–servant relationships and the economically and psychologically corrosive effects of an unreformed feudal system. Oblomov and Zahar are mutually dependent, and their constant bickering and deep-seated resentment brings out the worst in both of them. Their relationship symbolizes the political paralysis of tsarist Russia, which was caused mainly by the torpid serf-holding nobility who stood in the way of progress but also by the (possibly deliberate) inefficiency of their serfs. Oblomov, in this reading, epitomizes an outdated feudalism, faced with a rapidly changing world that will soon bring about its bloody demise.

Yet on another level, Goncharov's novel raises more profound questions about the meaning of life and the value of work and explores the philosophical origins of Oblomov's chronic state of exhaustion and his refusal to partake in life's ordinary trials and pleasures. At an early age, Oblomov gives up his (not particularly demanding) post as a collegiate secretary, justified by a doctor's note listing a range of questionable illnesses. He withdraws from public life and spends most of his days in bed, clad in his famous loose dressing gown. He sometimes tries to read and resolves to work on a master plan for his future, which entails the reform of his rapidly decaying inherited estate. Yet he never manages to finish his books, and he never commits his plans to paper. He suffers from panic attacks when forced to go out and is prone to bouts of nervous fear. He is also depressed and languorous, and often bored, and grows fat later in life.

Oblomov's apparent laziness, however, also has psychological and philosophical causes. He longs, above all, to re-create an earthly paradise, an idyllic Arcadian existence where all work is banned. There is an infantile, regressive dimension to this dream, as it closely resembles his early childhood experiences: in the country, cared for by his doting parents and their many servants, he was free from any responsibilities to manage his life; instead, he could roam the gardens and sleep, eat, and play at his leisure. Oblomov's dream of a life free from work and responsibility chimes with a desire with which all of us are familiar: a secret longing to return to the realm of childhood, where our energies were ours to spend as we saw fit; where the days were structured by a diet of pleasure, play, and sleep; and where there was no obligation to bow to the laws of productivity and efficiency. Many experience the transition to the world of work as trauma, as an expulsion from paradise, and memories of that paradise lost continue to haunt us throughout our adult lives.

Oblomov's best friend is a man called Andrey Stolz, who is in every respect his opposite: Stolz is inventive, productive, optimistic, taut, full of energy and vitality. Significantly, he was brought up by a German father, from whom he inherited his discipline, dedication, and apt hand at business, as well as all his other stereotypically Teutonic qualities. His dreamy Russian mother, however, a singer of songs and a teller of tales, nourished his imagination and thus equipped him with a passionate and spiritual dimension to his character. Stolz is the very embodiment of efficiency: he "went his way firmly and cheerfully; he lived on a fixed plan and tried to account for every day as for every rouble, keeping unremitting watch over his time, his labour, and the amount of mental and emotional energy he expended."[2] Stolz represents progress and capitalist inventiveness. Yet there is also a philanthropic and a patriotic dimension to his industriousness: he builds bridges, streets, schools, and houses and works tirelessly for the advancement of Russian industry and the education of its people. Stolz, in other words, is a model capitalist—a capitalist with soul.

Stolz repeatedly rescues Oblomov from bankruptcy and frees him from the clutches of various scroungers and financial exploiters, tirelessly trying to draw his friend out of his inertia. It is in various conversations with Stolz that Oblomov shares his philosophical reservations about living an active life. When Stolz praises the merits of socializing, for example, Oblomov objects: "All these society people are dead men, men fast asleep, they are worse than I am! What is their aim in life? They do not lie in bed like me, they dash backwards and forwards every day like flies, but what is the good?" Stolz eventually accuses his friend of "Oblomovism," a term he has invented to characterize Oblomov's turpitude and lack of ambition. But Oblomov defends himself:

> "What, then, is the ideal life, you think? What is not Oblomovism?" he asked timidly and without enthusiasm. "Doesn't everyone strive for the very same things that I dream of? Why," he added more confidently, "isn't it the purpose of all

your running about, your passions, wars, trade, politics—to secure rest, to attain this ideal of a lost paradise?"

On another occasion, the two friends discuss the merit of work:

"You will stop working some day," Oblomov remarked.

"Never. Why should I?"

"When you have doubled your capital," Oblomov said.

"I won't stop when I have squared it."

"Then why do you work so hard," Oblomov began after a pause, "if it isn't for the sake of providing for your future and then retiring to the country?"

"Oblomovism in the country!" Stolz said.

"Or to attain a high rank and social position and then enjoy in honourable inactivity a well-earned rest? . . ."

"Oblomovism in Petersburg!" Stolz said.

"When, then, are you going to live?" Oblomov asked, annoyed at his remarks. "Why slave all your life?"

"For the sake of work itself and nothing else. Work gives form, and completeness, and a purpose to life, at any rate for me. Here, now, you have banished work from your life, and what is the result?"[3]

The result of the permanent expulsion of work from Oblomov's life is both comic and tragic. Having been duped into a ruinous rental arrangement on the poor side of St. Petersburg, he eventually marries his destitute landlady, the widow Agafya Matveyevna, having fallen in love with her rapidly moving white elbows when she pounds cinnamon. In her benevolent and undemanding care, Oblomov grows fat and happy. Agafya accepts him just as he is and dedicates her life to cooking his favorite dishes and shielding him from unwanted exertion and excitements.

While he thus manages to create an albeit significantly less glamorous version of the earthly paradise of which he has always dreamed, his choices are also driven by a darker, more sinister force. In another conversation with Stolz, we learn about Oblomov's true thoughts on life: "It disturbs one, gives one no peace! I wish I could lie down and go to sleep . . . forever." The narrator also informs us that "with years, agitation and remorse visited him less and less often, and he settled down slowly and gradually in the plain and wide coffin he had made of his existence, like ancient hermits who, turning away from life, dig their own graves." And Oblomov's thinly veiled death wish is ultimately fulfilled. He not only succeeds in practicing a kind of death in life but also dies young—of a stroke brought on by oversleeping, lack of exercise, and too much vodka, wine, red meat, and rich and spicy dishes. Yet at least he passes away quietly, "like a clock that stops because it hasn't been wound up."[4] Oblomov's time, Goncharov seems to suggest, has run its course, as is true of everything he represents: the age of feudalist paralysis and a spirit that is profoundly anticapitalist and antiprogressive in its refusal to subscribe to the values of work, self-improvement, and productivity. Yet what also dies with Oblomov is the possibility of inhabiting a childhood-like state in a work-free land of milk and honey in adulthood.

❉ ❉ ❉

States of exhaustion, as we have seen in the previous chapters, have been theorized both as primarily physical and as primarily mental phenomena. In ancient humoral theory and current biomedical thinking, exhaustion's causes are explained in terms of imbalances in bodily economies: it may be triggered by a disequilibrium between the humoral fluids in the body, on the one hand, and a deficiency in serotonin levels in the brain, on the other. Psychoanalytic approaches, in contrast, shifted the focus onto formative childhood experiences revolving around loss and mourning, as well as onto repression and our drive to return to a state of death-like repose, where all toil and suffering ceases. In Oblomov's case, we can clearly observe the workings of the death drive—his vision of earthly paradise closely corresponds to the inorganic, Nirvana-like condition that Sigmund Freud describes in *Beyond the Pleasure Principle* (1920).[5]

Although these theories take into consideration the ways in which external factors may affect our inner lives, they are primarily concerned with processes that take place inside us—be that in our bodies or our psyches. A radically different explanatory model emerged in the eighteenth and nineteenth centuries that centers on the idea that the causes for what was perceived as an epidemic rise in cases of exhaustion are to be found predominantly on the outside. In the works of George M. Beard, Richard von Krafft-Ebing, and other physicians writing on neurasthenia, the focus shifted toward cultural and environmental factors as the key triggers of exhaustion. Chief among these are the pressures of the liberal market economy, urbanization, a different attitude toward time and work, and a faster, technologically enhanced pace of life.

Exhaustion is intricately bound up not just with our private inner lives and our physical health but also with wider social developments, in particular with more general cultural attitudes toward work and rest. In the Enlightenment, attitudes toward work began to undergo radical transformation, triggered by various factors. These include above all secularization, which was one of the key engines driving scientific progress. In the wake of scientific progress there followed rationalization, the division of labor, industrialization, and bureaucratization. The seventeenth, eighteenth, and nineteenth centuries also saw the rise of a new and increasingly more influential middle class. Most important, however, the modern period saw the advent of free-market capitalism, and the rapid spread of the capitalist system had serious consequences for the psyche of the individual, owing primarily to changing cultural conceptions of the value of work and an increasing commodification of time.

With the onset of industrialization and factory production, the rhythms of work changed. They were now no longer dominated by nature, the seasons, and the weather, as in agrarian societies, but were regulated by abstract rational principles, such as clock time and measurable productivity. Workers had to adapt their rhythms to those of the machines they were servicing; they had to perform the same repetitive movements over and over again, all day long. Karl Marx, too, had much to say about the exhausting nature of factory work. During the course of his lifetime, Marx radically changed his attitude toward labor: in his younger years, he considered work as identity generating, as the primary human activity that defines us as social beings. In his late works, however, he increasingly came to see labor as a burden, as a constraint on freedom and self-realization. As the historian Anson Rabinbach points out, while originally advocating emancipation through work, Marx eventually came to dream of emancipation from work.[6]

One of the most important texts on changing attitudes toward work in the modern period is *The Protestant Ethic and the Spirit of Capitalism* (1904–1905), by the German founding father of sociology, Max Weber.[7] It is significant that Weber was himself diagnosed with neurasthenia and suffered from bouts of prolonged mental and physical exhaustion and an inability to work. Weber was born into a wealthy family in 1864 and was adversely affected by tensions between his parents as a child: his father, a politically engaged lawyer, was a lover of earthly and sensual pleasures, while his mother adhered to a religious-ascetic lifestyle. Weber felt torn between these two poles. He studied law, history, philosophy, and economics and was made professor in Heidelberg in 1896. In 1897, he fell out with his father after a severe quarrel, and when his father died a few months later, Weber suffered a nervous breakdown and sank into depression. His breakdown is usually attributed to overwork, but the historian Joachim Radkau has recently suggested a more complex link between Weber's nervous exhaustion, his intellectual life, and his childhood experiences.[8] Radkau argues that Weber's life was marked by a struggle between his ascetic aspirations, on the one hand, and his erotic inclinations, on the other. Not just the age of modernity, then, but Weber himself is the hero of his famous study, his intellectual interest in the topic having been shaped both by the zeitgeist and by personal experience.

Weber spent five years unable to work and to sleep, moving into and out of sanatoriums and suffering numerous relapses. Eventually, having accepted the chronic nature of his ailment, he decided to give up his academic post for good. In November 1900, while recovering in a sanatorium in the Swabian Alps, Weber felt so weak and depleted that even the thought of writing to his wife, Marianne, seemed "dreadful." Always eager to assist her ailing husband and to remain informed about his physical and mental state, Marianne composed little ready-made cards for him that he simply had to complete. One of these cards read "sleep: 'reasonable'; Legs: 'weary'; Head: 'swimming.'"[9]

Weber was constantly haunted by fears of overstimulating his fragile nervous system. As a result, he was very much opposed to any cures that involved stimulation as a therapeutic strategy, including hydrotherapy and electrotherapy, which were popular measures for treating exhaustion at that time. Yet he fully embraced the dominant medical metaphors that doctors used to describe the phenomenon. He believed that all "overspending" of nervous energy would be "punished" with exhaustion. Nerve force, in his view, behaved just like capital and was governed by strict laws regulating the conservation and expenditure of energy. Exhaustion was nature's revenge for any forms of exertion that were out of the ordinary, including long walks, intense conversations, and even concentrated reading. In a letter to his friend Robert Michels in 1908, Weber wrote: "Exhausted nerve 'capital' (and you don't have a lot of that) behaves like exhausted capital in civil society: when it's gone, it's gone."[10]

In a letter in 1909 to the same friend, who also suffered from exhaustion and whose condition deteriorated, Weber wrote (overindulging in his characteristic fondness for italicized emphasis):

> *I wish I did not know with such eerie certainty* the fate that your style of life and work is storing up for you. . . . You have "cut down on" your *night work*, and that is supposed to help you? You are going to Paris "for relaxation," and that—a cure for over-tiredness through new *stimuli*—has (surprise, surprise!) done *nothing* to help? . . . Give up for a year *all* lecture trips abroad and *all* hurried work, go to bed every (*every*) day at 9.30, spend two weeks *at a time* in the summer relaxing without books (without *any* books) in the isolated German *forest* . . . , and you will know after a year *how much* work capacity/capital you have left; you will again have the security of feeling healthy and, in particular, know precisely how much you are able to work. But only then . . . Please forgive

me if you hear in this the know-all attitude of a "nerve specialist" more than the sympathetic interest of a friend, but
there are times when one *has to* get the truth off one's chest.[11]

The ways in which Weber imagines bodily economies of energy and
depletion are based on financial and theological models very similar to the ones he describes in his most famous work, the essays that
were published in 1904 and 1905 and that constitute *The Protestant
Ethic and the Spirit of Capitalism*. In this study, Weber establishes a
parallel between the Protestant religious ethos and what he calls the
"spirit" (*Geist*) of capitalism. Weber's argument is a radical one: he
explores the cultural and historical origins of a basic attitude toward
work that most of us have come to accept as natural: the importance
of being efficient and successful in one's chosen profession.

Today our profession has come to define who we are perhaps
even more than do our racial and class origins and our gender.
"What do you do?" is one of the first questions asked when we
meet someone. The aspiration to do well at work, and to rise
through the ranks of our chosen profession, is an aim that most
of us accept automatically and uncritically. Very few people today
choose not to partake in that process. Yet this has not always been
the case. Moreover, in the past century, and in particular as a result
of the shift from manufacturing to service industries in the majority of Western countries, the nature of many jobs has also radically changed, in that sociopsychologically exhausting tasks have
replaced physically draining ones.

Weber analyzes the cultural-historical origins of the German
concept of *Berufspflicht*, loosely translatable as "duty toward one's
profession." *Beruf* means "profession," but it is also related to *Beru-
fung*, which translates as "calling." One's *Beruf* can thus be seen not
just as a mere occupation but also as a vocation that has "called" or
claimed us. Weber's study begins with the observation that people
from a Protestant background occupy leading economic positions
much more frequently than do those from other religious denomi-
nations, and that they tend to dominate in market-driven economies. He wonders why this should be the case and argues that

there is something at the very heart of the Protestant worldview that drives people to do well in capitalist society.

The primary enemy of the capitalist spirit, Weber argues, is traditionalism. Economic traditionalists are not interested in multiplying their assets but only in covering their basic needs. Their concern is with the present rather than the future, and consequently they are more interested in working less than in earning more.[12] Creaturely pleasures are valued more highly than achievement. A parable about a Southeast Asian fisherman and an investment banker neatly illustrates the difference between the traditionalist worldview and the entrepreneurial spirit. It also raises some interesting questions about the very foundations of the capitalist frame of mind:

> An American investment banker went on a much-needed holiday to Thailand. Having worked hard all year trading in derivatives, he was exhausted and dying for a proper break. He booked himself into a luxury hotel, drank cocktails at the bar in the evenings, and spent his days fishing in the calm emerald-green waters that caressed the edges of the resort's sandy beach and that gently rocked the colorful small boats moored at the ramshackle pier of a nearby fishing village. On his first afternoon, the banker struck a deal with one of the local fishermen, who sat idly on the pier in the sunshine, and who agreed to take the banker to a good fishing spot in his little boat for a few hours each day. On the third day, as he sat in the boat fishing, the banker began to question the fisherman about his life.
>
> "How many fish do you catch on a good day?" he asked.
>
> "I never catch more than five."
>
> "Why?" the banker asked, astounded. He had been able to catch seven on his second day and was hoping to break his record that day.
>
> "Why not?" the fisherman replied. "We only need five. My family and I, we couldn't eat more than that, and fish don't keep."

"Why don't you sell the additional ones at the market, or to the hotel?"

"Why should I?" the fisherman shrugged.

"To make a profit, of course! In just a few weeks, you could earn enough to buy a second boat, and an employee, and together you could catch even more fish, and earn even more money. You could soon afford an entire flotilla of boats, build warehouses for storage and sell your fish at markets that are further away."

"But why would I want to do this?" The fisherman was genuinely puzzled.

"You would grow rich!"

"And then? What would I do with my money?"

The banker laughed. He thought the fisherman was pulling his leg. But when the latter remained silent, the banker tried to explain further: "You could buy Porsches, live in a big house with air-conditioning and a pool, wear fancy clothes, buy the latest technological equipment. You could drink champagne instead of water. You could eat oysters every day. You could buy your wife designer handbags and Manolo Blahniks. You could send your children to Harvard!"

The fisherman was not impressed. These things did not mean anything to him.

The banker started to become exasperated. But then he had an idea: "You could go on holidays to great places like this one, and spend all day enjoying the sun and fishing!"

"But I'm already doing that," the fisherman said, smiling, and then he rowed the banker back to the shore.[13]

Investing more energy in work in order to multiply one's money with the purpose of rendering life more enjoyable and comfortable, or of buying earlier retirement, would be a different version of the traditionalist attitude—a more systematic, future-orientated pursuit of pleasure. In communities driven by the Protestant work ethic, however, there is no such hedonistic, life- and fun-loving motivation behind the dedication to work—surplus capital gained is simply reinvested to earn more money. Earning money is merely a by-product of doing well in one's vocation, rather than the original aim, and the fruits of hard labor are not spent on creaturely comforts, which were considered sinful and base. Weber argues that Protestants save rather than spend and are therefore able to accumulate capital. But what is the driving force behind the desire to do well in one's profession, if pleasure and material wealth as values in their own right do not matter?

Weber explains this puzzling phenomenon with recourse to the essentially ascetic nature of the Protestant work ethic. Protestant reformers such as Martin Luther, John Calvin, and John Knox attempted to limit the role of intermediaries between believers and God, including priests and the church as an institution, and attacked established customs such as confession and indulgences. The reformists wished to get rid of what they considered "magical" sacramental practices that promised grace and salvation. Weber describes this process as the "disenchantment" of the modern world: the spiritual consequences of sinful behavior could no longer simply be forgiven if one expressed remorse in the confessionary or purchased one's salvation in the form of a letter of indulgence. Therefore, one's entire life had to be systematically managed so that believers could derive from it continual reassurance about their state of grace, on the one hand, and avoid even the occasional slipping into sin, on the other. As a result, asceticism (formerly practiced only by monks) took on a renewed importance. In Protestant cultures, Weber argues, asceticism was gradually transformed from a monastic spiritual practice into a worldly one, as it had become the principal way of controlling one's state of grace or, at least, the external signs that were thought to signal a state of grace. And one's complete dedication to the profession to which one has been called by God, as well as the rationalization of one's lifestyle, were the primary means of achieving this asceticism in a worldly setting.[14]

These, in a nutshell, are the processes that, according to Weber, explain how industriousness, frugality, efficiency, discipline, and a strong sense of personal responsibility became the very fabric of the Protestant moral code. The emphasis on the value of asceticism and industriousness also explains the condemnation of everything that stood in their way—above all, comfort, indulgence, sensual pleasure, waste, and rest. As a consequence, attitudes not just toward work but also toward rest and time changed dramatically. Weber argues that relaxation and the enjoyment of worldly possessions was seen as a dangerous distraction from a holy life. The saints' everlasting rest, he writes, is in the next world. Yet on Earth, humans above all have to fulfill God's calling:

> Not leisure and enjoyment, but *only activity* serves to increase the glory of God, according to the definite manifestations of His will.
>
> *Waste of time* is thus the first and in principle the deadliest of sins. The span of human life is infinitely short and precious in order to reassure oneself of one's calling. Loss of time through sociability, "idle talk," luxury, even more sleep than is necessary for health—six to at most eight hours—is worthy of absolute moral condemnation.[15]

Here, we can see that once again, wasteful (that is, nonproductive) activities and rest have been classified as sins—just as acedia had been defined as one of the Seven Deadly Sins in the Middle Ages. The sudden renewed increase in cultural anxieties about exhaustion and its effects occurred precisely at the historical moment when the values that exhaustion threatened (above all, activity, productivity, and progress) rose in importance and became an ineradicable part of our social fabric. In other words, exhaustion is the flip side of the dominant cultural values of the modern era. The more important these values became, the more their opposites were feared and vilified: wasting time and lack of energy and ambition became the primary secular sins of the capitalist age. The squandering of time and energy was considered as scandalous an act as the squandering of money itself.

And yet there is a further twist to be added to this argument: as Rabinbach has suggested, technological progress is also essentially driven by the hopes of redemption from labor, by the desire to avoid hard, crude, and unnecessary physical work and the bodily fatigue that comes in its wake.[16] Many innovations are the result of visions of less or easier work: think of such simple devices as washing machines, excavators, and suitcases on wheels; or imagine robots able to perform human tasks so that we no longer have to do them ourselves. Modernity, then, in a paradoxical move, causes exhaustion but is also driven forward by the desire to avoid exhaustion.

* * *

The German novelist Thomas Mann, just like Weber, describes himself explicitly as neurasthenic in his diaries and letters. Illness, particularly nervous ailments, and the connection between illness and genius more generally, is a topic that was to preoccupy him all his life. In his first novel, *Buddenbrooks* (1901), Mann reflects explicitly on the effects of work and capitalist competition on the body, mind, and spirit of the individual. The novel is set in the nineteenth century and chronicles the social, physical, and psychological decline of a German bourgeois merchant family, the descendants of which become increasingly unable to perform well in a new market-driven economic setting. The fall of the Buddenbrooks is contrasted with the rise of the nouveau-riche and economically much more adventurous Hagenströms, who signal a new era in which coarse and ruthless capitalists are victorious. The Hagenströms are blessed with a healthy appetite (both literally and metaphorically), and their children are vigorous and socially successful. The members of the Buddenbrook family, in contrast, battle with exhaustion, nervous weakness, hypochondria, melancholia, tuberculosis, bad teeth, and world-weariness.

The brothers Thomas and Christian Buddenbrook represent the generation in which the family's fortunes begin visibly to deteriorate. Christian, the younger of the two, is a clownish hypochondriac, obsessed with an increasing number of trivial nervous and bodily ailments. He squanders his wealth, time, and talents and ends up in an asylum. His reproachful brother Thomas describes him in medical terms as "a growth, an unhealthy pustule on the body of our family."[17] For Thomas, who takes over the family business, bourgeois existence turns into an increasingly difficult charade. His commercial dealings do not go well—he lacks the entrepreneurial ruthlessness and acumen of his competitors. The pressures of the changed economic landscape oppress him, as do the many misfortunes of his siblings. He grows weary of, and alienated from, his family and his profession and finds it ever more difficult to keep up the social masquerade. He becomes anxiously obsessed with his clothes, his appearance, and external symbols of status and wealth, precisely because he knows that beneath the surface everything is falling apart. When he reads Schopenhauer's *The World as Will and Representation*, the book has a devastating effect on him.

Mann's description of Thomas's state of psychological, physical, and spiritual exhaustion, which is brought on not just by the corrupting influence of Schopenhauer but also by too much hard work and the hopelessness of the task of trying to rescue the family's business in a radically transformed socioeconomic landscape, centers on the waning of engagement and commitment, a feeling of existential emptiness, and the excessive and increasingly impossible investment of energy that is necessary in performing simple tasks and upholding a socially acceptable façade:

And, in truth, Thomas Buddenbrook's existence was no different from that of an actor—an actor whose life has become one long production, which, but for a few brief hours for relaxation, draws on and consumes unceasingly all his energy [*beständig alle Kräfte in Anspruch nimmt und verzehrt*]. In the absence of any passionate, authentic interest, which would have engaged him, his inward impoverishment and desolation oppressed him almost without any relief, with a constant, dull chagrin, while he stubbornly clung to an inner duty and the tenacious determination to be worthily representative, to conceal his inward decline, and to preserve "the *dehors*" whatever it cost him. All this made of his life, his every word, his every motion, his every interaction with people, an artificial, self-conscious, forced, exhausting and nerve-wrecking act of histrionics.[18]

Thomas soon dies an ignoble death as a result of an infected tooth. His son Hanno, the last of the Buddenbrooks, is of a pale and weakly constitution, hypersensitive, effeminate, nervous, and completely incapable of performing ordinary worldly tasks. He fears pressure, work, and competition. The only areas of joy in his life are a homoerotic friendship with an aspiring young writer and improvising on the piano. Hanno dies young as a consequence of overexertion—after an emotionally draining session playing Wagner on the piano, he succumbs to tuberculosis.

In *Buddenbrooks*, Mann connects nervous weakness and world-weariness with modern culture and its discontents. These include the need for an ever more complex repression of sexual desires, a loosening of family bonds, and the shift from traditional values and an old-fashioned Protestant work ethic to a new, more cold-blooded type of competitive capitalism. The representatives of the old world suffer bankruptcy, marry badly, and fall from grace. Mann's novel suggests that there is something about artistic and sensitive people that is incompatible with the new world order. The decline of the family's social status and mental and bodily health is accompanied, or perhaps even caused, by an increase in sensitivity and artistic inclinations. Thomas's father, for example, is extremely religious; Christian spends most of his time in the theater and most of his money on entertaining actresses; Thomas marries an eccentric violinist and develops a fatal interest in metaphysics. It is no coincidence that Hanno, a sickly and hypersensitive artist figure, is deemed to have no chance of survival from the moment he is born.

Mann's alignment of nervous weakness and mental instability with the arts draws, as we have seen, on a much older topos: as far back as the fourth century B.C.E., Aristotle associated the melancholic temperament with scholarship, creativity, and genius, a link that Marsilio Ficino strengthened further in the fifteenth century. What Mann adds to this idea is that the competition-driven modern world has become so hostile to those who are born sensitive that their very survival is at risk.

✳ ✳ ✳

In our own times, the imperative to be productive and the desire to earn money have been stripped entirely of the spiritual dimension that Weber argues they possessed in the past. It is ironic that in many Western countries today (unlike in Japan, for example), hard work is no longer held a value in itself. Gone are the days when a long-term strategy for professional success—based on drudgery, long apprenticeships, and life-long learning—was considered admirable. Subjects that require a sustained cognitive effort, such as modern languages, are in danger of all but disappearing from higher education. "Get-rich-quick" schemes, the appeal of the promise of lotteries to create millionaires in two seconds, climbing the property ladder, risky investments, and reckless stock market trades are the new "magical" ladders leading to salvation. The figure of the investment banker, in particular, has attracted so much attention recently because it embodies the hope that we can all get obscenely rich without any long-term physical or intellectual effort. In many ways, the antifutural, impatient "maximum-results-with-minimum-effort" mentality that characterizes our age is the very opposite of the Protestant work ethic and more akin to the mind-set of the gambler and the drug addict: both desire instant bliss without exertion and pursue it without any regard for the long-term consequences.

It is no wonder, then, that our age has seen the advent of another phenomenon: capitalism fatigue. The idea that a drive to maximize profit, growth, and progress at all costs is a "natural" human desire, and that unregulated free-market capitalism is the only system that allows it to thrive, is one that still dominates economic policies in the West. However, the mantra of growth for growth's sake, the celebration of unfettered consumption on credit, and the basic premises of neoliberal market theories are increasingly being questioned, and not just by economists on the left. A discontent with the globalized version of capitalism is becoming ever more tangible, and it is taking many different forms.

In *The Price of Inequality: How Today's Divided Society Endangers Our Future*, the Nobel Prize–winning economist Joseph Stiglitz challenges the dogma of neoliberal and laissez-faire economic policies. He argues that a very small, very wealthy, and very powerful elite with vested interests determines economic policies in the West, all of which are designed to render them even richer. He challenges the "trickle-down myth": the economic activities of the super-rich elite are not productive and do not result in more jobs or investment in infrastructure, since they are mainly of a distributive, "rent-extracting" nature. Stiglitz provides compelling evidence for the fact that, as a result of deregulating the markets, the incomes of a small elite have exploded out of proportion while average incomes have fallen and inequality has increased. While Stiglitz does not argue against free-market capitalism as such, he recommends systematic government regulation as a cure for the rapidly growing chasm between rich and poor. Without such constraints, this chasm, and especially the gap between the 1 percent of super-earners and the rest of the population, will not just result in social problems but indeed threaten the stability of the market itself: excessive inequality of the kind we are currently witnessing, Stiglitz warns, creates volatility, undermines productivity, and hinders growth.[19]

The French economist Thomas Pikkety's best-selling *Capital in the Twenty-First Century* (2013) provides a painstakingly researched empirical-historical account of the evolution of inequality, showing that an ever smaller number of people control an ever larger concentration of capital, and that this tendency, if unchecked, will lead to the inevitable demise of the system in its current form.[20] The British economist Adair Turner goes even further. He argues that there is something fundamentally wrong with the ways in which "growth" is uncritically accepted as a value and pursued by Western governments as the ultimate aim of all economic policies.[21] Various so-called happiness economists, such as Kate Pickett, Richard Wilkinson, Richard Layard, Bruno Frey, and Alois Stutzer, have provided compelling statistic evidence that economic growth does not automatically translate into increased happiness.[22] On the contrary, growth, particularly in the Anglo-American version of capitalism, is generally accompanied by increased inequality, which diminishes human happiness and brings with it its own specific forms of exhaustion, on both a broader cultural and an individual-psychological level. Earning enough money to allow for all primary human needs (such as food, accommodation, education, and health care) to be covered comfortably does matter, of course. There is no doubt that poverty renders people unhappy. But there is no statistically measurable correlation between happiness and an income that exceeds this minimum level: beyond a basic living wage, there is a flattening of the relationship between income and well-being. One winter coat, for example, keeps you warm, but two do not keep you warmer. The added benefits of luxury, style, and status are marginal factors that cannot bring about or sustain an increase in contentment. The adverse and socially corrosive effects of inequality, in contrast, such as rising crime levels, falling education and literacy standards, health and addiction problems, obesity, and teenage pregnancy rates, are likely to be so severe that they outweigh the benefits of allowing a tiny proportion of the population to grow wealthier.

The numerous studies conducted by the happiness economists confirm a very simple and old idea: money cannot buy happiness. Stiglitz's, Pikkety's, Turner's, and many other studies attest to a growing disenchantment in the West with capitalism in its current neoliberal form. There is a steep rise in books and media reports dedicated to capitalism's night sides, ranging from the appalling conditions in Southeast Asian sweatshops and the grave environmental disasters such as oil spills and leaking nuclear power stations, to the mindboggling bonuses paid out to precisely the bankers who have gambled away the foundations of their own companies, and much else besides.

Capitalism fatigue finds its perhaps most visible expression in the Occupy movement, which emerged in Spain in March 2011 under the label *Indignados* and in the United States in the autumn of 2011 as the Occupy Wall Street movement and then spread to many other countries. The Occupy movement uses the slogan "We are the 99%" and protests against the mounting power of multinational global corporations over politics, growing social and economic inequality, and the failure legally to prosecute those responsible for causing the financial crisis. Yet the movement has been criticized for a lack of alternative goals—its advocates are, above all, negators, militating against the current system, rather than proposing concrete and realizable action plans. In addition, what renders this and other antiglobalization movements potentially less impactful than, say, left-wing protests in the 1960s and 1970s, is the fact that there simply appear to be no viable alternatives to capitalism. Following the demise of the last serious Communist regimes in the 1990s, we are left with only one, albeit deeply flawed, system. The situation is reminiscent of self-loathing, depressed people feeling strongly that they can simply no longer continue being themselves, yet there is nothing else they can be.

It is worth remembering, however, that there may at least be better, more humane versions of capitalism out there that acknowledge the importance of individual well-being and the quality of life of the many, insist on legislation to bring about a less exhausting work–life balance for its workforce, and place more emphasis on maintaining a reasonable equilibrium between the avoidance of obscene levels of inequality and the pursuit of growth. The Scandinavian model, for instance, demonstrates more concern for the general welfare of its citizens by prioritizing areas such as education, childcare, affordable housing, and a functioning benefit and health-care system, which contrasts starkly with the main aims of the exclusively growth-focused Anglo-American brand of capitalism. The pursuit of growth for growth's sake demands a high price—not just socially but also psychologically and physically, as the steep rise of neurasthenia, depression, and burnout in our century and the previous two shows.

Goncharov, Weber, Mann, and numerous other writers and thinkers have raised serious questions about the psychological, ethical, and experiential consequences of modern attitudes toward work and growth that many of us tend to accept uncritically. Turner and Stieglitz, too, argue that what is needed is, above all, a shift in priorities and a reintroduction of moral principles into economic policy making. They propose therapy rather than a radical revolution. Yet whether a gentle readjustment will be able to restore trust in what in many respects appears an exhausted model of organizing economic activities remains to be seen.

7

Rest

Rest is a state that is characterized by the cessation of labor and the absence of exertion of any kind. Rest structures our lives and furnishes them with rhythm—we constantly alternate between phases of activity and repose, which are manifest most notably in our waking and sleeping patterns but also in the ways in which we organize our weeks by distinguishing between workdays and weekends, and by interrupting longer periods of work with vacations. Rest is an interval of inactivity of a specific duration from which we expect to emerge restored, with our energy replenished and our spirit renewed. It is a necessary counterpoint to human activity, during which we recover both physically and mentally from life's exertions. The fact that our energies are exhaustible and that we need periodically to rest is precisely what makes us human and what distinguishes us from zombies and robots.

Many religions explicitly prescribe a specific day of rest. The fourth of the Ten Commandments, for example, states:

> Remember the Sabbath day, to keep it holy. Six days shalt thou labour, and do all thy work: But the seventh day *is* the Sabbath of the Lord thy God: *in it* thou shalt not do any work, thou, nor thy son, nor thy daughter, thy manservant, nor thy maidservant, nor thy cattle, nor thy stranger that *is* within

thy gates: For *in* six days the Lord made heaven and earth, the sea, and all that in them *is*, and rested the seventh day: wherefore the Lord blessed the Sabbath day, and hallowed it.[1]

The fact that the Sabbath rule features so prominently in the Decalogue, a list featuring only the most indispensable of laws (the others proscribing murder, theft, adultery, jealousy, and blasphemy), illustrates how seriously the human need for rest was taken in the past. Indeed, it suggests that even an almighty and omnipotent God needed a break after having created the heavens and Earth. The importance of rest in biblical times was probably motivated by the desire not so much to enhance people's productivity, which is the primary modern justification of rest, but to strengthen the bonds of community—when everyone rests on the same day, rest becomes an experience that brings people together, imposing a shared, communal rhythm on their lives.

Many theorists of exhaustion bemoan the loss of the natural rhythm of life in the age of modernity and look back nostalgically to periods when, they imagine, lives were structured by clearly demarcated periods of rest and activity. Agrarian societies, for example, are assumed to have been dominated by entirely natural rhythms: before the advent of gas lamps and electricity in the nineteenth century, the diurnal cycle of daytime and nighttime produced by Earth's orbital motion remained undisturbed by artificial interventions. Working hours ended naturally with the fading of daylight and the setting of the sun. The seasons, moreover, also dictated periods of increased activity at certain points in the year (for example, during planting and harvest time), which were counterbalanced by periods of relative inactivity (notably, the cold winter months during which nature itself rests and nothing grows). While nature appeared to dictate the patterns of rest and activity in the premodern era, modernity saw the introduction of artificial lighting and clock time. In the industrial age, the pace and rhythm of work were increasingly dictated by external factors, and workers had to bow to the dictates of productivity and efficiency.

Among other things, fatigue can be understood as a warning sign emitted by the body to indicate when it is being overtaxed.

It signals limits and that the body requires rest. In workplaces where the tempo of work is externally determined, such warning signs can often be ignored and the body's needs overridden. Many exhaustion theorists, moreover, have declared that the conditions of modernity more generally imposed an externally regulated pace on people's natural rhythms, a pace that many experienced as too fast and that relentlessly assaulted the individual with new stimuli and demands, no longer allowing for properly restorative periods of rest.

A characteristic feature of cases of chronic exhaustion is that they cannot be relieved by normal periods of rest. Many neuras-thenics, for example, experienced what we would now describe as postexertion malaise. Even the simplest, seemingly least taxing physical activities would result in states of complete exhaustion, from which it took them a disproportionally long time to recover. Yet, as the influential American physician Silas Weir Mitchell (1829–1914) points out, the problem becomes even more troubling when we consider the issue of mental exhaustion. Unlike the body, the mind very rarely sends clear fatigue signals, and it is more dif-ficult to determine when enough is enough and when the mind needs to rest. Moreover, "an excess of physical labor is better borne than a like excess of mental labor," since physical labor encourages positive collateral activities that mental labor discourages: physi-cal labor quickens the heart, drives the blood "through unused channels," hastens the breathing, and increases the secretions of the skin. Brain work, in contrast, impoverishes all these functions and requires a much higher "expenditure of nerve material."[2]

Paradoxically, the core symptom of the overworked brain, abused by too much activity and too little rest, is precisely that it becomes unable to rest. It is not surprising that sleeping disorders loom large in the list of symptoms that accompany exhaustion in various diagnoses, including neurasthenia, depression, burn-out, and chronic fatigue syndrome. Mitchell aptly describes this vicious circle in the following terms:

At last we stop and propose to find rest in bed. Not so, says the ill-used brain, now morbidly awake; and whether we will or not, the mind keeps turning over and over the work of the day, the business or legal problem, or mumbling, so to speak, some wearisome question in a fashion made useless by the denial of full attention. Or else the imagination soars away with the unrestful energy of a demon, conjuring up an endless procession of broken images and disconnected thoughts, so that sleep is utterly banished.[3]

Mitchell devised an infamous and highly influential therapeutic regime that would shape the treatment of the chronically exhausted for decades: it was appositely called the "rest cure."

✸ ✸ ✸

John is a physician, and *perhaps*—(I would not say it to a living soul, of course, but this is dead paper and a great relief to my mind)—*perhaps* that is one reason I do not get well faster.

You see he does not believe I am sick!

And what can one do?

If a physician of high standing, and one's own husband, assures friends and relatives that there is really nothing the matter with one but temporary nervous depression—a slight hysterical tendency—what is one to do?

My brother is also a physician, and also of high standing, and he says the same thing.

So I take phosphates or phosphites—whichever it is, and tonics, and journeys, and air, and exercise, and am absolutely forbidden to "work" until I am well again.

Personally, I disagree with their ideas.

Personally, I believe that congenial work, with excitement and change, would do me good.

But what is one to do?[4]

The woman who commits to paper this cautious disagreement with her physician-husband's recommendations experiences a form of nervous weakness that makes her feel exhausted and hopeless. Her ostensibly well-meaning husband, John, orders her to stay in bed and rest, deprived of all stimuli, company, and the activity she cares for most—writing. He ushers her away to a country manor for the summer months in order to isolate her from her familiar surroundings and friends, and he forces her to undergo an aggressive rest cure. In spite of his wife's protests, her husband compels her to occupy a room at the top of the house, which is decorated with yellow wallpaper on which are printed disconcertingly complex and flamboyant patterns.

Lonely, ailing, and deprived of all sensual and intellectual input, the woman becomes increasingly obsessed with the strange pattern of the yellow wallpaper. The wallpaper's color, a sickly and "smouldering unclean yellow," repels her.[5] It quickly turns into a source of delirious optic horror, its irrational structure morphing into a torturing puzzle she is desperate to solve.

Soon she thinks that she can detect a second layer of meaning behind the mystifying arabesques: at night in the silvery moonlight, she can make out the faint shapes of a woman behind the pattern. The wallpaper woman creeps and crawls to and fro and sometimes shakes the pattern as though it were bars through which she is trying to break. Eventually, the narrator decides to free the person behind the wallpaper, but when she has finished ripping it off the walls she finds that it is she herself who is liberated in a strange way—she has shed all pretenses and creeps along the walls of her room like an animal. When her horrified husband eventually finds his creeping wife and faints, she does not change her path and creeps right over him.

The plight of the exhausted woman, whose mental health declines sharply as a result of a wrongly administered "rest cure," is explored in Charlotte Perkins Gilman's (1860–1935) famous short story "The Yellow Wallpaper" (1892), one of the most influential feminist texts of the modern period. Like all great works of literature, the story invites various interpretations: Are we to understand the woman behind the wallpaper as a psychological projection, a symbolic representation of the narrator's pain and her sense of entrapment? Or does the text simply chronicle a descent into madness, a gradual loss of sanity that results in obsessive delusions and hallucinatory visions? Is the wallpaper woman a cipher for all women who are oppressed by an incomprehensible and stifling patriarchal system, a system that seems designed to prevent women from independent thought and the free play of the imagination? Is she an externalization not so much of the nervous narrator's psychological pain but of her socioeconomic plight, caused by unsympathetic and oppressive figures of authority, epitomized by her physician-husband?[6]

"The Yellow Wallpaper" can be interpreted in all these ways. Yet it is also an important semiautobiographical document detailing the horrors that patients in the late nineteenth century could suffer at the hands of insensitive physicians, who were not yet properly able, or indeed willing, to respond to the mental suffering of women. It is, above all, a textbook case study of a gender-biased misdiagnosis. It illustrated the plight of the female patient whose voice was being ignored, and it shows the dangerous consequences of medical arrogance. It also illustrates the ways in which theories of exhaustion and its origins translated into concrete medical practice, and how these could affect the lives of real people.

Gilman, who was an author, a feminist, and a social reformer, experienced both mental and physical exhaustion, as well as what might now be diagnosed as severe postpartum depression, after having given birth to her first and only child in 1885. She was treated by Mitchell, who was not only the inventor of the "rest cure" but also the author of *Wear and Tear: Or, Hints for the Overworked* (1871) and *Fat and Blood and How to Make Them* (1877). Mitchell and his cure are clearly the targets of "The Yellow Wallpaper"—he is even mentioned by name when the narrator's husband threatens to send his wife to Mitchell in the autumn if her condition does not improve. Mitchell's rest cure required the patient's complete isolation, strict bed rest, deprivation of any intellectual stimuli, and rapid weight gain. He wished to renew the vitality of feeble people by "a combination of entire rest and of excessive feeding." Conjecturing that the loss of fat impoverished the blood, he assumed that weight gain would improve "the color and amount of the red corpuscles." "To gain in fat," he declares, "is nearly always to gain in blood."[7] His rest-cure patients, most of whom were female neurasthenics, were confined to bed for a period of six to eight weeks.

Serious cases were not even allowed to relieve themselves or to turn over without the doctor's permission. During this period of enforced rest, they also had to consume large quantities of milk (at least four pints a day), mutton chops, beef tea, bread and butter, malt extract, and iron supplements.

After Gilman had spent nine weeks at his clinic, submitting herself completely to his rest regime, Mitchell sent her home to her husband with the following instructions: "Live as domestic a life as possible. Have your child with you all the time. . . . Lie down an hour after each meal. Have but two hours' intellectual life a day. And never touch pen, brush or pencil as long as you live."[8] Gilman attempted to follow his instructions for a while but, after her condition worsened, finally abandoned his advice, divorced her husband, dedicated herself fully to her various intellectual projects, and swiftly recovered.

Its dubious benefits notwithstanding, Mitchell's rest cure was soon prescribed to patients all over Europe. Virginia Woolf, for instance, who was also diagnosed with neurasthenia, was subjected to the same regime of bed rest, avoidance of excitement, and excessive milk and beef consumption by a doctor called George Savage, who followed Mitchell's theories.[9] Like Gilman before her, Woolf was certainly no fan of this cure. In 1910, in a letter to her sister Vanessa Bell, she complains bitterly about her treatment:

> I really dont think I can stand much more of this . . . you cant conceive how I want intelligent conversation—even yours. . . . However, what I mean is that I shall soon have to jump out of a window. The ugliness of the house is almost inexplicable. . . . Then there is all the eating and drinking and being shut up in the dark.
> My God! What a mercy to be done with it![10]

Throughout her adult life, Woolf battled with mental health problems and alternating states of extreme exhaustion and manic activity, until she committed suicide by drowning herself in the River Ouse in 1941. In 1922, she was (rather poetically) diagnosed with a "tired heart." In June of that year, she also had three of

her teeth pulled—this was supposed to lower the body temperature of "overheated" hysterics and neurasthenics, because it was
assumed that nests of germs were clustering under the roots of
the teeth, generating feverish excitement.[11] Like Gilman, Woolf
fiercely criticizes the male medical establishment and its attitudes
toward mental health in her writing. In *Mrs. Dalloway* (1925), for
example, she pens a scathing portray of an arrogant, judgmental
psychiatrist called Sir William Bradshaw, whose lack of sympathy ultimately leads to the suicide of a shell-shocked and severely
distressed war veteran. In her essay "On Being Ill" (1926), Woolf
defiantly sings the praises of the sick, whose unique sensibility and
imagination she contrasts favorably with the restless activity- and
project-driven "army of the upright."[12]

❊ ❊ ❊

Mitchell's rest cure has not just attracted the wrath of various
writers but also become a much-discussed case study in feminist
debates about the ways in which medical diagnoses can be bound
up with assumptions about "natural" and "unnatural" gender roles
and behavior. George M. Beard's neurasthenia diagnosis is based,
above all, on classist and racist beliefs—that is, the idea that only
refined, upper-class "brain workers," in particular American citizens and those of other "civilized" and "advanced" nations, can
fall prey to this disease. Mitchell's therapeutic regime, in contrast,
rests primarily on traditional conceptions of appropriate gender
roles. It is not difficult to see the dubious gender ideology that
lurks behind his "medical" recommendation to Gilman—a woman
is to return home to her husband, abandon all intellectual pursuits, focus on motherhood, and resume her "natural" place in the
kitchen and in bed.

These views are particularly evident in *Wear and Tear*, in which
Mitchell rails not just at the general "thoughtless sinners against the
laws of labor and of rest" but, above all, against the dangerous consequences of educating young women. Using metaphors very similar to those deployed by Beard, he articulates fears about exhausting "a capital of vitality" painfully accumulated by generations

of healthy, outdoor-living men. Mitchell, too, bemoans the "cruel competition for the dollar, the new and exciting habits of business, the racing speed which the telegraph and railway have introduced into commercial life," but he is particularly concerned with "the overeducation and overstraining" of girls. The various nervous ailments that result from submitting young girls to the pressures of an education that goes beyond teaching them about household economy, sewing, and cooking results in their failure to "fulfill all the natural functions of mothers." He is particularly worried about the age of puberty, during which girls should be kept away from school altogether.[13]

"Overuse," he sternly warns, "or even a very steady use, of the brain is in many dangerous to health and to every probability of future womanly usefulness." Education makes a girl "unfit for her duties as woman" and unable to deliver what "nature asks from her as wife and mother." This lack of "future womanly usefulness" has, of course, frightful consequences for the biological and psychological capital of the nation: "[T]here comes a time when the matured man certainly surpasses the woman in persistent energy and capacity for unbroken brain-work. If then she matches herself against him, it will be, with some exceptions, at bitter cost."[14]

Moreover, Mitchell generally seems strongly to dislike his female neurasthenic patients, as remarks such as the following indicate, in which he compares them to tyrants, malingerers, and vampires, as well as describing them as selfish and morally despicable: the female invalids who are destined for "the shawl and the sofa," we are informed, have produced "untold discomfort in many a household." These "self-made invalids" can make entire households "wretched," destroying "generations of nursing relatives" in the process.[15] He gravely alleges: "I have seen a hysterical, anaemic girl kill in this way three generations of nurses." The exhausted woman is "like a vampire, sucking slowly the blood of every healthy, helpful creature within reach of her demands."[16] The undisguised misogyny and hostility that is evident in these remarks render his resting and fattening regime even more sinister. By confining women to their beds and, above all, by suggesting that it was their attempt to seek an education and to compete with men in the workplace that made them ill in the first place, Mitchell is essentially trying to put a halt to a social process with which he clearly felt uncomfortable—the emancipation of women.

Various feminist critics have commented on gender-political assumptions that often influence the construction of medical diagnoses. Nervous weakness and, in particular, hysteria were at the forefront of ailments that were primarily associated with women. Lisa Appignanesi and Elaine Showalter, for example, argue that women whose views and behaviors were at odds with established norms were frequently medicalized—labeling their socially deviant actions or troubling opinions as "mad" was effectively a strategy designed to silence them.[17] Mitchell is, of course, not the only physician to have put forth dubious medical claims about the origins of nervous exhaustion in women. Beard, too, famously lists "the education of women" as one of the five main factors that led to the epidemic spread of neurasthenia. Even Richard von Krafft-Ebing constructs a similar argument: the emancipation of women, he writes, is a primary "source for the emergence of nervousness that is not to be underestimated":

> Although women might now be capable of competing with men in various fields, for millennia, their destiny has been a different one. Only over the course of many generations can the capacity of the brain that is necessary for succeeding in formerly exclusively male scientific or artistic professions be acquired by a woman. Only a few singular, unusually strong, and advantageously equipped female individuals can already successfully assert themselves in the intellectual work-place competition that is enforced by modern social circumstances. The vast majority of women who accept this fight risk losing it. The number of the defeated and the dead is simply mind-blowing.[18]

Although women were far from being the only group diagnosed with nervous exhaustion in the final decades of the nineteenth and the early decades of the twentieth centuries, there can be no doubt that conceptions of "natural" and "unnatural" gender behavior substantially shaped medical debates and diagnoses, and that certain diagnoses were used to submerge critical female voices and to stifle feminist activities. Moreover, Mitchell's case illustrates once again how cultural critique and medical diagnosis can be fused together, often in insidious ways. Many theories of exhaustion are used as vehicles to express fears about social transformation—be they technical, cultural, or sociopolitical in nature. Often, unwanted developments are held directly responsible for specific psychosomatic symptoms—think of the railway spine or, more recently, the wind turbine syndrome. Mitchell's rest cure articulates deep-seated anxieties about the emancipation of women, their entry into the world of work, and changing gender roles. Here, and elsewhere, culturally conservative views are presented in the guise of a medical treatise.

✳ ✳ ✳

Charles Darwin (1809–1882), the famous British naturalist who first articulated the idea of natural selection and whose work *On the Origin of Species* (1859) directly influenced theories such as Krafft-Ebing's that explained nervous exhaustion as a result of degeneration, experienced numerous physical ailments during his lifetime. These included attacks of dyspepsia, flatulence, vomiting, dizziness, and nausea and frequently resulted in extreme fatigue and prolonged states of exhaustion. Darwin suffered from severe seasickness during his five-year voyage on HMS *Beagle*, which took him to the shores of Brazil, Argentina, Chile, and the Galápagos Islands. His physical distress is well documented in the diary he kept during this journey, as well as in his correspondence. In a letter to his father, written in February and March 1832, Darwin complains:

My dear Father

Nobody who has only been to sea for 24 hours has a right to say, that sea-sickness is even uncomfortable.—The real misery only begins when you are so exhausted—that a little exertion makes a feeling of faintness come on.—I found nothing but lying in my hammock did me any good.[19]

It was while on board the *Beagle* that Darwin discovered a routine that enabled him to manage his physical ailments by alternating short periods of work with extended interludes of stillness and inactivity. Back on English soil, he would continue to follow a rigorous daily regime structured by carefully measured intervals of work and rest. After an hour of writing in the morning, for example, he would lie down on the sofa in the drawing room and listen to a member of his family reading out his correspondence or the papers. After another hour of work, he would go for a brief walk, withdraw to his bedroom to smoke and read novels, or lie immobile on the sofa once again.[20]

Many have speculated about the exact nature of Darwin's disease. Some consider his ailments to be primarily of a psychosomatic nature and have suggested hypochondria, depression, nervous exhaustion, neurosis, and neurasthenia as possible diagnoses. Others argue that he contracted Chagas disease as a result of having been bitten by a bug in the Argentine pampas in 1835; yet others conjecture that he may have suffered from arsenic poisoning. Even chronic fatigue syndrome (which did not, of course, exist as a diagnosis during Darwin's time) has been suggested as a retroactive explanation for his various malaises.

In addition to following his own personalized "rest cure," Darwin found some respite in hydrotherapy and returned numerous times to spa establishments offering aquatic treatments, including in Malvern in Worcestershire, Ilkley in Yorkshire, and Farnham in Surrey. In October 1849, he sent a letter to his friend J. D. Hooker, describing the workings of the water cure in detail:

My dear Hooker

You ask about my Cold Water Cure; I am going on very well & am certainly a little better every month; my nights mend much slower than my days.—I have built a douche & am to go on through all the winter, frost or no frost—My treatment now is lamp 5 times per week & shallow bath for 5 minutes afterwards; douche daily for 5 minutes & dripping sheet daily. The treatment is wonderfully tonic, & I have had more better consecutive days this month, than on any previous ones.— The vomiting I consider absolutely cured. I am allowed to work now 2½ hours daily, & I find it as much as I can do; for the cold-water cure, together with 3 short walks is curiously exhausting; & I am actually *forced* always to go to bed at 8 oclock completely tired.—I steadily gain in weight & eat immensely & am never oppressed with my food. I have lost the involuntary twitching of the muscles & all the fainting feelings &c black spots before eyes &c &c Dr Gully thinks he shall quite cure me in 6 or 9 months more.—

The greatest bore, which I find in the Water Cure, is the having been compelled to give up all reading, except the newspapers; for my daily 2½ hours at the Barnacles is fully as much as I can do of anything which occupies the mind: I am consequently terribly behind in all Scientific books.[21]

The water cure, alongside the rest cure, electrotherapy, tonic tinctures, and strict dietary regimes, was one of the most popular treatments prescribed to those experiencing nervous exhaustion. Darwin, like Woolf and Gilman, was forced to limit intellectual stimulation and "brain work" as part of the therapeutic regime to which he subscribed. However, in contrast to Woolf and Gilman, he seems to have been more or less at peace with the idea that he had to manage his energies carefully by permanently restricting his working hours, living a relatively secluded and quiet life, and building long periods of regular rest into his daily routine in order to avoid the dangers of more persistent states of exhaustion. Unlike Woolf and Gilman, he chose his own personal rhythm of work and rest—one that was tailored to fit with and enhance his own energy levels. It was, perhaps, precisely the "one-size-fits-all" recipe of Mitchell's rest cure that jarred with so many of his patients, all of whom had unique needs, rhythms, and sensibilities.

✻ ✻ ✻

The most obvious form of rest in which we regularly engage is, of course, sleep. We spend roughly one-third of our lives asleep. Sleep disturbances frequently accompany and sometimes cause states of exhaustion. Sleep scientists have established that a short-term lack of sleep can adversely affect mood, judgment, and concentration and may increase the risk of accidents. Chronic sleep deprivation can lead to much more serious problems, including cardiovascular diseases, obesity, diabetes, and even early mortality. In the 1990s, 20 percent of the American workforce slept for six hours or less, while the number of people not obtaining enough sleep on a regular basis had risen to 30 percent in 2007. Over the past century, the quality and quantity of our sleep has radically diminished.[22] When sleeping, we normally cycle through different phases and vacillate between two types of sleep—rapid-eye-movement (REM) sleep, during which our brain is relatively active and we dream most intensely, and non-REM sleep, which is deeper, and during which our brain is at its least dynamic.

One of the key hypotheses about why humans need sleep is the "energy conservation theory." When we are asleep, our metabolism is significantly reduced, and we are less receptive to external stimuli. Our body temperature drops, our breathing becomes regular, our heart rate and pulse slow down, and we need fewer calories than when we are awake. A group of Harvard sleep scientists explain the theory in Darwinian terms: "[O]ne of the strongest factors in natural selection is competition for and effective utilization of energy resources. The energy conservation theory suggests that the primary function of sleep is to reduce an individual's energy demand and expenditure during part of the day or night, especially at times when it is least efficient to search for food."[23]

Another theory about why humans need sleep is the "recuperation hypothesis," which is based on the idea that we undergo physical renewal during sleep and that our bodies repair the damage that occurs during waking hours. Aristotle was the earliest proponent of this theory, and recent studies have shown that there is some truth to it. Animals deprived of sleep, for example, lose all immune functions and die in the course of a few weeks. Moreover, the Harvard sleep scientists argue that this theory is further supported "by findings that many of the major restorative functions in the body like muscle growth, tissue repair, protein synthesis, and growth hormone release occur mostly, or in some cases only, during sleep."[24] We also feel much more cognitively able and mentally alert after a good slumber, while cognitive abilities such as concentration are significantly impaired when we merely toss and turn in bed. Sleep, finally, is also vital in the development and structural changes of the brain.

It is interesting to note that formerly held assumptions about sleep, such as the idea that the brain is "switched off" and is completely inactive during sleep, have not proved to be correct. In fact, electroencephalograph scans have shown that sleep is actually a rather dynamic behavior: REM sleep, in particular, is characterized by high-frequency brainwave activity and anarchically broadcasting neurons and is associated with the production of a vivid and vibrant dream life. Psychoanalysts, moreover, would argue that the production of dreams is the very opposite of a restful or passive activity—Freud explicitly writes of "dream *work*" (*Traumarbeit*) when referring to the complex coding processes in which the unconscious engages when translating unconscious desires into dream imagery, and which include condensation, displacement, and symbolization.

Finally, it is also worth noting that the currently favored pattern of sleeping during darkness for an ideally uninterrupted period of eight hours, which most Westerners consider "natural" and healthy, is in fact both culturally and historically specific. In various cultures, in particular those in hot climates, sleeping in the afternoon is a common practice—think of the siesta tradition in Italy, Spain, and Mexico, for example, where many shops close during the afternoon and where people go home to their families to eat and then sleep, to avoid exhausting their energies during the hottest part of the day.

The historian Roger Ekirch, moreover, found ample evidence that the dominant form of human sleeping–waking cycles before the Industrial Revolution and the advent of artificial lighting was segmented, which means that two or more periods of sleep were punctuated by periods of wakefulness during the course of a day.[25] In the Middle Ages, for example, it was common to sleep in two shifts and to get up for an hour or so in the middle of the night to pray, think, meditate on dreams, have sex, or even visit neighbors. Ekirch believes that this biphasal sleep model is in fact more "natural" than the eight hours of consecutive sleep model that we currently follow. The growing number of insomniacs who wake repeatedly during the night, he thinks, may simply be experiencing a return to the preindustrial manner of sleeping. Yet, since most of us consider waking up in the middle of the night as unhealthy, we become anxious and agitated, which then keeps us awake for too long and leads to genuine sleep disturbances and all their dire medical consequences.

* * *

Jonathan Crary's 24/7: Late Capitalism and the Ends of Sleep is a telling example of a present-day polemic against new technology and its perceived adverse impact on our lives and our energy reserves.[26] Crary, who is a cultural theorist and an art critic at Columbia University, argues that new technologies, especially the Internet, have eroded the natural rhythms of life, including those related to night and day and to the boundaries between work and rest. We have never slept as little as now in human history, Crary claims—average sleeping hours having slumped from ten in the nineteenth century, to eight at the beginning of the twentieth, and to six and a half in the early twenty-first century. He uses "24/7" as shorthand for the core evils of the global techno-capitalist machine, and especially for the process of incessant consumption and production of goods made possible by nonstop Internet connectivity and commerce. We can now shop twenty-four hours each day, no matter where we are, as online trading never sleeps. What is worse, it is of course the late capitalist workforce who have to keep this process going. As a consequence, the demands on workers have intensified: we are expected to be continuously connected and productive, in synchronicity with the nonstop networks of trade and surveillance.

The world of 24/7 consumerism, Crary argues, has created a new temporality that is continuous and therefore socially corrosive: it is no longer marked by communal caesura such as dawn and dusk, weekdays and weekends. We no longer share mutual patterns of work and rest, nor do we congregate in communal spaces when we do cease work. Instead, we all stare at the screens of our high-tech devices in isolation and for far too long. Experience itself, Crary argues, is restructured by this continuous, incessant, rhythmless rhythm of 24/7 culture, and not in a good way. We are the victims of a dull sameness that assaults us without any pause.

Sleep, Crary argues, has become the true enemy of capitalism, as the capitalist economy envisages a machine-like, willingly sur-veillable citizen who is always productive and perpetually engaged in the circulation and consumption of goods. Sleep is therefore the true nemesis of unlimited productivity and presents one of the last remaining forms of possible resistance to capitalist consumerism. The sleeping subject can neither produce nor consume and thus becomes useless to the capitalist economy. Sleep alone cannot be commodified.

While many of Crary's micro theses are convincing, it is striking just how similar his high-theory, twenty-first-century jeremiad is to earlier exhaustion theories. Crary, too, assumes that ours is the most sleepless, and therefore most exhausted, age—a claim that many of the exhaustion theorists we have so far encountered also embrace. Second, he, too, is a traditionalist at heart, who looks back nostalgically to a lost past when life could be lived in a more natural, less exhausting way. The period that Crary romanticizes most is the 1960s, as this decade was marked by a wide range of anticonsumerist and countercultural activities that, he believes, posed a genuine threat to the capitalist system. Third, he blames the evils of the present on new technologies—above all, the Inter-net, which, he believes, not only drives the 24/7 global culture but insidiously restructures our modes of attention, our experiences, and even our perceptual faculties. Finally, his account also resem-bles those of George Cheyne, Krafft-Ebing, Mitchell, and Oswald

Spengler, to name just a few, in that its tone is apocalyptic, diagnosing colossal paradigm shifts that have horrifying outcomes, which, if unchecked, will lead to the decline of the West. Looked at cynically, these overblown claims could, of course, be seen as simple rhetorical gestures aimed at securing attention, but it is certainly remarkable that many exhaustion theories are driven by visions that are ultimately nostalgic, apocalyptic, technophobic, and conservative in spirit.

8

The Death Drive

During the course of his long career, Sigmund Freud (1856–1939) developed three major theories to explain the exhaustion of human energy: the first concerns the loss of energy arising from an individual's interaction with the sociocultural environment; the second presents a biophilosophical explanation of exhaustion revolving around the controversial concept of the "death drive"; and the third suggests that our energies can be used up internally in battles between the id, the ego, and the superego. It is, above all, Freud's theory of the death drive—the first ever attempt to explain exhaustion in metaphysical terms—that is the focus of this chapter. All activity, Freud suggests, is anathema to a significant part of us, as one of our core drives (Thanatos, the counterpart to Eros, the life drive) wishes to return us to an inanimate state.

Freud's first theory, his intervention in the neurasthenia and exhaustion debates at the close of the nineteenth and the beginning of the twentieth century, was simple but dramatic. He brushed aside the idea that these conditions were caused by the faster pace of modern city life, "brain work," new technologies, or the unrelenting exposure of the modern subject to sensory overload. Instead, he argued that neurasthenia and the other "functional" neuroses had an entirely different cause: harmful sexual behavior, either too much of it or too little.

In his earliest paper on the topic, "On the Grounds for Detaching a Particular Syndrome from Neurasthenia Under the Description 'Anxiety Neurosis'" (1895), Freud argues that neurasthenia and anxiety neuroses (which he later described as the "actual" or "functional" neuroses) differ from the psychoneuroses in that their cause is somatic rather than psychogenic. Neurasthenia and anxiety are linked to present and ongoing sexual problems rather than to the aftereffects of repressed infantile sexual traumas, which cause the symptoms of the psychoneuroses. Like many eighteenth- and nineteenth-century medical men before him, Freud believed that the fragile energy-economy of the human body could be severely damaged by masturbation and the careless waste of sexual energy (libido), which he considered the cause of neurasthenia. The anxiety neuroses, in contrast, are the product of pent-up sexual energy resulting from dissatisfying or insufficient sexual experiences, above all *coitus interruptus* and sexual abstinence.[1]

In "Sexuality in the Aetiology of the Neuroses" (1898), Freud revisits the topic and agrees with George M. Beard, Richard von Krafft-Ebing, and Wilhelm Erb that there has indeed been a sharp increase in cases of neurasthenia. He also concedes that civilization and wider cultural developments play a significant part in the etiology of the condition—but for reasons very different from those indicated by his colleagues: Freud argues that neurasthenics are not victims of modernity or heredity but quite simply "people who are crippled in sexuality" (*Sexualkrüppel*).[2] In the lecture "The Common Neurotic State" (1917), Freud goes further still, asserting that neurasthenia is essentially a toxicological problem caused by disturbances in the sexual biochemistry of the organism. Like the other functional neuroses, it is therefore a predicament to be examined by biologists and not by psychoanalysts.[3]

In "'Civilized' Sexual Morality and Modern Nervous Illness" (1908), a precursor to his better-known late work *Civilization and Its Discontents* (1930), Freud once again attacks the models of Beard and other then-famous theorists of modern exhaustion and nervousness. In this essay, he introduces the troubling idea that the rapid spread of the neuroses (both the functional and the psychogenic varieties) is the price we pay for living in a culture that is essentially based on the ever-more complex repression of the individual's instincts. The rise of the neuroses is the direct consequence of the cultural command permanently to sublimate our sexual and aggressive drives, and of channeling these energies into socially acceptable activities, such as work, art, science, and the pursuit of love, beauty, and material goods.

According to Freud, civilization feeds on the energy derived from sublimated drives. The sexual drive, in particular, "places extraordinarily large amounts of force at the disposal of civilized activity."[4] In his model, the drives thus fulfill a precarious double function: on the one hand, they are the very energy that fuels all the achievements and activities that constitute "culture." On the other hand, the very act of their repression and sublimation causes an alarming number of illnesses and neuroses that threaten to destabilize our culture from within.

Freud identifies heterosexual intercourse sanctified by marriage as the only form of sexual behavior that is considered morally legitimate in the framework of the prevailing "sexual morality" of his age. Yet this severely limited form of monogamy, he argues, has disastrous consequences for the libidinal economies of the individual, who is forced to forsake the gratification of his or her drives. He gloomily predicts that, at some point, the rapidly declining mental health of the sexually impaired modern subject might undo all the advantages associated with repressing the drives in the first place, and he raises the question "whether our 'civilized' sexual morality is worth the sacrifice which it imposes on us."[5] Modern cultural demands to repress our desires have become more restrictive, on the one hand, and there are also far more external and internal stimuli with which the modern subject has to cope on a daily basis, on the other. All this sublimation and repression requires the expenditure of tremendous amounts of energy—more energy, indeed, than many possess.

Freud takes these ideas further in what is perhaps his darkest work, *Civilization and Its Discontents*.[6] The pursuit of happiness, he gloomily informs the reader, is always already doomed to fail: true happiness can never be achieved, since our fragile bodies, an essentially hostile nature, and the inherent vicissitudes of human relationships will always frustrate our efforts. What we identify as happiness, moreover, is either simply the absence of pain and dis-pleasure or the lessening of tension that comes in the wake of drive satisfaction, which is in its very nature episodic and short-lived. It is for this reason that so many of us turn to drink and drugs, or else to religion, which Freud describes as a collective delusion that is erected on systematic intellectual intimidation and that propels us back to an infantile stage in which magical thinking reigns.[7]

Moreover, culture fails spectacularly to deliver on its key prom-ises, thereby casting doubt on the original justification of the individual's permanent drive-gratification sacrifice. Freud under-stands culture as the sum total of the achievements and institu-tions that distinguish our mode of life from that of our animal ancestors, and that serve two main purposes: to protect us against nature and to regulate our relationships with other humans. Gen-erally speaking, individuals bow to the demands of the cultural contract in exchange for stability, safety, and order. Or, as Freud laconically puts it: "Civilized man has exchanged a portion of his possibilities of happiness for a portion of security." However, ever more people consider culture itself—the very institution that was to offer them protection—their true enemy. A rapidly increasing number of people have become disenchanted with progress and its failed promises: the newly acquired technological mastery over space and time, the increased control of nature, the fulfillment of all kinds of cravings for extravagant luxuries and sensory stimula-tions have not rendered them happier. On the contrary, modern man becomes ever more neurotic, "because he cannot tolerate the amount of frustration which society imposes on him in the service of its cultural ideals." Freud writes:

> Here, as we already know, civilization is obeying the laws of economic necessity, since a large amount of the psychical energy which it uses for its own purposes has to be withdrawn from sexuality. In this respect civilization behaves towards sexuality as a people or a stratum of its population does which has subjected another one to its exploitation. Fear of a revolt by the suppressed elements drives it to stricter precautionary

measures. A high-water mark in such a development has been reached in our Western European civilization.[8]

Freud's argument—that which is repressed and sublimated (that is, unacceptable sexual and aggressive desire) is precisely what functions as fuel for all higher cultural activities—is based on a simple mechanical energy-transfer model: the sublimated energy of the individual is converted and then put to work in a different form in another system, culture. This culture, in turn, allows the individual to save energy in other areas: since social relations are (ideally) regulated by intelligible laws in civilized societies, people do not constantly have to fear for their personal safety and their possessions. They can direct elsewhere the energies that someone in a less-stable environment would have to invest in keeping safe. So far, so reasonable. Yet Freud argues that something goes very wrong in the course of this exchange: the energy return no longer matches the original investment, such that the individual's energy reserves are not protected but instead gradually exhausted by the arrangement. This, in turn, has negative consequences for culture, too: the amount of available energy in the overall system grows smaller, since the exhausted are no longer properly able to supply the energy that culture needs to thrive. A vicious circle of energy depletion thus ensues.

The image of the oppressed tribe that Freud uses in the quoted passage is telling: he compares culture to a colonial oppressor no longer able to exploit a once subjugated tribe. Putting the tribe to work originally freed up the oppressor's time and energies, as the subalterns were forced to undertake the hard physical labor that the oppressor would otherwise have to perform. But then something changed: now all the oppressor's energies are used up in the act of oppression itself, rendering the energy investment futile. The oppressor could just as well set the slaves free.

Unsurprisingly, Freud does not suggest a return to more primitive forms of social organization but instead takes up a defeatist and nihilistic position, unable or perhaps unwilling to propose a way out of the predicament he describes. At times, he appears troubled by his own argument and even apologizes to the reader

that he is unable to offer any kind of solace.⁹ Freud's late works
grew ever more pessimistic, his own increasingly declinist vision
of humankind and its hazardous, energy-depleting cultural institutions no doubt affected by the rise of Nazism and the rapid dark-
ening of the sociopolitical climate in Europe during the 1930s.

✳ ✳ ✳

Freud presents his second big theory on the mechanisms of
human energy exhaustion in his groundbreaking essay "Beyond
the Pleasure Principle" (1920). Here, Freud modifies his previous
positions on the human drives (*Triebe*) by introducing the idea of
an antagonistic dual-drive model. Underlying all his drive theories
is an essentially economic model of the psychic apparatus, based
on the idea of a limited amount of instinctual-libidinal energy
circulating in the human subject. This energy has to be managed
wisely and distributed carefully so as to maintain a state of psychic
equilibrium. Generally speaking, Freud understands the drives as
internal forces that are partly somatic and partly psychogenic in
nature. They differ from temporary external stimuli in that they
are internalized and constant.¹⁰ The psychic apparatus largely follows the dictates of the so-called pleasure principle, the core aim
of which is the avoidance of displeasure and the attempt to keep at
bay any tension caused by the demands of the drives.

The idea of the drives lies at the very heart of Freud's psychoanalytical model of the mind, and yet, surprisingly, they remain
curiously ill-defined in his oeuvre. In "Instincts and Their Vicissitudes" (1915), he defines them in the following terms:

> If now we apply ourselves to considering mental life from a
> *biological* point of view, an "instinct" [*Trieb*] appears to us a
> concept on the frontier between the mental and the somatic,
> as the psychical representative of the stimuli originating from
> within the organism and reaching the mind, as a measure
> of the demand [*Maß der Arbeitsanforderung*] made upon
> the mind for work in consequence of its connection with
> the body.¹¹

Here, then, the drives are presented as a diffuse form of inner-somatic stimuli or tension that originates in the organs and is subsequently "represented" or symbolized by the psyche. Of particular interest here is the formulation *Maß der Arbeitsanforderung* (measure of the amount of required work): the force of a given drive can be measured by the amount of work that is required by the psyche to manage it. The stronger the drive, the more energy is required to repress it. Freud is slightly clearer about what can happen to the drives: as we have seen, they can be sublimated and repressed, but they can also be turned against the self. As for what the drives actually are and where they come from, however, Freud remains evasive: "The study of the sources of instincts lies outside the scope of psychology. Although instincts are wholly determined by their origin in a somatic source, in mental life we know them only by their aims."[12]

In "Beyond the Pleasure Principle," he emphasizes repeatedly that we know nothing about the drives: "This is the most obscure and inaccessible region of the mind." Indeed, he describes the drives as "at once the most important and the most obscure element of psychological research" and insists again and again on the "obscurity that reigns at present in the theory of the instincts." Almost melancholically, he states: "No knowledge would have been more valuable as a foundation for true psychological science than an approximate grasp of the common characteristics and possible distinctive features of the instincts. But in no region of psychology were we groping more in the dark."[13]

Although the drives are the very foundation on which Freud's entire theory rests, they remain the true "dark continent"—a strange lacuna at the very heart of his oeuvre. Energy (*Energie*), too, remains an ill-defined concept: it is a term deployed in many of his texts, both on its own and, for example, in the compounds *Energiebetrieb* ("energy mechanism" or "energy work"), *Besetzungsenergie* ("cathectic energy" or "energy investment"), *Energievorrat* (energy reserve), and *Energieumsetzung* ("energy deployment" or "energy transformation").[14] Freud famously compares the ego to a parasitical rider, who simultaneously tries to control and to feed on the energy of the id: "The functional importance of the ego is manifested in the fact that normally control over the approaches to motility devolves upon it. Thus in relation to the id it is like a man on horseback, who has to hold in check the superior strength of the horse; with this difference, that the rider tries to do so with his own strength while the ego uses borrowed forces."[15] We are told little about the true nature of human energy, however, except that it is somehow derived from the id.

One of the reasons for Freud's remarkable reluctance to define the nature of the drives and of human energy might be his aspiration to make use of biological concepts for phenomena of that kind, while holding to the belief that the language and methods of biology cannot describe or capture them.[16] In "Beyond the Pleasure Principle" in particular, he frequently appears to yearn for the biochemical certainties of the empirical sciences but finds himself compelled to use the imagery and metaphors of psychology instead, for otherwise he could not describe the phenomena that interest him. Furthermore, Freud is of course a child of his times, suspicious of anything that reeks of vitalism or of plain esotericism. He shares the tendency of many modern Western scientists and theorists to shy away from defining what human energy really is. Yet, like many of his contemporaries, Freud sought to explain the ways in which human energy—whatever its true nature might be—can be exhausted.

The notion of intrapsychological conflict is central to Freud's structural model of the human psyche: he argues that our energies can be depleted from the inside, in fierce battles between various psychic agencies as well as between various drives. The notorious dual-drive model introduced in "Beyond the Pleasure Principle" is based on the assumption that two kinds of drive with conflicting aims are engaged in a perpetual battle within us. In addition to what he alternately calls libido, Eros, and the life or sexual drive, which aims at the perpetuation of the human species, there is also the death drive (often referred to as Thanatos, although Freud himself never uses this term). The death drive aims to return us to a state of tranquility where no disturbances can upset our psychic equilibrium. Both the life and the death drive are conservative, seeking to replicate a former state of being: the life drive seeks fusion with another, while the death drive seeks to return us to a homeostatic state approximating the inorganic.

Freud's explanation of the death drive is biological in origin and based on a stimuli–response model as well as the idea of homeostasis: the psychic apparatus, he writes, wants above all else to avoid "un-pleasure" (*Unlust*). It seeks to reduce tension, to maintain calm in the house of the psyche by getting rid of all excitation. He calls this the "principle of constancy" (*Konstanzprinzip*) or, more evocatively, the "Nirvana principle" (*Nirvanaprinzip*). Tensions can be reduced either by satisfying a pressing drive demand or by avoiding the stimuli that produce upheaval in the first place:

> The dominating tendency of mental life, and perhaps of nervous life in general, is the effort to reduce, to keep constant or to remove internal tension due to stimuli (the "Nirvana principle," to borrow a term from Barbara Low)—a tendency which finds expression in the pleasure principle; and our recognition of that fact is one of our strongest reasons for believing in the existence of the death instincts.[17]

Freud's conceptualization of the death drive is the first great metaphysical theory of exhaustion, and it has wide-ranging consequences: it suggests that all activity is essentially anathema to one of our two core drives, as it is associated with displeasure, tension, and exertion. A very strong part of ourselves longs for nothing but a state of permanent physical and mental rest, the cessation of all feeling and of all movement. It also explains one of the mechanisms of intrapsychological conflict, which can deplete our energies from within. Freud offers the following image of these contradictory impulses: "It is as though the life of the organism moved with a vacillating rhythm [*Es ist wie ein Zauderrhythmus im Leben der Organismen*]. One group of instincts rushes forward so as to reach the final aim of life as swiftly as possible; but when a particular stage in the advance has been reached, the other group jerks back to a certain point to make a fresh start and so prolong the journey."[18]

Another way in which our energy can be exhausted internally is related to Freud's argument in *Civilization and Its Discontents*:

because culture constantly urges us to repress our aggressive impulses, we tend to internalize them, turning them against ourselves rather than outward, in the form of guilt and self-hatred. Our superego can become a persecutory and even a sadistic agency, viciously lacerating the ego, constantly berating it for its failures. It can even drive a person to abandon the will to live altogether, leading him or her to give in to the lure of the death drive.[19] The melancholic is a classic example of a patient tormented by a cruel superego in overdrive.

* * *

Freud's third and final contribution to the corpus of exhaustion theory revolves around the ancient concept of melancholia, which he redefines as being characterized, above all, by the notion of loss. When neurasthenia disappeared from the medical handbooks in the second decade of the twentieth century, a modern version of melancholia entered the diagnostic stage, and one of Freud's most important essays, "Mourning and Melancholia" (1917), contributed substantially to the renewed interest in the condition. In the 1930s, "depression" began to replace the older term and was increasingly regarded as a syndrome that could explain a host of other physical and mental symptoms that are structured around exhaustion.[20] Although Freud still uses the term "melancholia," he defines some of the core features of depression as we understand it today. As in the case of traditional melancholia, these symptoms include causeless sorrow and fear but also a new category: self-hatred: "The distinguishing mental features of melancholia are a profoundly painful dejection, cessation of interest in the outside world, loss of the capacity to love, inhibition of all activity, and a lowering of the self-regarding feelings to a degree that finds utterance in self-reproaches and self-revilings, and culminates in a delusional expectation of punishment."[21]

Moreover, melancholia is associated with loss—in a complex psychological procedure, the melancholic transforms emotions originally triggered by the loss of a love object into the loss of a stable sense of self. The melancholic internalizes the lost love object and then turns all the hatred and the reproaches that were originally aimed at this object back against the self. Above all, Freud famously writes, the melancholic experiences a "delusion of inferiority":

> In mourning it is the world which has become poor and empty; in melancholia it is the ego itself. The patient represents his ego to us as worthless, incapable of any achievement and morally despicable; he reproaches himself, vilifies himself and expects to be cast out and punished. . . . This picture of a delusion of (mainly moral) inferiority is completed by sleeplessness and refusal to take nourishment, and—what is psychologically very remarkable—by an overcoming of the instinct which compels every living thing to cling to life. . . . [The patient] really is as lacking in interest and as incapable of love and achievement as he says. But that, as we know, is secondary; *it is the effect of the internal work which is consuming his ego.*[22]

The melancholic's energies are expended, then, on sadistic attacks inflicted on the vulnerable ego by a judgmental superego; in other words, they are literally consumed by self-hatred. "The complex of melancholia," Freud writes, "behaves like an open wound, drawing to itself cathectic energies . . . from all directions, and emptying the ego until it is totally impoverished."[23]

Freud, then, presents three groundbreaking theories on the ways in which human energy can be exhausted. The first concerns the interaction of a person with the cultural environment. The energy return that the modern subject receives from the renunciation of immediate drive satisfaction in exchange for living in a safe, orderly, and civilized communal structure is no longer great enough to merit the original sacrifice. The sublimation of one's sexual and aggressive drives results in an energy vacuum both in culture at large and in the psychic apparatus of the neurotic individual. The second theory suggests that one of our two core drives has as its aim a state in which all exertion, tension, and activity cease. The wish to die—perhaps the most extreme form that psychological exhaustion can take—would thus not so much be an act of giving up as an act of giving in.[24] The third theory, finally, demonstrates that our energies can be used up internally in battles between the superego, the ego, and the id, and of course by maintaining a set of complex psychological defenses.

One might read Freud's entire oeuvre as focusing at a deeper level on human energy and its exhaustion. Yet given that the idea of exhaustion constitutes one of the core concepts of his thought, it is all the more surprising that he fails clearly and convincingly to define its opposites: energy and the drives. While his theory of the death drive is no longer accepted uncritically even in the psychoanalytic community, the idea that our psychological energy can be used up in ongoing battles between different parts of our psyche with conflicting aims and objectives is still convincing as an explanation of the origins of chronic mental exhaustion, the origins of which are internal rather than exogenic.

✳ ✳ ✳

While the idea of the death drive may no longer have much purchase in analytical practice, it is a concept that can illuminate representations of otherwise inexplicable self-destructive and suicidal behavior of the existentially exhausted in the world of fiction. Herman Melville's short story "Bartleby, the Scrivener: A Story of Wall-Street" (1853), for example, provides a beautiful *avant la lettre* illustration of the workings of the death drive. The story opens with the narrator informing us that he has employed a man called Bartleby as a law copyist. A conflict-shy solicitor, the narrator describes himself as an "eminently *safe* man" and a "man of peace," who cherishes above all tranquility and the easy life. For many years, he has put up with two insolent copyists, Turkey and Nippers, repeatedly excusing their severe shortcomings for the sake of harmony. Turkey suffers from anger, impatience, and recklessness, and Nippers from indigestion, "nervous testiness and grinning irritability." The two spend their time eating and drinking, blotting important papers, and taking out their frustration on their desks and colleagues. The narrator's offices are also "deficient in what landscape painters call 'life'": all windows look out onto brick walls, shafts, and dead ends. Into this deathly environment wanders Bartleby, "pallidly neat, pitiably respectable, incurably forlorn!"[25] He is placed at a desk facing a viewless window with very little light.

At first, he copies assiduously but refuses to perform any tasks beyond copying. Whenever the narrator asks him to help with something else, Bartleby responds mildly: "I would prefer not to," which becomes his trademark phrase. Indeed, he says little else throughout the story. He prefers not to do an increasing number of things and finally informs the narrator that he has given up copying altogether. Instead, he spends his days in "dead-wall reveries," gazing dull-eyed at the "dead brick wall" onto which his window looks.[26]

Unable to address conflict openly, and vacillating between charitable and hypocritical impulses, the narrator finally decides to fire Bartleby. But Bartleby prefers not to quit the premises, in which he has taken permanent residence. His ghostly presence in the offices is disconcerting, and, fearing for his own reputation, the narrator eventually decides to quit the premises himself. Yet even after the narrator has moved out, Bartleby refuses to leave the office, and when the new tenants forcibly remove him, he continues to haunt the landing and stairwells of the building. Finally, Bartleby is carried off to the "Tombs," the local jail, where he stops eating and gradually wastes away. The narrator tries to alleviate his bad conscience by visiting his gentle nemesis and by paying a "grub man" to feed him, but when he calls on him a second time he finds Bartleby dead, rolled up in a fetal position in front of one of the prison walls. Strangely "huddled at the base of the wall, his knees drawn up, and lying on his side, his head touching the cold stones," Bartleby has finally succeeded in literally wasting away.[27]

The story is permeated by imagery of walls and claustrophobic, dead-end spaces. Bartleby is described as "motionless," "mild," and "cadaverous," and his ghost-like paleness is repeatedly emphasized. He appears to be dead in life, devoid of any desires, defined only negatively by what he would "prefer not to" do. Turkey and Nippers, by contrast, are characterized by their appetites—both literally and metaphorically. They eat and drink excessively, and their dominant moods are wrath and irritability. Bartleby, though, remains as lifeless as a statue and uncannily even-tempered. He never speaks but to answer. By starving himself to death in jail, he expresses his mental decline physically. However, the process of his gradual emotional, affective, and physical death appears to have begun long before he took up the post as the narrator's copyist. Choosing to become a law copyist, a particularly "dull, wearisome, and lethargic affair," and taking up permanent residence in the soulless, prison-like offices, appear not only to precipitate Bartleby's decline but also represent apt externalizations of his inner state.[28]

The narrator, who has already proved himself to be incapable of asserting his authority with his other copyists, is entirely at a loss about what to do with Bartleby. Torn between pity, charity, and anxieties about his own reputation, he finally admits that the melancholy presence of Bartleby inspires fear and repulsion in him:

> My first emotions had been those of pure melancholy and sincerest pity; but just in proportion as the forlornness of Bartleby grew and grew to my imagination, did that same melancholy merge into fear, that pity into repulsion. So true it is, and so terrible too, that up to a certain point the thought or sight of misery enlists our best affections; but, in certain special cases, beyond that point it does not. They err who would assert that invariably this is owing to the inherent selfishness of the human heart. It rather proceeds from a certain hopelessness of remedying excessive and organic ill.

Common sense, the narrator asserts, much in the spirit of Freud's Nirvana principle, bids the soul to avoid pain. Witnessing weakness can inspire a fear of contagion. The narrator becomes convinced that the scrivener is "the victim of innate and incurable disorder." He realizes that while he might give alms to his body, it is Bartleby's soul that is ailing and that his soul would remain unreachable. When he recognizes that his own reputation is beginning to suffer as a result of the strange creature living in his offices,

he turns more forcefully against Bartleby, thinking of him no longer as a "poor, pale, passive mortal" but as a gloomy apparition and
an "intolerable incubus."[29]

Bartleby essentially refuses to live, and in the end his death wish
is fulfilled. Lonely, isolated, and alienated, he is unable to derive
pleasure from anything. He declines to take an interest in anything
and refuses to accept help. When the narrator discusses possible
alternative jobs with him, Bartleby dismisses all of them, in spite of
his assertion that he is not particular. Apart from a rumor, which
the narrator shares with us at the end of the story, that Bartleby
used to work in a "Dead Letter Office" before he came to be a scrivener, we know nothing about either his circumstances or the origins of his profound weariness with life. This lacuna has allowed
critics to project various theories onto the figure of the scrivener.
Marxist commentators have argued that it is the creativity-killing
and soul-destroying mechanical labor that led to Bartleby's death
wish, this argument being supported by the fact that the law offices
are situated on Wall Street, the symbolic center of capitalism. Others consider Bartleby's grand refusal to be an act of revolutionary,
or else infantile, resistance against the utilitarian imperative to act
reasonably and to behave with common sense. Others still have
interpreted his existential exhaustion as spiritual, as a reaction to
the secular and materialistic dictates of his soulless age, and many
have interpreted his behavior in clinical terms, as a case study in
severe depression.

Bartleby is, of course, also a perfect example of someone giving in to the death drive: he refuses to change anything in his
dire circumstances; ceases to accept spiritual, mental, and physical nourishment; becomes literally and metaphorically immobile;
and declines to leave his shelter. He becomes incapable, or perhaps
unwilling, of working, an ambiguity captured in the beautifully
understated phrase "I would prefer not to," and he deliberately
allows his body and his soul to wither. He is drawn to brick walls
and dead ends, which function as external symbols of his state
of hopelessness. He is an accusation but also a nuisance, inspir-
ing pity and fear in equal measure. In the end, the narrator wonders whether Bartleby "was billeted upon me for some mysterious

purpose of an all-wise Providence," but he fails to understand what that purpose might have been.[30] His charitable impulses remain too feeble and are often driven by self-interest, and, ultimately, they are all rejected by Bartleby, as though he was able to see through the hypocrisy of it all.

* * *

Freud's exhaustion model centers, above all, on a conflict that is both intra- and extrapsychological in nature: the neuroses are caused by conflicting internal drives, such as the contradictory demands of the life and the death drives, and of the id, the ego, and the superego, as well as by the need to repress sexual desires, the realization of which would be in conflict with social norms. By contrast, the French psychologist and psychiatrist Pierre-Marie-Félix Janet (1859–1947), one of Freud's contemporaries and, later, adversaries, developed an alternative model of the psychoneuroses that was based on the concept of energy insufficiency. Janet was chosen by Jean-Marie Charcot (who was also an important influence on Freud) to direct the psychological laboratory at the Salpêtrière hospital in 1890, a position he held for fifty years. In 1902, he was appointed professor of psychology at the Collège de France, and he published numerous important studies on hysteria and other mental pathologies. Yet he is perhaps best known for coining the term "psychasthenia," a diagnostic category that he introduces in *Les obsessions et la psychasthénie* (*Obsession and Psychasthenia*, 1903). Unhappy with the concept of neurasthenia, as it implied the presence of material neurological defects that could not be empirically verified, Janet proposed psychasthenia as an alternative. Like neurasthenia, psychasthenia is an umbrella category, a syndrome that comprises various symptoms and symptom clusters, including obsession, mania, states of mind related to self-doubt and low self-esteem, tics, phobias, delirium, anxiety, neurasthenia, and conditions related to feelings of alienation and depersonalization. According to Janet, all these symptoms are united by the fact that they are marked by "the feeling of effort and the feeling of fatigue" (*le sentiment de l'effort et le sentiment de la fatigue).* Psychasthenic symptoms are caused, above all, by a "lowering of psychological tension" *(abaissement de la tension psychologique),* or, in other words, a loss of psychological energy.[31] In turn, energy insufficiency results in a loss of the "function of the real" *(la fonction du réel),* which Janet describes as the ability to adapt to one's physical and social environment and to react appropriately to external demands.[32] Psychasthenics thus become alienated, isolated, and apathetic. Prone to rumination, obsessive thoughts, states of emotional extremes, or even mania, they lack psychological energy, which results in a weakening of the will, the cognitive faculties, and the ability to dwell in the present, as well as in severe self-doubt.[33]

Janet differentiates between higher- and lower-level cognitive and psychological functions. When our psychological energy is on the wane, the higher-level functions are affected first, and these include attention, cognition, rational judgment, and the ability to synthesize and analyze our perceptions. They give way to obsessive rumination, restlessness, tics, exaggerated emotions, and a range of other symptoms. Janet believes that human energy levels vary greatly and are determined partly by heredity and partly by external causes such as conflict, trauma, past experiences, education, and disease.

Freud was initially complimentary about Janet's work, acknowledging his ideas and influence, but he later turned against him when Janet accused him of plagiarism. He thought Janet's model too simplistic, and in 1910 he uncharitably compared Janet's psychasthenic "to a weak woman who is so overburdened with packages that she is always dropping one and no sooner grasps that one than she drops another."[34] Janet's theory of psychasthenia was never integrated into mainstream psychology and to this day remains hardly known outside France. Interestingly, Janet, like Freud, never really defines what "psychological tension" actually is—he only lists behaviors that emerge when it is absent. Ultimately, psychological tension is just another metaphor, like Freud's concept of libido, or Galen's *pneuma* and animal spirits, or the *élan vital* theorized by the vitalists, or the Chinese *qi.* Although all exhaustion theories center on models describing the depletion of human energy and the physical, mental, affective, and behavioral consequences of this depletion, hardly anyone supplies a concrete definition of what human energy actually is. Chemists and physicists, as well as nutritionists, are the only scientists today who operate with clearly defined and measurable concepts of energy—albeit, of course, not of human energy.

❋ ❋ ❋

Discrepancies in human energy levels—whether they are caused by internal battles and conflicting drives, as Freud would have it, or are the result of hereditary and external factors, as Janet believes—can have extremely serious consequences for those who find themselves positioned at the lower end of the energy spectrum. In *The Drowned and the Saved* (1986), the Italian Auschwitz survivor Primo Levi reflects on the phenomenon of the "Muselmann" in the Nazi concentration camps, those who provide an extreme and tragic example of the potential consequences of low constitutional and/or environmentally influenced levels of human energy, as described by Janet. *Muselmann* is German for "Muslim," and the term was used to designate the "irreversibly exhausted, worn-out prisoner close to death" in the camps. While the exact origins of the name are uncertain, Levi proposes that it may have been inspired by the fatalism of the terminally exhausted or by the head bandages they wore, which resembled turbans.[35] Another theory suggests that the designation was coined on account of the fatigued postures of the moribund: bent over, too weak to hold themselves upright, they resembled a Muslim praying on his knees with his face on the floor.

In *If This Is a Man* (1947), Levi writes that the Lager was "preeminently a gigantic biological and social experiment."[36] He argues that there were two fundamental categories of men in the camps: the saved and the drowned. The Muselmänner, belonging to the latter group, were doomed because they lacked the energy and the adaptability that was necessary to survive in the camps:

Their life is short, but their number is endless; they, the Muselmänner, the drowned, form the backbone of the camp, an anonymous mass, continually renewed and always identical, of non-men who march and labour in silence, the divine spark dead within them, already too empty to really suffer. One hesitates to call them living: one hesitates to call their death death, in the face of which they have no fear, as they are too tired to understand.

They crowd my memory with their faceless presences, and if I could enclose all the evil of our time in one image, I would choose this image which is familiar to me: an emaciated man, with head dropped and shoulders curved, on whose face and in whose eyes not a trace of thought is to be seen.[37]

Levi describes a "pitiless process of natural selection"—only the strong, energetic, or otherwise exceptionally skilled managed to survive the camps: "To sink is the easiest of matters; it is enough to carry out all the orders one receives, to eat only the ration, to observe the discipline of the work and the camp. Experience showed that only exceptionally could one survive more than three months in this way."[38] He suggests that it is only those with extraordinary energy resources, with a strength and willpower that exceeded the norm, who stood a chance of surviving the horrors of the camp. While the camps were unparalleled regarding the extreme atrocities, cruelty, and pressures to which they exposed the interned, Levi considers the psychological dynamics operating within them as representative of more general human behavior. Like Bartleby, the Muselmänner elicited not only pity but also fear of contagion: they served as unwanted and potentially infectious reminders to the others of just how easy it was to succumb to the urge to give in to the lure of the death drive.

9

Depression

When my grandfather returned from Russia, where he had been a prisoner for over five years following the end of the Second World War, he was a physical and mental wreck. For weeks, he lay in his darkened bedroom, too traumatized to speak about his experiences on the eastern front and in the prisoner-of-war camp, where he survived solely because of his skills as a carpenter and where he saw the majority of his fellow prisoners starve to death or succumb to the harsh Russian winters. His eyes were always open, even at night, but they did not focus on anything—like limpets that have lost suction and become playthings of the waves, they slid off the walls and off the people who came to visit. After he had vegetated like this for three months, refusing all my grandmother's dishes and growing even thinner than during his time in the camp, my grandmother called in the family doctor. A country physician and an eminently pragmatic man, he was not in touch with current medical and psychological thinking and had never heard of anything called the psyche. When he had listened to my grandmother's description of the situation, and then found my grandfather in bed at midday, he sternly shook his head and, turning to my grandfather, declared:

"You have two choices, young man: either you pull yourself together, get up, and be a good husband to your wife, or else you should do us all a favor and die."

My grandfather sighed and responded: "I'd very much like to. But I'm too tired to die."

My grandfather found himself trapped between two medical paradigms. Although the impact of Freud's work on intellectuals, artists, and writers had been significant from the early decades of the twentieth century onward, his ideas about trauma and forms of suffering that are located in the borderland between the mind and the body took much longer to trickle down to medical professionals, and especially those in nonmetropolitan surroundings. Suspended in a diagnostic no-man's-land, in an era that was moving from psychoanalytical to biological explanations of mental pain, there was thus no cure at hand for my grandfather's posttraumatic exhaustion in rural Germany in the 1950s.

*　*　*

After the First World War, the medical establishment in western Europe and the United States increasingly dismissed neurasthenia—one of the most popular diagnoses of the final decades of the nineteenth and the first decade of the twentieth century—as malingering and shirking. Following neurasthenia's progressive disappearance from the medical handbooks, a twentieth-century version of melancholia entered the diagnostic stage in the 1930s: the concept of depression. Gradually, depression began to be regarded as a core syndrome that could explain a host of physical and mental symptoms that were clustered around exhaustion. At first, depression was considered to be a subcategory of neurosis. Indeed, although Sigmund Freud still used the term "melancholia," he defines what were to become some of the main features of depression in his essay "Mourning and Melancholia" (1917). As in the case of traditional melancholia, these symptoms include causeless sorrow and fear, but also—and this is new—self-hatred. Melancholics, Freud claims, suffer above all from a "delusion of inferiority." They present their egos as worthless, as incapable of any achievement, and as morally despicable: "The distinguishing mental features of melancholia are a profoundly painful dejection, cessation of interest in the outside world, loss of the capacity to love, inhibition of all activity, and a lowering of the self-regarding feelings to a degree that finds utterance in self-reproaches and self-revilings, and culminates in a delusional expectation of punishment."[1]

Moreover, as explored in chapter 8, Freudian melancholia is associated with loss: in a complex psychological procedure, the melancholic transforms emotions originally caused by the loss of a love object into the loss of a stable sense of self. Melancholia thus "behaves like an open wound," and all the melancholic's energies are consumed in an inner struggle between the punishing, sadistic superego and the ego.[2]

Freud's model was based primarily on the ideas of guilt and conflict: on struggles between the incompatible needs of the id, ego, and superego, and the constant demands that civilization places on individuals to repress their desires. These psychological conflicts could use up all one's energy. Yet in the second half of the twentieth century, and especially after the countercultural revolution of the 1960s, the influence of institutions and traditional sources of authority policing sexual behavior weakened, including that of the family, the church, the state, and educational institutions, and formerly more rigidly hierarchical ways of interacting in public and at work were challenged. Yet paradoxically, when these social structures and pressures became more lax, the French sociologist Alain Ehrenberg argues, we began to internalize the laws, assumptions, and expectations that used to be imposed on us from without. Consequently, a shift took place in the postwar decades such that the Freudian guilt–conflict model was replaced by the idea of insufficiency and personal responsibility.[3]

It is significant that the idea of depression became as important and ubiquitous as it is today only when pharmacological "cures" for some of its symptoms became available.[4] Much more so than its historical predecessors, the depression syndrome was shaped by commercial considerations and, in particular, the interests of what has come to be known as "big pharma." This process began in the 1950s, when two scientists discovered independently from each other that a drug originally developed to treat tuberculosis (Iproniazid) produced an elevation of mood. The Swiss scientist Roland Kuhn and his team found that changing the levels of neurotransmitters—chemical molecules that regulate emotions, our reactions to external events, and our physical drives—led to euphoric states in some patients. Kuhn subsequently developed a tricyclic (a three-ringed chemical compound) drug called Imipramine (marketed as Tofranil) as a treatment for depression. He understood these drugs primarily as mood correctors. The American scientist Nathan Kline also conducted research in this area. Unlike Kuhn, however, he considered the psychoactive drugs he developed to be "psychic energizers"—that is, "doping" and performance-enhancing rather than mood-correcting substances. He understood depression primarily as a deficiency in psychic energy.[5] However, Kline's Iproniazid drugs were withdrawn from the marked in 1961 owing to their lethal side effects.

The second wave of antidepressant research concentrated on a specific neurotransmitter—serotonin. Selective serotonin reuptake inhibitors (SSRUI) were first developed in the 1980s, and SSRUIs are still the basis of many antidepressants on the market. Serotonin is a molecule that transmits signals between the synapses in the brain, and low serotonin levels are a symptom of depressive moods. It is, however, still unclear whether low serotonin levels also actually cause depression, or whether they are simply one of its biochemical consequences. SSRUIs were first sold under the trade name Prozac, developed by Eli Lilly & Company, in 1987. Prozac became a blockbuster prescription drug, earning its developers $350 million in just two years. Annual sales now exceed $1 billion, and Prozac is still the most frequently prescribed antidepressant. Significantly, it was when Prozac first became available on prescription that the diagnosis of depression spiraled. It is now assumed that 25 percent of adults in the Western world suffer from a depressive episode at some point in their lives. Depression is the most commonly treated mental disorder, and the World Health Organization (WHO) has warned that depression is the single largest public-health problem after heart disease and the leading cause of disability worldwide. It estimates that globally 350 million people of all ages suffer from depression.[6]

* * *

The music journalist and writer Elizabeth Wurtzel was one of the first people to have been prescribed Prozac when it came on the market in 1987. Wurtzel's memoir *Prozac Nation: Young and Depressed in America* (1994) explores her battle with severe depression and her various experiments with drugs, both legal and illegal. Wurtzel's narrative is often contradictory and rambling and remains curiously devoid of epiphanies: strangely affectless, it evokes feelings as dreary as depression itself. *Prozac Nation* reads like the account of someone who still cannot really make sense of her experiences and who has not found a reconciliatory explanation for her own suffering. Wurtzel's excursions into psychology and her reflections on her own past remain oddly superficial. Yet her repeated vacillations between self-pity and self-loathing are probably an apt representation of how a depressed person might view and narrate her or his life story, and her memoir thus primarily enacts rather than analyzes the state of mind she attempts to describe. However, self-pity and self-loathing are also precisely the two characteristics of Wurtzel's account that make it hard for the reader fully to sympathize with her plight.

At the age of twenty, Wurtzel was diagnosed with "atypical" depression—the kind that begins in early adolescence and that is chronic and severe. Depressives of her type, she writes, are the "walking wounded," those "who are quite functional, whose lives proceed almost as usual, except that they're depressed *all* the time, almost constantly embroiled in thoughts of suicide even as they go through their paces."[7] Atypical depression is manifest, above all, in a lack of energy, interest, and initiative, alongside a great sensitivity to rejection. Wurtzel first tried to kill herself when she was only twelve years old, and throughout her book she voices resentments about her parents, who did not get on, divorced, and then fought over who was responsible for paying her psychiatry bills throughout her teens and her time at Harvard.

She often takes a curious pride in her own suffering, repeatedly emphasizing that its gravity and relentlessness exceed those of everyone else around her: "Harvard was full of nut cases, and we'd all managed to find each other, as if by centrifugal force. Still, no one's desperation came close to matching mine." There is even an undisguised moment of Prozac-pride at the end of her account:

> Every so often, I find myself with the urge to make sure people know that I am not just on Prozac but on lithium too, that I am a real sicko, a depressive of a much higher order than all these happy-pill poppers with their low-level sorrow. Or else I feel compelled to remind people that I've been on Prozac since the F.D.A. first approved it, that I've been taking it longer than anyone else on earth, save for a few laboratory rats in cages, trapped but happy.[8]

At Harvard, she consumes a plethora of drugs and suffers numerous breakdowns, panic attacks, and psychotic episodes, regularly visiting the medical emergency room. But her manic periods alternate with exhausted ones, and it is the descriptions of her lethargic phases that are most interesting. "I often didn't even have the energy to get to therapy sessions, so Dr. Sterling [her therapist] would have to talk to me by phone. I didn't have the energy to eat and, strange as this may sound, I didn't have the energy to sleep. All I could manage was lying in my bed." "Bathing," she writes, "seems like an exercise in futility, like making my bed or brushing my teeth or combing my hair. Clean the slate, then let it get sullied once more. Wipe it down, and wait for more filth. This inevitable pattern of progress and regress, which is really what life is all about, is too absurd for me to continue."[9]

During one of her many stints in an emergency ward, she describes herself as too tired to die:

> I don't want any more of life's vicissitudes, I don't want any more of this try, try again stuff. I just want out. I've had it. I am so tired. I am twenty and I am already exhausted.
>
> The only reason I agree to go to Stilman [the Harvard infirmary] . . . is that I am too tired to do anything else. It takes energy and will to commit suicide, and I don't have either. . . .

Madness is too glamorous a term to convey what happens to most people who are losing their minds. That word is too exciting, too literary, too interesting in its connotations, to convey the boredom, the slowness, the dreariness, the dampness of depression.

Elsewhere, she writes: "Depression is about as close as you get to somewhere between dead and alive, and it's the worst."[10]

After ten years of extreme psychological distress, and having taken almost all the psychopharmaceutic drugs available at that time to treat her condition—including lithium, desiprameine, Desyrel, Xanax, and Mellaril—Wurtzel's moods finally begin to stabilize with Prozac. However, the arrival of the wonder drug does not usher in a happy ending, nor does it result in positive character transformation or lead to any significant insights into her suffering: like everything else in her memoir, the Prozac-moment remains strangely underwhelming and anticlimactic: "And then something just kind of changed in me. Over the next few days, I became all right, safe in my own skin. It happened just like that."[11] Perhaps this is exactly how being on Prozac feels—limp, damp, and curiously lifeless.

❋ ❋ ❋

What is the role of exhaustion in depression? Is it a primary condition—that is, a trigger? Or is exhaustion the result of depression? Or is it merely one of its many symptoms? There are as yet no clear answers to these questions, partly because the nature of depression is by no means as clear-cut as it might appear. As with many mental health diagnoses, the emphasis on specific symptoms and behaviors not only changes through time but also depends on the methodological and ideological convictions, as well as the vested interests, of those who define it. The discovery of various psychopharmacological "cures" for depression, moreover, has led to the focus shifting ever more from psychological concepts such as guilt, loss, childhood traumas, and sadness to behaviors such as inhibition, slowing, inactivity, and inefficiency.

In 1980, the condition was labeled "major depressive disorder" in the *DSM-III*, the American Psychiatric Association's *Diagnostic and Statistical Manual of Mental Disorders*, which is as influential as it is controversial. The *DSM-III* and its successor volumes aim to be primarily descriptive and consequently concentrate on listing behaviors, at the cost of eliminating patients' personal histories, as well as any psychological explanations of mental suffering. In the most recent edition of the manual, the *DSM-5*, the principal features of depression are defined as depressed mood and the loss of interest or pleasure in nearly all activities for a period lasting at least two weeks. In addition, the individual must also experience at least four of the following additional symptoms: "changes in appetite or weight, sleep, and psychomotor activity; decreased energy; feelings of worthlessness or guilt; difficulty thinking, concentrating, or making decisions; or recurrent thoughts of death or suicidal ideation or suicide plans or attempts." The *DSM-5* also informs us that fatigue and insomnia are often the "presenting complaint," the most frequently cited reason why sufferers first consult general practitioners about their condition: "Decreased energy, tiredness, and fatigue are common. . . . A person may report sustained fatigue without physical exertion. Even the smallest tasks seem to require substantial effort. The efficiency with which tasks are accomplished may be reduced. For example, an individual may complain that washing and dressing in the morning are exhausting and take twice as long as usual."[12]

The WHO's *International Statistical Classification of Diseases and Related Health Problems (ICD-10)*—another important diagnostic manual—specifies three typical symptoms of depression: lowering of mood, reduction of energy, and decrease in activity. In addition, "capacity for enjoyment, interest, and concentration is reduced, and marked tiredness after even minimum effort is common. Sleep is usually disturbed and appetite diminished. Self-esteem and self-confidence are almost always reduced and, even in the mild form, some ideas of guilt or worthlessness are often present."[13]

Although the definitions of depression in the *DSM-5* and *ICD-10* are primarily behavioral and appear to be written in a factual, objective style, it is striking how similar they are to earlier descriptions of diagnostic entities structured around exhaustion. Low mood, hopelessness, difficulty concentrating, cognitive impairment, inactivity, and of course the essential lowering of energy levels have also featured prominently in theories that we have encountered in the previous chapters: think of Galen's melancholic, who viewed everything through a glass darkly; John Cassian's moping monks, unable to focus on their prayer or to perform their monastic duties; Marsilio Ficino's dull-spirited, slow-blooded children of Saturn; or George M. Beard's and Richard von Krafft-Ebing's irritable and lethargic neurasthenics. There is, then, a core cluster of symptoms that are regularly grouped together in the historically changing constellation of exhaustion-related diagnoses. These core symptoms are essentially all cognates of the affective, behavioral, emotional, and physical consequences of exhaustion. What changes, in addition to a list of variable and less significant secondary symptoms, is the way in which the etiology of these symptoms is explained and narrativized.

❋ ❋ ❋

In *The Noonday Demon: An Anatomy of Depression* (2001), his autobiographical account of his struggle with the illness, Andrew Solomon provides a range of descriptions of the experiential dimension of depression that are both poignant and beautiful. These examples demonstrate the power of metaphor to describe states of mind and physical experiences in such a way that others can get a strong sense of how the condition may feel. Those of us who have been spared the experience of depression firsthand can fathom its insidious workings only via analogy and simile, the apt deployment of which is Solomon's particular gift. Just like Sylvia Plath's haunting descriptions of depression in her novel *The Bell Jar* (1963), Solomon's precise, lyrical eloquence enables readers to step into the shoes of a depressed person and to see the world from that person's point of view.

One particularly memorable image that Solomon deploys is that of a huge vine gradually smothering an oak tree around which it has twisted itself and on which it feeds. From a distance, the vine leaves seem to be identical to those of the tree—it is almost impossible to tell the two apart:

> My depression had grown on me as that vine had conquered the oak; it had been a sucking thing that had wrapped itself around me, ugly and more alive than I. It had had a life of its own that bit by bit asphyxiated all of my life out of me. At the worst stage of major depression, I had moods that I knew were not my moods: they belonged to the depression, as surely as the leaves on that tree's high branches belonged to the vine. When I tried to think clearly about this, I felt that my mind was immured, that it couldn't expand in any direction. I knew that the sun was rising, and setting, but little of its light reached me. I felt myself sagging under what was much stronger than I; first I could not use my ankles, and then I could not control my knees, and then my waist began to break under the strain, and then my shoulders turned in, and in the end I was compacted and fetal, depleted by this thing that was crushing me without holding me. Its tendrils threatened to pulverize my mind and my courage and my stomach, and crack my bones and desiccate my body. It went on glutting itself on me when there seemed nothing left to feed it. . . .
>
> I would have been happy to die the most painful death, though I was too dumbly lethargic even to conceptualize suicide. Every second of being alive hurt me. Because this thing had drained all fluid from me, I could not even cry. My mouth was parched as well. I had thought that when you feel your worst your tears flood, but the very worst pain is the arid pain of total violation that comes after the tears are all used up, the pain that stops up every space through which you once metered the world, or the world, you. This is the presence of major depression.[14]

The vine imagery that Solomon uses is telling and reveals much about the author's conception of the condition. Creepers are external rather than internal threats. Their victims are selected randomly, in that they afflict trees through no fault of their own: weak or strong, old or young, rare or common trees can all find themselves targeted. Creepers like the one Solomon describes are energy-draining parasites, which vampirically feed on their hosts, slowly smothering and depleting them, literally sapping their life energy. But worse, at some point the parasite and the host merge, and it becomes ever more difficult to tell them apart. And at some point, the tree is so weakened that even removing the vine will not save it:

> Drug therapy hacks through the vines. You can feel it happening, how the medication seems to be poisoning the parasite so that bit by bit it withers away. You feel the weight going, feel the way that the branches can recover much of their natural bent. Until you have got rid of the vine, you cannot think about what has been lost. But even with the vine gone, you may still have few leaves and shallow roots, and the rebuilding of your self cannot be achieved with any drugs that now exist. With the weight of the vine gone, little leaves scattered along the tree skeleton become viable for essential nourishment. But this is not a good way to be. It is not a strong way to be. Rebuilding of the self in and after depression requires love, insight, work, and, most of all, time.[15]

The cure for depression, Solomon believes, lies in love, which he defines as the capacity to give and receive affection, the ability to be passionate about projects, as well as a sense of purpose (combined with psychopharmacological medication and the talking cure):

> Depression is the flaw in love. To be creatures who love, we must be creatures who can despair at what we lose, and depression is the mechanism of that despair. When it comes, it degrades one's self and ultimately eclipses the capacity to give or receive affection. It is the aloneness within us made manifest, and it destroys not only connection to others but also the ability to be peacefully alone with oneself. Love,

though it is no prophylactic against depression, is what cushions the mind and protects it from itself. Medications and psychotherapy can renew that protection, making it easier to love and be loved, and that is why they work. In good spirits, some love themselves and some love others and some love work and some love God: any of these passions can furnish that vital sense of purpose that is the opposite of depression. Love forsakes us from time to time, and we forsake love. In depression, the meaninglessness of every enterprise and every emotion, the meaninglessness of life itself, becomes self-evident. The only feeling left in this love-less state is insignificance.[16]

Burnout, too, as we will see in chapter 11, is increasingly defined by its opposites, by what it is not—that is, the absence of the ability to engage, to care, and to feel part of anything beyond the self. Similarly, the French theorist Roland Barthes has described acedia in terms of "a loss of investment" in life: "Acedy (modern acedy): no longer being capable of investing in other people, in living-with-several-other-people and yet at the same time being incapable of investing in solitude. Throwing it all away, but without even somewhere to throw it: waste without a waste bin."[17] In the final sentences of the quoted passage, Solomon also evokes the same idea as Lars von Trier in the film *Melancholia*: that most nondepressed people are simply protected by a shield of illusions that act as a buffer between them and the disconcerting truth about the fundamental insignificance of human existence and all human pursuits. The depressed person lacks this protective shield and, according to Solomon, thus loses above all the ability to love and to derive pleasure from experiences others find enjoyable, the clinical term for which is "anhedonia." The term "anhedonia," deriving from the Greek *an* (without) and *hedone* (pleasure), denotes a state of chronic lack. The anhedonic experience chronic feelings of emptiness, hopelessness, and isolation. They lack interest and motivation and are unable to experience joy.

✳ ✳ ✳

The debate about how best to treat depression and how to understand its causes, continues to this day. Many general practitioners and psychiatrists promote a reductive biochemical view of depression, based on the idea that the origins of depression (rather than its consequences) can be fully explained by chemical imbalances in the brain. It is undoubtedly the case, however, that antidepressants are not a "cure" for depression but instead merely control some of its symptoms. They do not promote healing but present a well-being and life-management solution, comparable to taking aspirin to combat chronic pain or injecting insulin to control the symptoms of diabetes. It is, of course, perfectly legitimate to take drugs to alleviate strongly debilitating symptoms, and antidepressants help many to live relatively normal lives. In this sense they are, like pain killers, a blessing. But when patients stop taking the drugs, their symptoms almost always return, suggesting that none of the underlying causes of the condition have been addressed. A backlash against the ever more frequent prescription of antidepressants is already taking place. Recently, numerous studies have been published on that topic, some complaining about a careless medicalization of "normal" sadness, some proposing a return to the talking cure, some radically questioning the efficacy of antidepressants, and some emphasizing the highly problematic influence of the pharmaceutical industry on the marketing and shaping of diseases.[18]

Some doctors also propose a variety of psychological treatments for depression, including psychoanalysis and various forms of psychotherapy, especially cognitive behavioral therapy (CBT). CBT is the most goal-orientated, purely behaviorist, and superficial form of psychotherapy, focusing as it does on cognitive reprogramming—that is, on identifying and eliminating negative thinking patterns. As it is also much cheaper than deeper, long-term forms of treatment, it is the state-sponsored therapy of choice in many Western countries.

Yet other theorists reject both biochemical and psychological cures and explanations, insisting instead on the social causes of the condition. Alain Ehrenberg, for instance, argues that depression should be viewed as a direct consequence of the political and moral autonomy of the modern individual. "Depression," he writes, "is melancholia plus equality, the perfect disorder of the democratic human being. *It is the inexorable counterpart of the human being who is her/his own sovereign.*"[19] In an age in which we are no longer bound by moral and religious law, or restricted by tradition in the way we used to be, and especially before the 1960s countercultural revolution, we have, theoretically at least, unlimited freedom to become anything we wish to be. But this newfound autonomy comes at a high price: given that freedom, personal choice, self-ownership, individual initiative, self-development, and self-improvement are now among our most cherished values, failure in any area of life has become a matter of personal responsibility. "Liberation," Ehrenberg writes, "might have gotten us out of the drama of guilt and obedience, but it has taken us straight into the demands of responsibility and action. And so the weariness of depression took over from the anxiety of neuroses."[20] According to Ehrenberg, we are weighed down by the possibilities inherent in the idea of a theoretically unlimited freedom: almost everything is allowed, but very little is actually possible. We all wish to be exceptional, and most of us find that we are not. And when we fully realize this, we break down.

What is more, we have also internalized the demands and assumptions that in the past figures of authority articulated. One of Franz Kafka's aphorisms neatly illustrates the troubling mechanism of internalizing concepts that used to be enforced on us from the outside and that are not necessarily to our advantage: "The animal wrests the whip from the master and whips itself in order to become master, and it does not know that this is just a fantasy, created by a new knot in the whiplash of the master."[21] This aphorism expresses the perversity inherent in the internalization of the values of the oppressor by the oppressed. The objects of disciplinary control become the monitors of their own behavior; the superego takes over from the authority figure; the depressed shoulder all responsibility for their own misery and blame themselves.

The expectation of constantly having to reinvent and fashion ourselves has turned into a terrifying responsibility: the very idea of absolute freedom is exhausting and paralyzing. As Ehrenberg writes: "Depression presents itself as an illness of responsibility in which the dominant feeling is that of failure. The depressed individual is unable to measure up; he is tired of having to become himself." Contemporary depression is, then, essentially bound up with feelings of failure, inadequacy, and inhibition. It is a disease of exhaustion, weariness, and slowing, above all manifest in a lack of initiative and the breakdown of action.[22]

The inhibited depressed person, moreover, stands in direct opposition to our most cherished values: "The depressed person has trouble forming projects; he or she lacks energy and the minimum motivation to carry them out. . . . With no project, motivation, or communication, the depressed person stands in exact opposition to our social norms."[23] Ehrenberg also poses some difficult questions about the difference between medication and personality enhancement: When do drugs such as antidepressants cease to "cure" specific pathological behavior, and when do they start to alter a person's temperament or personality? When do they become the equivalent of psychic doping or mind-altering drug taking? For example, antidepressants might lower the inhibitions of people who may in fact be shy and retiring by nature. The antidepressants act like alcohol, but their effects are more long lasting, affecting the person's character.

As convincing as many of Ehrenberg's ideas are, he, too, follows a by now familiar pattern, in that he turns the analysis of an exhaustion-illness into a vehicle for social critique, ultimately delivering a grander narrative about the perils of bourgeois individualism. In this and in other respects, his theory resembles that of other theorists of exhaustion, who single out specific sociocultural transformations that they hold responsible for depleting our energies. Like George Cheyne, Beard, Krafft-Ebing, Jonathan Crary, and many others, Ehrenberg situates the causes for an increase in exhaustion-related illnesses primarily in the cultural field. It is the neoliberal, bourgeois-individualist environment that, to return to Solomon's image, acts as the vine that slowly saps us of our energies, growing ever stronger as we waste away.

10

Mystery Viruses

Parallel to the rise of depression in the second half of the twentieth century, an even more explicit concern with exhaustion began to emerge under the label chronic fatigue syndrome (CFS), once again under the banner of somatic diseases. It was first named and defined in the 1980s and is also known as myalgic encephalomyelitis (ME), postviral fatigue syndrome (PVFS), and chronic fatigue immune dysfunction syndrome (CFIDS).[1] Mental and physical fatigue, postexertion malaise, a perceived sense of effort that renders many everyday activities impossible, and difficulties with concentrating, cognitive tasks, and short-term memory are among its cardinal symptoms. It remains a controversial diagnosis and has in recent decades prompted fierce debate among medical practitioners and patients.[2] It has also attracted considerable media attention: the press contributed substantially to the popularization of the condition and polarized the debate further by repeatedly reporting on allegedly "groundbreaking" medical discoveries of definitive organic causes, on the one hand, and by coining unsympathetic labels such as "yuppie flu" and "lazy cow syndrome," on the other.[3] Some physicians, researchers, and the majority of patients with CFS argue strongly for the somatic origins of the condition. Most commonly, viral infections, immune dysfunctions, and central nervous system or metabolic disorders are thought to trigger the illness. Others, however, have dismissed the validity of these biological explanations and argue that CFS is primarily a psychosomatic or a behavioral problem, closely related to depression and anxiety, and should therefore be classified as a psychiatric disorder.[4]

The prehistory of CFS began in the United States and Great Britain in the 1950s with reports of epidemic episodes of viral infections. These included "polio-like" outbreaks of viral illnesses in a psychiatric hospital near Washington, D.C., in 1953, and in Punta Gorda, Florida, in 1956. There had also been a previous outbreak at the Los Angeles County Hospital in 1934, during which similar symptoms were described. Patients complained about motor and sensory symptoms, fatigue, muscle pain, and cognitive impairment.[5] In 1955 in Britain, an infectious epidemic struck 192 members of the medical staff in the Royal Free Hospital in London. They experienced extreme fatigue and severe muscle pain, as well as stiff necks and abdominal tenderness. The syndrome was initially called encephalomyelitis in Britain and, in 1956, benign myalgic encephalomyelitis. The medical historian Edward Shorter explains: "It was 'benign' because nobody died and there were no pathological findings, 'myalgic' because of muscle pain, and 'encephalomyelitis' because the brain (encephalo-) and spinal cord (myelo-) were presumably inflamed."[6] However, the adjective "benign" was later dropped, and the condition became known as ME. Rheumatologists referred to a very similar symptom cluster as fibrositis, or fibromyalgia. They, too, assumed that the condition was caused by organic and/or external factors, such as viral infections. Yet even the discussion of these early epidemics in the 1950s was already polarized: some researchers considered them instances of mass hysteria, while others argued fiercely for the organic and infectious origins of these outbreaks.

In the 1960s and 1970s, patients who had not been directly exposed to these epidemics began to report similar symptoms. While the earlier epidemic cases were deemed infectious and acute, the newly emerging sporadic cases tended to be noncontagious and chronic. In the 1980s and 1990s, media interest in the condition surged dramatically, partly in response to medical papers published on the illness and partly to widely read patients' illness accounts, which chimed with the personal experiences and symptom perception of many readers.[7] Support, lobbying, and activist groups soon began to proliferate, and physicians were confronted with a rapidly growing number of patients who were convinced that they had CFS.[8]

In 1964, Michael Epstein and Y. M. Barr discovered a virus that came to be called Epstein-Barr virus (EBV). The symptoms produced by this virus include lassitude, aching legs, fatigue, and mood disorders, and it was later established that it causes mononucleosis. In the 1980s, many researchers assumed the existence of a direct causal connection between EBV and CFS, but the evidence linking the two was subsequently problematized. Many researchers still believe that viral infections, such as EBV, hepatitis, and meningitis, trigger the onset of CFS symptoms, but they also propose that psychological, behavioral, genetic, and immunological factors play a significant role in the development of the illness.[9] At present, most researchers in the field accept that CFS is the result of a complex and heterogeneous network of causes and agree that there is no persuasive evidence for any of the definitive monocausal explanations of the condition that have been suggested in the past, and nor are there any conclusive biomarkers.[10]

The Centers for Disease Control and Prevention (CDC) case definition from 1994, which many clinicians still use to diagnose the illness, states that in order to be diagnosed with CFS, patients must meet three criteria. First, they must have experienced severe chronic fatigue for six or more consecutive months, and the fatigue may not be explained by ongoing exertion or other medical conditions associated with fatigue. Second, the fatigue must interfere significantly with their daily activities and work. Third, the individual must also suffer from four or more of the following eight symptoms: postexertion malaise lasting more than twenty-four hours, unrefreshing sleep, significant impairment of short-term memory or concentration, muscle pain, joint pain, headaches, tender lymph nodes in the neck or armpit, and a frequent or recurrent sore throat.

The currently most widely accepted clinical understanding of CFS is that the syndrome often has a microbiological trigger (such as EBV), but that social, behavioral, and psychological factors may contribute to perpetuating the illness and to a patient's inability fully to recover from the viral infection. Patients frequently cite viral infections as having caused the condition, and recent research has also established that many CFS patients have immunity dysfunctions, endocrine abnormalities, and cardiovascular irregularities.[11] CFS is generally considered a syndrome with either potentially many causes or a single cause that has not yet been established. The latter option is, of course, a genuine possibility, and one in which many CFS patients believe firmly. Many feel extremely frustrated about the lack of progress in identifying the underlying organic factors and blame the government and the medical establishment for failing to direct more funds to CFS research. At present, the only available (and moderately efficacious) therapeutics offered to those with CFS include cognitive behavioral therapy (CBT) and graded exercise, both of which focus on symptom relief only.

* * *

How does living with chronic fatigue actually feel? How do those who experience it describe their illness, their everyday life, and their ongoing struggle with this often highly debilitating and chronic condition? The Scottish writer Nasim Marie Jafry has turned her own illness history into a fictionalized narrative, *The State of Me*, which allows readers glimpses of the experiential dimension of the condition. Jafry's semiautobiographical heroin Helen Fleet, a promising, active, and energetic student, falls ill on her year abroad in France and, after months of being in the dark about her disconcerting condition, is finally diagnosed with the rare Coxsackie B4 virus in 1984, and later with chronic postviral ME. The narrator tells us: "Her symptoms have signed a lease behind her back and moved in permanently. They like living in her muscle tissue. It's nice and warm there."[12]

Helen suddenly finds herself transformed from an ambitious student into a housebound, permanently exhausted woman dependent on disability allowance and the care of others, for whom ordinary mental and physical activities require a superhuman effort. She constantly has to economize her very limited supply of energy:

> I'm always measuring out my energy behind the scenes, but people don't see it. They see you at a party and think you're fine, they don't see you resting all day to be able to go, and being wrecked all next day because you went. They don't see you leaning on walls at bus stops because you can't stand for more than five minutes. They don't see how tired your arm gets after beating an egg. They don't know you almost always have poison in your calves when you wake up. They don't see you weeping because you're so tired of it all.

Helen, however, gradually learns to live with her condition, finds love, and generally approaches her difficult life with a healthy and often humbling dose of humor. Moreover, she learns to find pleasure in the more mundane aspects of life: "[I]f you're chronically ill you just survive it. You start to appreciate small things. It's what gets you through."[13]

Jafry vacillates between using a first- and a third-person voice to describe Helen's experiences, showing her struggle alternately from the inside and the outside, and includes various imaginary dialogues with interested strangers, who quiz Helen on her mystery illness. These "frequently asked questions by well-meaning strangers in the late 80s" include:

> STRANGER: What did you do today?
> ME: I had a shower and made a cup of tea.
> STRANGER: Is that all?
> ME: I tried to wash my hair but my arms were too weak to lather.
> STRANGER: That's a shame. Are you able to read to pass the time?
> ME: Sometimes, but my arms get exhausted holding the book. They feel like they're burning. And my head feels like it's being sawed. . . .

STRANGER: I feel tired all the time. I think I've got the mystery illness.

ME: It's much worse than feeling tired all the time. You feel like toxic waste and you have to have the symptoms for six months before they'll diagnose you. . . .

STRANGER: Is it like flu?

ME: It's like flu (without the mucus) PLUS glandular fever PLUS a vile hangover every day. You have to stay in bed. Your life stops and you can't function. There are subsets of symptoms within symptoms. You discover new kinds of pain, new kinds of weakness, neurological sensations you didn't think possible. And if you're lucky, you might have irritable bowel syndrome, allergies and tinnitus thrown in. . . . [I]f you climb the stairs you feel like you've run a marathon—your muscles burn, they think they've done much more than they actually have. And they don't recover normally.[14]

In addition to struggling with her symptoms, Helen struggles with the unsympathetic views of "non-believers." She reacts particularly scathingly to medical professionals who suggest psychiatric treatments:

STRANGER: Why do some doctors not believe you?

ME: I honestly have no idea. Maybe because there's no single diagnostic test and because they're arrogant. They don't understand it, so it's easier to blame the patient, label them as depressed, neurotic, lazy *etc.* They say people are jumping on the ME bandwagon, but how can you jump on a fucking bandwagon that you didn't know existed?! . . . I think there should be a mass crucifixion of all the GPs, psychiatrists and journalists who don't believe it is a physical illness. These people are so powerful and are causing so much damage by not believing us. They should be made to pay. They're making people *more* ill, forcing them to keep going.

STRANGER: Do you feel that strongly?

ME: Well, I'm against the death penalty but I'd be happy if they all got ME themselves. That would be enough. They would soon believe in it, within twenty-four hours of having it. I'll tell you that for nothing.[15]

Jafry has no time for Freudian or even only remotely psychological explanations of her illness—all such approaches are anathema. A strong, at times even violent, antipsychiatric and antipsychoanalytical stance is in fact a defining characteristic of many CFS patients and activist groups. Jafry not only wishes that doctors who suggest graded exercise or CBT would fall ill with ME themselves but also includes a passage in which she appears to mock the idea that childhood experiences or infantile trauma may have contributed to her illness in some way:

I'm reading one of Sean's psychology books, about traumas in childhood causing problems later on. I think of my childhood traumas and wonder if my immune system could've been damaged. Possible events were:

1) The sofa with the swirly brown and orange cover. I hated the feel of the nylon against my skin, but I would make myself rub my hands along the cushions.

2) Shitting myself in primary one because I was too scared to tell the teacher that I needed the toilet—I sat at my desk playing with rods (the colourful wooden units we learned to count with) and said nothing. I waddled home, a navy gusset sticking to me.

3) Sean peeing on me from halfway up the Michael tree. I can still feel the warmth of my brother's urine on my scalp. He cried later and denied it.

4) Divorce of Rita and Peter.[16]

Although on the surface the passage appears to satirize psychoanalytical narratives, many would consider the final point to be a potentially traumatizing event for a child. Has the divorce of her parents crept unconsciously onto her list, or is its inclusion a gentle hint that, perhaps, Helen's fiercely antipsychiatric and anti-psychoanalytical rhetoric may function as a defense mechanism designed to shield her from confronting painful and unwelcome emotions and experiences? Her parents' divorce is the only one of the four points on which she does not elaborate.

※ ※ ※

At the center of the controversy surrounding the CFS diagnosis is the question of whether psychiatric factors contribute to, or even cause, the development of the condition, or whether depression, anxiety, somatization, and other affective and mood disorders, which often accompany CFS, are merely a secondary reaction to the chronic and often debilitating illness. Just like Helen, many patients react angrily, and some violently, to suggestions that their illness might not be organic in nature and feel that the offer of CBT and graded exercise as the only viable therapeutics is demeaning. Most patient pressure groups embrace fiercely antipsychiatric rhetoric and sometimes attack and insult psychiatrically oriented researchers who, they feel, call into question the reality and severity of their suffering by suggesting that it is "all in the head." Psychiatrists have responded to this challenge of their authority by declaring that the firm belief in the organic origins of their illness, as well as antipsychiatric attitudes, are in fact to be counted among the characteristic "illness beliefs" of this particular patient cohort.

Jafry, for example, who also writes a blog, fiercely objects to the "psychosocial brigades" and even the label CFS, which she considers to be a nebulous term preferred by a "psychiatrically" oriented school of physicians and which denies the neuro-immunological nature of ME. In her view, the cardinal features of ME are postexertional malaise, or postexertional neuro-immune exhaustion, which are caused by viral triggers. "If I were mentally ill," she writes, "I'd happily be referred to a psychiatrist, but I'm not, so I prefer to stick with neurologists, virologists, immunologists, etc.—the people who may actually be able to help me." She is particularly scathing about the British psychiatrist and professor of psychological medicine Simon Wessely, one of the most important CFS researchers in Britain, accusing him and his followers of "stealing neurological illnesses and labelling them as psychiatric." According to Jafry, they "will do anything to prevent biomedical research into ME, they desperately want to keep it all to themselves—with their loveable, eccentric and conflating notions of 'false illness beliefs' and 'chronic fatigue syndrome.' . . . It truly beggars belief that an individual doctor can seek—with catastrophic results—to overturn the reality of so many patients, and the reality of other doctors and researchers."[17]

Others with CFS/ME, and pressure groups, too, have targeted Wessely, who has even received death threats. It is ironic that Wessely should have become such a hated figure in the CFS/ME community, as he repeatedly emphasizes that the label "psychiatric" pertains to symptoms and does not in any way include a judgment on the patients' culpability or responsibility. And neither does the label suggest that the symptoms that patients experience are made up, hysterical, or "all in their minds." His position is much more nuanced. He does not even deny the possibility that external factors cause CFS:

> We suggest that agents such as EBV or viral meningitis can lead to the experience of abnormal symptoms, such as fatigue, malaise, and myalgia. However, the transition from symptoms to disability may be more closely linked to cognitive and behavioural factors. Hence interventions such as CBT designed to reduce disability and counteract maladaptive coping strategies ought to be more effective in reducing disability than symptoms. The evidence so far supports this model—many patients do show considerable improvements in disability and everyday functioning, but are not rendered symptom free by cognitive or behavioural interventions.[18]

Here and elsewhere, Wessely proposes that, since it has so far not been possible to identify and treat any potential underlying microbiological causes of the condition, it should instead be a priority to help patients with this chronic and debilitating disease to cope better with and to regain some control over their symptoms.

Other researchers and theoreticians would have been more understandable targets for the wrath of the patient lobby. The literary critic Elaine Showalter, for example, discusses CFS alongside other syndromes and phenomena as a modern version of hysteria in *Hystories: Hysterical Epidemics and Modern Media* (1997).[19] The medical historian Edward Shorter is certain that CFS is a purely psychosomatic disorder and that patients "choosing" this label deliberately adopt highly subjective symptoms such as fatigue and muscle pain because they cannot be medically disproved. He, too, considers CFS to be a twentieth-century successor of classical hysteria and its motor-sensory symptoms, such as fits, convulsions, and paralysis. Shorter proposes that somatizing patients always adapt their symptoms to fit with the medical thinking of their times, so that they conform to what medical professionals consider "legitimate" diseases. CFS symptoms correspond to what "doctors under the influence of the central-nervous paradigm expected to see," and its predominantly sensory symptoms were also "almost impossible to 'disprove.'" "The saga of chronic fatigue syndrome," Shorter writes, "represents a kind of cautionary tale for those doctors who lose sight of the scientific underpinning of medicine, and for those patients who lose their good sense in the media-spawned 'disease-of-the-month' clamor that poisons the doctor-patient relationship."[20]

He describes CFS as an "epidemic of illness attribution," or "epidemic hysteria." "A whole subculture of chronic fatigue has arisen," he asserts, "in which those patients too tired to walk give each other hints about how to handle a wheelchair and exchange notes about how to secure disability payments from the government or from insurance companies." This remark, and the implication that CFS patients might be malingerers and benefit scroungers, is very reminiscent of the antishirker rhetoric that was used in the 1920s to dismiss the cases of shell-shocked veterans and of neurasthenics. Shorter seems particularly disturbed by CFS patients' disrespect for medical expertise and the fact that they appear to elevate the "subjective knowledge of their bodies to the same status as the doctors' objective knowledge." He emphasizes that the rejection of psychiatric diagnoses by chronic fatigue patients is much more violent than "are the normal reactions of medical patients to psychiatric consultation, and is itself a characteristic of the illness."[21] In other words, he turns the antipsychiatric rhetoric into a full-fledged CFS symptom in its own right.

CFS patients, in Shorter's view, are particularly susceptible to media reports and willing constantly to change their symptom attributions to make them fit with new diagnostic fads. He concludes his unsympathetic account of the CFS "subculture" with the socially conservative diagnosis that loneliness and a general loosening of familial and social bonds in our modern, anticommunal, and self-centered age are to blame for a widespread loss of common sense regarding the perception and interpretation of bodily symptoms. Lonely people, he suggests, have significantly higher rates of somatization because they are deprived of "feedback loops"—that is, access to the collective wisdom on health and illness of others, who might be able to correct or challenge their perhaps exaggerated subjective fears and anxieties. Our age, marked by the "triumph of the desire for individual self-actualization over commitment to the family as an institution," fetishizes above all personal growth, to the detriment of communitarian objectives. Pain and fatigue, then, are the characteristic and entirely logical complaints that define our times:

> It is the lonely and disaffiliated who give us the image of our own times, who are the latter-day equivalent of the hysterical nineteenth-century woman in her hoop skirts and fainting fits. . . . The development of psychosomatic symptoms can be a response to too much intimacy or too little. And if our forebears of the "modern" family suffered the former problem, it is we of the postmodern era who endure the latter.[22]

While there might be truth in Shorter's remarks on the power of the media in shaping and perpetuating symptoms, and in a resulting transformation of the doctor–patient relationship, it is very noticeable that he—just like George Cheyne, George M. Beard, Jonathan Crary, Alain Ehrenberg, and many other theorists of exhaustion syndromes before him—essentially subscribes to a nostalgic, idealized vision of a better, more community-oriented past. It is clear that he mourns the decline of traditional social structures and despises the rise of a new brand of individualism, which focuses, above all, on self-realization and personal growth. Ultimately, he holds these wider postwar developments responsible for the spread of fatigue illnesses such as CFS and, like his predecessors, thus pathologizes specific sociocultural changes that he deems problematic.

❊ ❊ ❊

Chronic fatigue syndrome rose to prominence in the 1980s and continued to attract considerable media coverage in the 1990s. Although the actual number of CFS patients has not lessened in the twenty-first century, media attention has now shifted to other exhaustion syndromes, above all depression, stress, and burnout. The British ME Association estimates that 250,000 people in Great Britain are affected by CFS, and the CDC estimates that more than 1 million Americans are currently experiencing the illness. CFS thus still affects more people in the United States than multiple sclerosis, lupus, and various forms of cancer.[23] But why did CFS preoccupy the cultural imagination in the final decades of the twentieth century, and with which historically specific anxieties and preoccupations did it chime? What are the dominant metaphors, imagery, and scientific concepts that are deployed in the popular writings on the syndrome?

In both Britain and the United States, the 1980s saw the rapid rise of neoliberalism. The governments of Margaret Thatcher and Ronald Reagan sought to implement a range of policies to ensure a free-market economy that could become global in its scope. A reduction in government spending, tax cuts, privatization, the disempowerment of the unions, and a privileging of economic growth over social equality lay at the heart of a socioeconomic revolution. In popular culture, the 1980s were often represented as the age of greed, in which materialism became a universally acceptable raison d'être, and in which figures such as the ruthless investment banker Gordon Gecko (*Wall Street*, 1987) were either openly or covertly venerated. In some ways, then, CFS can be viewed as an (albeit unconscious) form of protest or backlash against the prevailing ethos of achievement, constant high-level performance, and the pressures of self-optimization.[24] Statistics do indeed show that the majority of typical CFS patients used to be unusually active, successful, and perfectionist before they fell ill.

The 1980s were also marked by growing concerns about the environment, and in particular about nuclear energy, the ozone layer, climate change, dwindling natural resources, and large-scale industrial pollution—concerns reflected in anxieties about pollution and purity, chemical sensitivities, allergies, food additives, the adverse effects of antibiotics, and auto-intoxication in many popular accounts of CFS. Patients frequently voice fears about modern "toxic lifestyles"—poisonous substances to which they are exposed in their daily lives and that they may even ingest in the form of food and drugs. An anonymous commentator, for example, claims: "Never in history have people been exposed to greater assaults on their bodies by environmental pollution. Food additives and drugs may also harm the body and adversely affect the immune system. Certain doctors even claim that long term antibiotics depress the immune system."[25] In addition, yeast infection, or candida, was a very popular topic in the CFS community for many years. It was thought to be promoted by the use of antibiotics, and patients were advised to cut out various food groups that were presumed to aggravate yeast-based toxicity.

In *Chronic Fatigue and Its Syndromes*, Wessely and his coauthors establish some fascinating parallels between CFS and neurasthenia. Those who theorized both syndromes claimed that the conditions were absolutely modern and new, and the result of specific sociocultural developments: "Just as CFS today is the price paid for pollution, exhaust fumes, food additives, aerosols, antibiotics, and so on, neurasthenia was the price to be paid for industrialization, the rise of capitalism, and the consequent strains to which the business and professional classes were exposed."[26] Both conditions also feature a list of similar associated symptoms, and even some of the therapeutic suggestions are alike in that CFS activists, too, argue that rest is the only effective coping strategy for those affected by the illness, thus evoking the ghost of Silas Weir Mitchell and his infamous "rest cure." The ME Action Campaign 1989, for example, suggests: "For the majority of M.E. sufferers, physical and mental exertion is to be avoided, and adequate rest essential. Important: if you have muscle fatigue do not exercise, this could cause a severe relapse."[27]

The big new medical paradigm of the postwar decades was immunology, in part as a result of the discovery of human immunodeficiency virus (HIV) and the anxieties associated with the epidemic spread of AIDS. Shorter describes immunology as the new "queen bee of the medical sciences," a medical holy grail, which became invested with high hopes and quickly turned into a symbol of all that was new and groundbreaking.[28] References to defective immune systems appear repeatedly in the CFS debate, and many commentators were keen to embrace immunological explanations of their condition. A patient writes, for example: "ME is very much a disease of our time—an attack on the immune system exacerbated by stress, pressure and the demands of twentieth century life."[29] One often encounters military metaphors in immunological arguments—the words "attack" and "pressure" are often used. Within the immunological paradigm, the body is frequently imagined as a battlefield invaded by viral or toxic enemies, while the immune system is seen as a kind of "patriotic defense unit."[30]

Wessely and his colleagues draw attention to yet another link between CFS and neurasthenia, and their observations apply to many other exhaustion-based diagnoses, too: most popular writings on fatigue-related syndromes draw on metaphors and concepts borrowed from the latest scientific and medical discourses. While Beard's texts on neurasthenia were written in the wake of a general preoccupation with nerves and electricity, CFS commentators frequently reference the latest immunological and virological concepts, as well as pollution, toxicity, and allergies.[31] The medieval theorists of acedia, in contrast, structured their arguments around free will, divine grace, and demonic influences, while Marsilio Ficino presented a mélange of humoral, astrological, and magical explanatory models that were popular in his age.

It is, of course, not entirely surprising that commentators should adjust their jargon and pepper their accounts with references to the latest medical discoveries; after all, these are simple strategies designed to enhance credibility and to make them sound up-to-date. All of us, moreover, operate within certain scientific paradigms and within the limits of what Michel Foucault describes as "epistemes." Epistemes are configurations of knowledge and discursive structures that determine not just which propositions are deemed acceptable (scientific or otherwise) at a given historical moment but what kind of ideas can be developed in the first place: each episteme entails limits that are based on a set of fundamental ideological assumptions specific to a historical moment, which might not always be obvious.

What is perhaps most surprising about the CFS controversy is that many patients consider a "psychiatric" diagnosis and the offer of "psychiatric" therapeutics as anathema to and an attack on the legitimacy of their experience. Regardless of the evidence for and against the organic origins of the illness, one would have thought that the bias against the perceived stigma that comes with mental health diagnoses would have substantially declined after Sigmund Freud, especially in the Western world. Yet the fiercely antipsychiatric stance of the patient lobby is reminiscent of the nineteenth-century neurasthenia debates, in that all causation is assigned exclusively to external or organic factors. In some ways, this position represents a distorted reflection of the current state of a strictly biomedically oriented psychiatric and medical establishment. After the Second World War, a second "biological turn" took effect, which reinforced an outdated nineteenth-century mind–body dichotomy, a neo-Cartesian splitting that many hoped had been overcome and that repressed rather than sublated the achievements of the psychoanalytical paradigm. Once again, mental illness was (and in many cases still is) seen purely as a disease of the brain, an idea first introduced by the German neurologist and psychiatrist Wilhelm Griesinger in the mid-nineteenth century.

Many other patient groups readily accept psychogenic theories about their conditions. The relative openness to psychosomatic explanatory models may also partly be determined by different personality types and cognitive and attributional styles—some patients, for example, do not mind self-identifying as depressed, while others prefer diagnoses structured around external agents, such as CFS, stress, and burnout, as they are thought to carry less stigma and suggest blamelessness. Wessely and his coauthors argue that the belief in external causes for patients' conditions may serve the function of protecting self-esteem, guarding them against self-blame and guilt (which are key symptoms of depression and notably absent in CFS), "but at the cost of increased helplessness in the face of an invisible, external adversary." Avoidance behavior, the reduction of mental and physical activity, and certain illness beliefs, they argue, are not what triggers CFS but precisely what keeps it going.[32]

✳ ✳ ✳

The debate over the biological or psychogenic origins of CFS may sound academic, even obscure. However, the ways in which we imagine and represent our illnesses, the narratives we tell ourselves and others about them, and the etiological theories in which we believe do matter. Beliefs, internal representations, and metaphors affect how symptoms are experienced, how we cope with them, and how we interpret bodily signals. Such beliefs can, of course, also be damaging or self-perpetuating; for example, the assumption that one's condition is incurable and possibly even fatal, and that rest is the only way to manage one's symptoms, can become the cause of anxiety and depression and perpetuate behavior that may aggravate or complicate the development of an illness.[33]

In *Why Do People Get Ill?*, Darian Leader and David Corfield present compelling evidence for the ways in which our minds can affect our bodies and the symptoms we develop. They explore some unsettling research on the impact of psychological factors on what we tend to think of as purely physical illnesses. Patients who are less able than others to engage with and express loss and trauma, they argue, often translate their losses directly into certain diseases: "*The body responds here with an answer when the symbolic universe doesn't.*" As they observe, a symptom "can be a form of language, an appeal which aims to make someone else recognize one's distress." The compelling evidence they present in their study questions the monocausal, antiholistic illness models and the fragmented view of the body that is dominant in the Western world and that the CFS patient lobby appears to have embraced with particular eagerness. Leader and Corfield relate this Cartesian splitting to the fact that modern medicine is largely determined by economic interests, and that two-thirds of clinical studies are funded by drug companies, which have no interest in promoting psychological techniques.

They analyze the bacterial-infection model as an example of a monocausal illness theory and present evidence on various bacterial illnesses that show that the matter is, in fact, more complicated: a surprisingly large percentage of children and adults, for example, carry the bacteria that cause tuberculosis, malaria, ulcers, and gastritis. However, a significantly smaller number actually develop the diseases. Psychological factors play a crucial role in whether the body is able to fight off these bacteria: "The bacterial model, after all, conceives of illness as a single, discrete entity, and it is suspiciously close to the ancient idea of illness as an autonomous entity which is visited upon one, like a demon. The discovery of microscopic organisms and infection processes did not dispel these archaic fears but rather gave them a new, scientific veneer." The belief in purely external agent–driven illness models, Leader and Corfield argue, constitutes a form of splitting. Moreover, it is in fact a defense mechanism aimed at shielding not only patients but also culture as a whole from certain troubling insights: as they observe, the split between mind and body "is in fact itself *a defence mechanism against recognizing how disturbing, excessive or unprocessable ideas affect us.*"[34]

Shorter, too, suggests that in the case of psychosomatic illnesses, our unconscious plays a major role in the shaping of our symptoms: it is the unconscious that orchestrates our bodies' responses to unhappiness or stress. But the unconscious mind is influenced by the surrounding culture and is able to read current medical models of "legitimate" and "illegitimate" symptoms. According to Shorter, most organically based symptoms would currently fall into the former, and most psychogenic symptoms into the latter category. Medical discourses shape symptoms, in that they provide culturally determined templates, or a "symptom pool," of legitimate illness behavior on which the unconscious draws. The unconscious wishes to ensure that the patient's distress will be considered sympathetically: "The unconscious mind desires to be taken seriously and not be ridiculed. It will therefore strive to present symptoms that always seem, to the surrounding culture, legitimate evidence of organic disease. This striving introduces a historical dimension. As the culture changes its mind about what is legitimate disease and what is not, the pattern of psychosomatic illness changes."[35]

It seems that CFS patients occupied a contested liminal space from the very start, one that even today challenges the cultural and medical limits of that which is considered legitimate and illegitimate illness behavior. While many diagnoses located in the mind–body borderland fall from favor at some point and are subsequently replaced with different ones, no other diagnoses have been greeted with so much hostility and disbelief from the outset. Ironically, it is precisely the insistence on the organicity of their condition—originally, of course, a strategy to secure a sense of legitimacy and proper medical recognition—that has backfired spectacularly: in the age of the biomedical paradigm, only measurable biomedical evidence is considered legitimate proof of organic disease. Until that is discovered, it is unlikely that the CFS controversy will be resolved.

11

Burnout

While the regular motions of the heavenly bodies commanded the patterns of rest and activity in the premodern era via the seasons and the circadian rhythm, in the industrial age the pace, frequency, and duration of work were increasingly imposed from the outside, dictated by the demands for measurable productivity and the rigid temporality of machine-determined processes. Nineteenth- and twentieth-century factory workers had to submit to the rhythm of the machines they were servicing. The soul-destroying impact of assembly lines, first introduced in 1913 by Henry Ford, is famously represented by Charlie Chaplin in *Modern Times* (1936), in which his alter ego fails tragically in his desperate struggle to complete an endless succession of monotone, one-movement tasks presented relentlessly by a conveyor belt. It was precisely this loss of control over the speed and the rhythm of their work that many workers experienced as particularly stressful and exhausting.[1]

As the historian Anson Rabinbach has shown, modern modes of mass production and the emergence of Taylorist—that is, scientifically enhanced—work-optimization programs stimulated a physiological "science of fatigue" that blossomed in the late nineteenth and early twentieth centuries. Many owners of the means of production became increasingly concerned about their chronically exhausted workforce, or, more specifically, the potential losses of earnings resulting from its diminished productivity. Fatigue scientists such as the Italian physiologist Angelo Mosso (1846–1910), who wrote the study *Fatigue* in 1891, measured the impact of repetitive movements on muscles and the pulse under laboratory conditions. Other scientists also turned their attention to the conditions of physical labor in order to establish the optimal number of hours of the workday, as well as the ideal length of breaks, the most efficient tempo of work activities, and the impact of wage incentives. Time-motion experts assessed repetitive movements to identify the most efficient working behaviors. Many of these studies were conducted with a view to optimizing to its utmost capacity the productivity of the workforce, as well as to avoid industrial accidents and demands for compensation, which began to pose a serious problem for factory owners. It became apparent that accidents in the workplace were directly related to fatigue and that they were much more likely to occur toward the end of a workday, when laborers were exhausted.

Just as in the late nineteenth and early twentieth centuries, the present cultural preoccupation with stress and burnout—the two related concepts that are the focus of the final chapter of this study—is driven not just by a concern for the well-being of the post-Fordist twenty-first-century workforce but also by economic considerations, particularly the desire to maintain and optimize said workforce's continuing productivity and efficiency. The WHO estimates that loss of productivity resulting from sick leave related to mental diseases such as depression and stress-related disorders costs Western economies billions each year.[2] And just as nineteenth-century theorists of neurasthenia blamed the epidemic of nervous exhaustion they were witnessing on a faster pace of life, too many stimuli in the urban environment, and the specific stresses of "brain work," late-twentieth- and early-twenty-first-century discourses on stress and burnout are also frequently characterized by a culturally critical agenda that raises concerns about the psychosocial consequences of postindustrial capitalism, technological acceleration, the specific stresses of globalization and neoliberal market policies, the transition from a manufacturing to a service industry, and the subjectivization of work. Like other exhaustion theorists before them, many commentators on stress and burnout assert that the specific stressors with which we are currently battling are unparalleled regarding their energy-draining nature, intensity, and damaging long-term effects.

Stress and burnout are distinct but interrelated concepts. At the most basic level, burnout is often considered the result of chronic stress in the workplace, manifest in a set of specific mental and physical symptoms.[3] The most influential physiological and endocrinological stress model was developed by the Austrian-Hungarian-Canadian biochemical and medical researcher Hans Selye (1907–1982), and it is largely due to him that "stress" became as ubiquitous a concept as it is today. Indeed, as the historian Patrick Kury points out, shorthand and coping strategy at the same time, the word "stress" has become cultural code for a whole range of diffuse modern discontents and allows for the thematization of diverse ailments encompassing subjective as well as broader sociopolitical complaints.[4]

A researcher at McGill University in Montreal, Selye first theorized a physiological response mechanism to a sudden increase in demands on the organism under the label "general adaptation syndrome" (GAS) in the 1930s. After the war, he merged his own ideas on the mechanisms of adaptation with the stress concepts developed by the American physiologist Walter B. Cannon (1871–1945) and by military medical researchers who investigated the resilience of fighter pilots.[5] It was Cannon who first used the word "stress" in a medical context, and who associated stress with the concept of homeostasis—that is, the organism's perpetual attempts to self-regulate autonomic processes in order to maintain a state of inner equilibrium by counterbalancing all disturbances to body temperature, the fluid economy, the metabolic rate, and the respiratory system. Cannon argues that the body strives, above all, for constancy and seeks to reestablish a state of normalcy after either external or internal disturbances upset its fragile equilibrium—an argument that has, of course, already been presented, in slightly different form, by physicians working in the Galenic tradition, who also emphasize the significance of balance, harmony, and constancy among the four bodily fluids.[6] Previously, the word "stress" had been deployed in physics and the metal industry to describe the interaction between a force and resistance against this force. Derived from the Latin word *stringere* (to press together), the term was used to designate the act of stretching, straining, and putting material under pressure.

Differentiating between stressor (the agent that causes stress) and stress (the body's biochemical adaptive reaction), Selye defines stress as "*the non-specific response of the body to any demand made upon it.*" Confronted with an external threat, for example, the organism's natural reaction is fight or flight, actively to attack the aggressor or passively to submit to it or to flee. Yet regardless of whether the stress-producing factor or activity is pleasant or unpleasant, the body's reaction is always exactly the same. According to Selye, "all that counts is the intensity of the demand for readjustment or adaptation." Whether stressors are excessive cold or heat, danger, drugs, nervous irritation, sorrow, or joy, they all produce the same adaptive biochemical response. Therefore, Selye specifies the "nonspecific demand for activity as such" as the very essence of stress.[7]

He proposes that the organism's general response to all kinds of stressors is characterized by three stages: "(1) the alarm reaction; (2) the stage of resistance; and (3) the stage of exhaustion." During the alarm reaction, the organism releases adrenalin and other hormones and increases the blood flow and respiration, such that additional physical and mental energy is made available to enable the organism adequately to deal with the sudden intense challenge. During the phase of resistance, the body adapts to the stressor but is unable to uphold the heightened state of alert for a longer duration—hence, "eventually, exhaustion ensues."[8]

Crucially, the triphasic model suggests that the "body's adaptability, or *adaptation energy*, is finite." Recognizing the importance of this observation, Selye reflects on its repercussions in various studies. In *Stress Without Distress* (1974), for example, he admits that he, too (just like Sigmund Freud and many others before him), is unable further to define "adaptation energy" and resorts to the deployment of metaphors instead:

We still do not know precisely just what is lost, except that it is not merely caloric energy, since food intake is normal during the stage of resistance. Hence, one would think that once adaptation has occurred, and energy is amply available, resistance should go on indefinitely. But just as any inanimate machine gradually wears out, even if it has enough fuel, so does the human machine sooner or later become the victim of constant wear and tear. These three stages are analogous to the three stages of man's life: childhood (with its characteristic low resistance and excessive responses to any kind of stimulus), adulthood (during which adaptation to most commonly encountered agents has occurred and resistance is increased) and finally, senility (characterized by irreversible loss of adaptability and eventual exhaustion) ending with death.[9]

Interestingly, Selye uses two distinct metaphors here: the first is the popular nineteenth-century trope of the body as a machine, which suggests a mechanical view of the body as something that can wear out through continuous use. The second image, in which he draws an analogy to the stages of life, comparing the stage of exhaustion with old age and physiological senility, is equally based on the "wear-and-tear" principle, although one of a natural, organic nature.[10] Selye also uses financial similes to illustrate the finite nature of our adaptation energy that are strikingly similar to those deployed by the nineteenth-century physician George M. Beard, who invented the neurasthenia diagnosis:

Our reserves of adaptation energy could be compared to an inherited fortune from which we can make withdrawals; but there is no proof that we can also make additional deposits. We can squander our adaptability recklessly, "burning the candle at both ends," or we can learn to make this valuable resource last long, by using it wisely and sparingly, only for things that are worthwhile and cause least distress.[11]

Again, this simile suggests that appropriate stress management is ultimately the individual's responsibility: just as it is in our power to make financially prudent decisions, it is also our personal duty to manage our energy resources wisely. However, the amount of adaptation energy an individual has at his or her disposal varies and depends largely on hereditary and genetic factors.

Like Freud, Selye openly admits his frustration about the fact that he is unable further to define adaptation energy: "No doubt, inestimable advantages would accrue to the practice of medicine if we succeeded in identifying 'adaptation energy.'—So far we can report no progress along these lines."[12] Rest and vacations "can restore our resistance and adaptability very close to what it was before." Yet Selye cautions: "I said 'very close to,' because complete restoration is probably impossible, since every biological activity leaves some irreversible 'chemical scars.'"[13] These "chemical scars" are again mainly related to the natural loss of energy that occurs during the process of aging.

Selye also distinguishes between "superficial" and "deep" adaptation energy, once again deploying economic metaphors to illustrate his claims:

> Superficial adaptation energy is immediately available upon demand, like money in a bank account that is readily accessible by writing out a check. On the other hand, deep adaptation energy is stored away safely as a reserve, just as part of our inherited fortune may be invested in stocks and bonds, which must first be sold to replenish our checking account, thus furnishing another supply of immediately usable cash. Still, after a lifetime of constant expenditure, even our last investments will be eventually exhausted if we only spend and never earn. I look upon the irreversible process of aging as something very similar. The stage of exhaustion, after a temporary demand upon the body, is reversible, but the complete exhaustion of all stores of deep adaptation energy is not; as the reserves are depleted, senility and, finally, death ensue.[14]

Selye was able to draw on groundbreaking new insights in the fields of endocrinology: the British physiologist Ernest H. Starling discovered hormones in 1905, and much research has been conducted regarding the precise function of these chemical messengers since. Yet it is striking to observe that, in spite of the new medical concepts and information available to him, Selye developed theories about energy and exhaustion, and chose metaphors to describe them, that are almost identical to those proposed by nineteenth-century physicians. As the quotations demonstrate, the progression from the neurological to the endocrinological paradigm has not resulted in a radically new conception of the exhaustion of human energy. In fact, there seems to be a persistent tendency in modern Western medicine to think of the body as a vessel filled with a finite amount of energy that can be terminally exhausted. In Eastern medical models, in contrast, life energy (such as the *qi* and the *prana*) is conceived as something that can be temporarily blocked, but the free flow of which can be reestablished.

In *The Stress of Life* (1956), Selye admits that, paradoxically, the holy grail of stress research also remains its dark continent—the concept of energy. He speculates about the exciting new avenues for future research that would open up if only it were possible to extract and even transmit vital energy:

> By learning more about the body's adaptation energy, the life-span could probably be greatly improved. The diseases of old age become constantly more important as more and more people live to be old, thanks to medical progress. . . . Still, we have not fully excluded the possibility that adaptation energy could be regenerated to some extent, and perhaps even transmitted from one living being to another, somewhat like a serum. If its amount is unchangeable, we may learn more about how to conserve it. If it can be transmitted, we may explore means of extracting the carrier of this vital energy— for instance, from the tissues of young animals—and transmitting it to the old and aging.[15]

The fantasy about the extraction and transmission of vital energy from young animals in order to renew and prolong the natural life span of the aging is reminiscent of the habits of a much older figure, who has haunted the cultural and literary imagination for centuries: the vampire. It also demonstrates why vampire literature and films, which hook into the age-old human dream of eternal life, perpetual youth, and constantly renewable energy, hold such a long-lasting appeal over our culture at large.

Finally, Selye, too, is unable to resist the temptation of presenting his medical research on stress and the exhaustion of life energy without cultural commentary. In *Stress Without Distress* and other writings, he even presents a "code of conduct" based on "natural laws." Again, he sounds suspiciously like his nineteenth-century predecessors in his lament against the evils of his present times and his nostalgic longing for a past in which religion, the state, and social hierarchies were still respected:

> For the greatest problem of our time is not atmospheric pollution, nor overpopulation, nor even the atomic bomb, but the lack of motivation by generally acceptable and respected ideals. Science has shaken our blind faith in virtually every traditional value and "infallible authority." Our young are no longer willing to believe blindly in the sanctity of purity in soul or body, of the family structure and responsibilities, the fatherland, the security offered by capital, social status, or the loyal submission to the will of our prophets and rulers, whether the divine rulers of the east or our Western kings and presidents. The authority of the clergy, and indeed the existence of God, have been called into question. An attitude of pessimism and doubt seems to have settled upon mankind; violence, drug abuse, and aimless destructive aggression appear more and more to replace constructive behaviour as an outlet for our need of self-expression and creation. Virtually every code of law inspired by human logic or divine inspiration has been flaunted with contempt, and often impunity, at some time, by some people, except one: the code of the eternal laws of Nature. To develop and disseminate this code strikes me as the greatest contribution that research on the stress of life could make to humanity.[16]

✳ ✳ ✳

Stress research took a psychosocial turn in the 1960s and 1970s, the focus gradually shifting from biochemical-physiological adaptive mechanisms to the role of sociocultural, environmental, and psychological stressors and their draining effect on our energy resources. This phase also coincided with the wider popularization of the stress concept. Stress research of that period was often combined with a reformist ethos and went hand in hand with reflections on work–life balance, occupational health, quality of life, debates about the role of the state in ensuring the mental and physical well-being of its workforce, ecological anxieties, and a new conception of the relationship between the individual and the environment.[17]

Researchers Harold G. Wolff, Richard S. Lazarus, and the Swedish doctor of medicine Lennart Levi wrote extensively on the psychosocial conception of stress. Levi became Sweden's first professor of psychosocial medicine at the Karolinska Institute in Stockholm in 1978. In 1959, he had founded the Karolinska's Department of Stress Research, which in 1973 became the first World Health Organization center in this field. Although inspired by Selye's work, Levi was particularly interested in the role of the sociocultural environment as a stress-response trigger. His research concentrated on the subjective judgment of what constitutes a stressor. Levi argues that in many cases, stress reactions are purposeful and adequate. But in some cases, people react not just to the actual experience of physical danger but also to threats and symbols of danger experienced in the past, to maintain a certain degree of "preparedness." Moreover, this preparedness can also be elicited "by the many socio-economic pressures and emotional conflicts in to-day's life. In such cases of 'emotional stress,' the stereotyped reactions of the body often are clearly inadequate and may even be actually harmful." At least one-third of sick leave in Western culture, Levi estimates, is due to stress reactions of that kind, which creates "a situation characterized by a great deal of human suffering, not to mention the enormous losses in production and efficiency sustained by society in general."[18]

Levi problematizes repeatedly the perceived malignancy of "modern man's rapidly changing psychosocial environment."[19] He

counts mechanization and automation, the fragmentation of production processes, shift work, and low wages among the primary
new psychosocial energy-draining stressors:

> People are asking whether some work processes, although
> economically and technically justifiable at first sight, do not
> constitute an insult to man's intellectual capacity. Similarly, it is
> conceivable that a great deal of our urbanized, industrialized
> environment constitutes an insult—and a trauma—to man's
> neuroendocrine system, giving rise to mental and/or psycho-
> somatic disease. . . . Modern society functions on the principle
> that steady economic growth must be maintained *ad infini-
> tum*. We seldom ask what mental and physical price we pay for
> this economic evolution. Should not physicians combat such
> a one-sided ideology of *wealth* with an ideology of *welfare*?[20]

The state, Levi argues, has to ensure that all conditions of life are
optimal, not just economic ones, and politicians must find an
appropriate balance between fostering trade and gross national
product, on the one hand, and their citizens' psychological well-
being, on the other.

While Levi subscribes to the basic principles of Selye's endocrinological stress model, he puts a reformist political spin on it,
calling for the implementation of specific occupational health
policies, such as the avoidance of quantitative over- or understimulation. Much in harmony with the 1968 ethos and the general principles of the social-democratic Swedish welfare state, he
presents traditional Marxist arguments on the specific stressors of
the postwar period, such as the alienation of the workers from the
mass-produced end-product of their labor, owing to the breakdown of the production process into "narrow and highly speci-
fied sub-units." Automated production systems result not just in
the fragmentation of the work process but also in a decrease in
workers' control over it, all of which "usually results in monotony,
social isolation, lack of freedom, and time pressure, with possible long-term effects on health and well-being." The long-term
effects of such chronic occupational stress are a host of mental and

physical symptoms caused by the gradual depletion of the work-force's energy. Levi gloomily predicts: "With the striving toward maximum automation, man may again become the tool—of his own tools!"[21]

Unlike Beard and Selye, then, Levi shifts the burden of responsibility for stress-related exhaustion from the individual to the state. He cautions, above all, about an increasingly problematic gulf between humans' "psychobiological programme," which has remained essentially unchanged for the past ten thousand years, and environmental demands on this program, which have changed dramatically.[22] Epidemiological, psychophysiological, and psycho-endocrinological studies, he claims, have all proved that "man's phylogenetically old adaptation patterns, preparing the organism for fight and flight, have become inadequate, and even harmful, in response to the predominantly psychological or socioeconomic stressors prevalent in modern society."[23] Levi thus calls not for the optimization of an individual's adaptation responses to external stressors but for a reform of the increasingly malign and energy-draining occupational and wider political environment.

✳ ✳ ✳

The critical and popular burnout debates, particularly in Germany, the Netherlands, and some Scandinavian countries, have much in common with Levi's principal arguments on the adverse health effects of new, predominantly socioeconomic stressors, which are the result of a radical restructuring of the world of work associ-ated with the transition from an industrial to a service industry. In these discourses, however, Levi's classical 1960s Marxist vocab-ulary is replaced with new critical theory–inspired catchwords, which include, above all, acceleration, the subjectivization of work, the achievement principle, the dissolution of work–life boundar-ies, self-optimization, self-exploitation, self-realization, and flexi-bilization.[24] Two paradoxical scenarios are repeatedly flagged as the root causes of the twenty-first-century workforce's chronic exhaustion: first, we live in a techno-capitalist age dominated by technological inventions, in particular in the communication sector, which, theoretically speaking, should allow us to save great amounts of time and energy by rendering various processes faster, easier, and more efficient. However, these time-saving technologies have introduced a host of new psychosocial pressures and a more insidiously controlling temporal regime, which means that our time and rhythms are more externally regulated than ever. Technology and its associated new patterns of interaction thus drain more of our energy than they save.[25] Second, while many of the reformist demands of the 1960s and 1970s regarding flexible working hours, employee initiative, and more autonomy in the workplace appear to have been implemented, precisely that new flexibility and its associated responsibilities have turned into a curse in their own right: a terrible kind of freedom manifest in the permanent pressure to optimize the self and to monitor one's own performance, resulting in chronic feelings of inadequacy.[26] Moreover, workers are increasingly expected to commit to their jobs in a way that draws explicitly on their subjective resources and responses, such as their initiative, creativity, emotions, ability to empathize, and ability to be self-motivating.[27]

The term "burnout" emerged in the 1970s in the United States as a popular metaphor for mental exhaustion among social-sector workers. It was first used in a mental health context by the New York–based (and German-born) psychotherapist Herbert J. Freudenberger in an article entitled "Staff Burn-Out," in which he describes his own experiences with the phenomenon.[28] Burnout originally surfaced in the context of human services, or "helper," jobs (such as street workers, teachers, psychotherapists, hospital counselors, and probation officers)—professions that are often chosen by people who are driven primarily by idealistic rather than materialistic motives.[29] In the 1980s, self-report inventories appeared on the market, most importantly the Maslach Burnout Inventory (MBI), which allowed individuals to measure their personal susceptibility to the new syndrome. The description of burnout by the inventor of this inventory, the American social psychologist Christina Maslach, proved to become one of the standard definitions: "Burnout is a syndrome of emotional exhaustion, depersonalisation, and reduced personal accomplishment that can occur among individuals who do 'people work' of some kind."[30] "Depersonalisation" is evident, above all, in a cynical, callous, or indifferent attitude toward the people with whom one works, be they patients, students, clients, or customers.

Although burnout was originally thought to be specific to the human-services sector, it was soon diagnosed in other professions, too, and is now recognized as a serious occupational health problem in most sectors. Burnout was subsequently defined more broadly as "a state of exhaustion in which one is cynical about the value of one's occupation and doubtful of one's capacity to perform."[31] In the 1990s, Maslach and Michael Leiter offered yet another definition of burnout. Rather than defining it as a negative state of mind, they viewed it as the erosion of a positive state of mind, as the waning of engagement. In other words, burnout was reconceived as the decline of commitment, a state in which "energy turns into exhaustion, involvement turns into cynicism, and efficacy turns into ineffectiveness."[32]

An alternative behaviorist burnout theory drawing on positive psychology models also emerged in the late 1980s and early 1990s: the conservation of resources (COR) theory, first proposed by the American psychologist Stevan E. Hobfoll. COR theory focuses on work engagement and vigor "as the positive counterparts of burnout and away from the deficit and pathology models."[33] According to Hobfoll and Marjan J. Gorgievsky,

> COR theory is a motivational theory that rests . . . on the basic tenet that individuals strive to obtain, retain, foster, and protect resources. Resources are entities that have intrinsic or instrumental value, including objects (e.g. car, house, but also luxurious objects), conditions (parental roles, being embedded in supportive social networks), personal resources (personal characteristics and skills), and energy resources. There is something quite central and primitive biologically in the acquisition and maintenance of resources.[34]

Within the COR framework, stress can occur under three conditions: "(1) when individuals' key resources are threatened with loss, (2) when resources are lost, or (3) when individuals fail to gain resources following significant resource investment. Burnout is one such stress outcome and typically follows from a process of slow bleed out of resources without counterbalancing resource gain or replenishment." Energy is a key resource that can be lost either directly or as the side effect of the depletion of other important resources. Once again, the concept of energy is central to this model but not defined any further. COR theorists consider burnout as an affective state that is marked by feelings of emotional exhaustion, physical fatigue, and cognitive weariness, all of which "denote the depletion of energetic resources resulting from cumulative exposure to chronic work and life stresses."[35]

Gorgievsky and Hobfoll argue that "exhaustion is generally accepted as the major component of burnout, with less agreement about the other elements of burnout." They consider the process of "resource loss, gain, and protection as primary in explaining burnout and work engagement" and define burnout as "the end state of a long-term process of resource loss that gradually develops over time depleting energetic resources . . . , whereas engagement is the resultant of the inverted process of real or anticipated resource gain *enhancing* energetic resources." They also argue that the fear of resource loss is a stronger motivational force than expected resource gain, and that losses of any resources usually result in avoidance strategies as well as in loss of self-confidence. People have to invest resources in order to protect against resource loss, to recover from losses, and to gain resources. Yet many of the strategies they employ "to offset resource loss may lead to other, secondary losses. If the situation becomes chronic, the resources people employ may get depleted."[36] Like Cannon and Selye, they maintain that people (as well as systems) generally seek stability and homeostasis and that, while adaptable in theory, they tend to be upset by most forms of change. This hard-core, highly schematic, and reductive behaviorist model makes human beings sound like little more than greedy and anxious squirrels, preoccupied with nothing but collecting and safeguarding an array of different types of nuts.

The WHO's *ICD-10* classifies burnout as a "life management difficulty" problem. In Sweden and the Netherlands (two countries that benefit from highly developed social security systems), burnout is an established medical diagnosis. In most other countries, it is still mainly a nonmedically accepted but widely used term for a cluster of symptoms related to mental and physical exhaustion originating in the workplace. It tends to be viewed as carrying less stigma than depression, although it shares some of its symptoms. Unlike depression, burnout is thought to be caused strictly by external and, more specifically, work-related factors and is neither treated psychopharmacologically nor thought to have a genetic basis. Sebastian Beck, writing in the German newspaper *Die Süddeutsche*, describes burnout as "socially accepted luxury-version of depression and despair, which leaves one's self-image unharmed even during moments of failure," and asserts: "Only losers become depressive. Burnout is a diagnosis for winners, or, more specifically: for former winners."[37] But burnout can also be regarded as a social form of depression, a systemic dysfunction that is directly related to the work environment and one's role and position in it. The individual is thus not responsible for falling prey to the condition but can be considered a victim of its alienating work environment and broader psychophysically damaging sociocultural developments, which are beyond his or her control.

Occupational health psychologists, health policy advisers, insurance companies, and management coaches tend to emphasize that burnout not only is of concern to the individual but also presents a serious economic problem. Among burned-out staff, there is an increased risk of absenteeism, diminished productivity and efficiency, poor qualitative performance, and dissatisfied patients, students, clients, or customers. All these can have severe financial repercussions for organizations, companies, and even national economies. The potentially damaging financial consequences of burnout are one of the reasons it is currently attracting so much attention, and it is notable that an explicit preoccupation with "staff well-being," "work–life balance," "workload," "stress management," "engagement," "institutional values," "corporate identity," and even "mindfulness" is becoming ever more prevalent in companies and organizations across Europe and the United States. These concepts are all related to a wider cultural fear of burnout and its adverse

economical consequences, and, having trickled down into managerial manuals and workshops, are shaping managerial practice
and thus directly affect the everyday lives of employees.[38]

* * *

It is interesting to note that burnout is a highly topical issue in Germany, where it continues to attract much media attention, but is
much less prominently debated in England and the United States,
for example. Germany, in particular, has seen the publication of
numerous popular self-help manuals, autobiographies by burnout
victims, as well as academic studies, and important newspapers and
journals continue to represent the syndrome as a highly worrying
Volkskrankheit, a national epidemic of terrifying proportions.[39] It
is also noticeable that the German burnout discourse, especially
of the academic-sociological variety, tends to be politicized and
frequently combines psychomedical arguments with criticism of
the damaging psychosocial repercussions of neoliberalism, globalization, and acceleration. In contrast, burnout self-help books in
general, and English ones in particular, tend to follow a much less
socioculturally oriented trajectory, redirecting responsibility for
the management of energy resources to the individual and subscribing to a simple biochemical adrenal-exhaustion model.[40] In
The Essential Guide to Burnout: Overcoming Excess Stress, Andrew
and Elizabeth Procter, for example, write that if we live in a state
of ongoing arousal, our constantly raised cortisol levels "eventually
cause a depletion of the circulating steroids in the blood. These
steroids maintain our energy levels and our ability to resist stress.
When stress is constant and chronic, even the body's store of cortisol becomes empty. Then our energy and immunity reduce and
we become very susceptible to viruses and feel fatigued. If nothing
is done, this ultimately leads to complete exhaustion."[41]

Their suggestions for curing the condition are equally down-
to-earth: they propose that sufferers "take a breather," visit wildlife
centers, do something creative or cultural, and work on deepen-
ing their relationships. As did Beard, they also reassure burnout
victims that they are part of a select and, ultimately, elect few, as

people affected by burnout are traditionally "conscientious, hard-working, and highly motivated with drive and commitment," or else "people with high levels of compassion and concern for others, who have high ideals and are willing to sacrifice the self in order to help others."[42]

The metaphors that burnout victims use to describe their condition attest to the broader technical and medical discourses by which they are influenced: while melancholics complained about the adverse effects of black bile in their systems and referred to clouded vision and adustion, and neurasthenics bemoaned the state of their overstrained nerves, the burned-out use predominantly endocrinological imagery that relates to the idea of high levels of stress hormones being pumped around in their bloodstream that are doing long-term organic damage. Furthermore, they bemoan the lack of an "off-switch" and talk about "running out of steam" and "running on past empty." They feel "overloaded" and "unable to switch off" and to "unwind," or they report feeling dead inside like "zombies" or "robots."[43]

The Australian pastor Steve Bagi, author of *Pastorpain: My Journey in Burnout*, admits to being "tired of being tired" as well as to "struggles with the boss." He writes:

> Physical, mental and emotional exhaustion can creep up on anyone. Burnout goes beyond tiredness—it's one step up. Tiredness is the battery wearing out. Burnout is the battery that has worn out and gives no light. This is not the tiredness that will fade with a good night's sleep or a holiday. It's a deep fatigue in which I feel that the last of my reserves have been sapped out. I guess that it's natural to feel tired in a job where you are giving out all the time. If the transfer of energy is always in output then of course, the batteries will die. I know I should have attached myself to the Ultimate Recharger more and not revved the engine all the time.[44]

The empty-battery image is a popular evergreen in modern exhaustion discourses, already frequently used by nineteenth-century theorists, although the idea of rechargeable ones is more recent. Bagi, too, seems to subscribe to the idea of the human body as a kind of machine that can, quite simply, run out of fuel.

Donna Andronicus, self-help author and life coach, deploys another popular image of depleting and parasitical energy transfers: that of the psychological "energy vampire." She warns that these, "unlike traditional vampires with their distinctive fangs, anaemic complexion, bloodshot eyes and funky hair," can be hard to spot. "They come in various forms and can be very cunning in their ability to exist in your life without you even realizing that they're there, bleeding you of our precious energy reserve." They tend to be people with a victim mentality who indulge in self-sabotaging behavior:

> As your energy vampire recounts his or her latest drama, you start to feel listless, your brain begins to ache, and a creeping numbness paralyses you to the spot (much the way a spider will stun its intended victim before immobilizing and eating it). The energy extraction has begun with a schlucking sound that's inaudible to the human ear, and you feel powerless to stop it. . . . Before you know it, it's all over. Having gained their emotional pay-off sympathy, understanding and attention from you, and with their energy levels replenished, they leave you in a sluggish and bewildered state as you wonder what on earth hit you. All you can do is watch them skip off into the sunset as they seek out their next unsuspecting victim.[45]

Yet perhaps the most dominant mind–body metaphor of our times is that which conceives of the brain as a computer and the body as its hardware. The German professor of communication studies Miriam Meckel uses it repeatedly in her autobiographical account of her burnout-related breakdown. While recovering from chronic exhaustion in a sanatorium in the Allgäuer Alps, at which patients are subjected to treatments including a modern version of the rest cure, yoga, and hypnotherapy, she reflects on her life and on the causes that led to her burnout. What is most noticeable about her account is that Meckel, like many patients who embrace the burnout diagnosis rather than depression, remains curiously antipsychological in her analysis, in spite of the fact that it is presented as a confessionary, illness-as-opportunity-to-begin-anew narrative. Her story is strangely devoid of proper soul-searching (apart from a short reflection on the impact of her mother's death), and instead Meckel blames her breakdown on chronic communication overload and on wider structural changes in the world of work. In the increasingly regulated, measured, and preprogrammed "functional achievement-oriented society," she claims, people live to work, rather than work to live. A problem at work thus affects the person as a whole, not just his or her professional life. She calls this phenomenon "alienation 2.0" and presents arguments reminiscent of those of Alain Ehrenberg and of Luc Boltanski and Eve Chiapello: "We currently witness the most extreme forms of individualization and flexibilization of the subject as a result of technological developments and the multioption society, while at the same time experiencing a maximum amount of external control through all-encompassing and continuous demands and constraints. Our freedom is only an illusion."[46]

It appears to be a characteristic trait of the academic and even some of the popular burnout debates in Germany that the burden of responsibility is frequently shifted away from the individual toward more general sociopolitical developments and wider structural issues. The German sociologist Greta Wagner suggests that this tendency (which can also be observed in some Scandinavian countries) is related to the type of welfare state from which these discourses emerge. It is predominantly in the conservative and the social-democratic welfare states that citizens expect the state to play a more active, reformist, and interventionist role in protecting them not just from physical but also from psychosocial stressors (for example, by changing occupational health legislation).[47] Or, viewed differently, one could also consider this tendency as an attempt to undo the transfer of responsibility for one's own psychophysical welfare from the state to the individual, which theorists like Michel Foucault, for example, consider a core characteristic of the neoliberal project.

Putting a digital communication–age spin on the old strained-nerves tale, Meckel writes: "I suffer from too much information input. 'You are completely overstimulated,' my doctor told me. Stimuli are the impulses that render possible the transfer of information. . . . My brain's memory software and its processors are overloaded. Often I find myself wishing that I could use the option 'filter messages' or 'cancel conversation' for my thoughts, just as for a computer program." She further develops the analogy between the brain as computer, relationships as exchanges of information, and burnout as a functional disturbance that is essentially communication-based in nature, in various other passages:

> It is the messenger hormones serotonin, adrenalin, dopamine, and endorphins that are responsible for the transportation of information between nerve cells. They are the media of chemical communication in the human brain. In the case of burnout or in other forms of depression it is, then, the brain's communication mechanism that is disturbed. For me, that is a particularly exciting insight. I suffer from a disturbance of my key professional competency: communication. Mind and body know rather well how to raise the alarm such that their message is heard.[48]

Meckel complains about feeling isolated and unable to communicate with others, again using communication-age imagery by referring to incompatible "transmission protocols." Blaming her burnout on information overload and too much traveling, and particularly on the "energy-robber" e-mail, she admits to a significant flaw in her strategy to combat her growing exhaustion: by trying to counter the strain quantitatively, by working harder and longer and sleeping less, she found that she became slower, less productive, increasingly unable to concentrate, and emotionally more volatile. In addition, she found herself suffering from bouts of causeless sadness and loss of faith in her work. "I have become a victim of my existential categorical error. By trying to combat the negative consequences of quantitative over-strain via a quantitative performance increase, I was programmed to fail." In the final chapter of her book, she addresses her life directly in a letter and writes:

I have texted my life story, sent chapters of my life into the world as attachments, planned my days and years in Outlook, and surfed around in myself—all too rarely without strategy and aim. . . . Without pause, you blinked and hummed and jingled inside me. You wanted attention, true attention. . . . But I only ever touched your user interface, behind which you remained hidden. I know your sounds, your smells, your colors and forms, the warmth of your bustling activities, your small messages and streams of information. I understood your user interface, but not your operating system. I never asked what really drives you.[49]

What are the implications of perceiving the mind as a computer and the body as its hardware, as Meckel and many others do? Mind–body metaphors such as this one are not just ornamental figurative illustrations that can be translated into clear-cut factual language, or that point to a definitive "reality" of mind–body interactions hidden behind the layers of discourse. In the arena of mind–body debates, metaphors and their associated narratives are not just all we have, as the interaction between the two entities cannot yet properly be studied and measured empirically, but they are also reality-generating. Metaphors do not just influence the way in which patients might experience and make sense of their symptoms but, as the historian James J. Bono points out, even have the ability to influence the shape of future research. Bono cites the example of the seventeenth-century physician William Harvey, who in 1628 for the first time compared the heart to a machine. Harvey, Bono argues, ushered in a paradigm shift that transformed the religious, social, cultural, and psychological meanings associated with the heart, primarily by facilitating conceptual exchanges between different discourses (in this case, the technical and the medical), and thereby opening up highly fruitful avenues for new research.[50]

One of the many repercussions of the "brain is a computer" metaphor is no doubt the present popularity of cognitive behavioral therapy and other therapeutic schools of thought, such as neuro-linguistic programming (NLP), that are essentially based on the idea of "reprogramming" the mind, just as one would reprogram a dysfunctional information technology system. In Britain, for example, CBT is now the only psychotherapy regime offered through the National Health Service. Yet to think about ourselves with recourse to concepts such as information overload, input–output imbalances, program error, memory defects, and dysfunctional feedback loops not just reduces the complexity of interpersonal interactions to mere data exchanges but also stifles any potential for explorations and conceptualizations of deeper, more irrational or emotional human responses and reactions. In other words, these metaphors dehumanize us, turning us into little more than substandard and dysfunctional robots. It is time to turn to some literary works that engage with burnout-like states, as they engage precisely with the flawed, unique, and irrational human responses to work-induced exhaustion that are eliminated in the brain-as-computer-based accounts.

❖ ❖ ❖

As in many of Graham Greene's novels, a lapsed Catholic features as the main protagonist in *A Burnt-Out Case* (1960): in his late fifties and at the height of his fame, the celebrated ecclesiastical architect M. Querry loses faith in both his religion and the merit of his buildings. Although written in 1960 (that is, fourteen years before the burnout diagnosis was born), Greene's book describes some of the phenomenon's core symptoms. Querry feels as though he has come "to the end of everything," a mental state that he seeks to express physically and spatially by traveling to the remotest place he can find on the map—a leper colony in the Congo, chosen simply because the boat that took him down the khaki-colored African river would go no farther. Querry is exhausted and no longer able to feel anything at all, including pain; he has ceased to desire anything, including women; he is alienated, disconnected, and unable to empathize; and he is cynical and disenchanted about the value of his work. Having lived exclusively for his profession most of his life, he informs Dr. Colin, the atheist doctor who runs the leprosery and who becomes Querry's friend and confidant, that he has now abandoned it for good: "A vocation is an act of love: it is not a professional career. When desire is dead one cannot continue to make love. I've come to the end of desire and to the end of my vocation."[51]

Although showered with accolades and awards, Querry feels that the real significance of his architectural work has always remained unappreciated, and that it was even regularly ruined and destroyed: "And in a year they had cluttered [the churches] up with their cheap plaster saints; they took out my plain windows and put in stained glass dedicated to dead pork-packers who had contributed to diocesan funds, and when they had destroyed my space and my light, they were able to pray again, and they even became proud of what they had spoilt."[52]

As a cynical reaction to the vacuity of the praise he received for the buildings about which he genuinely cared, Querry built more frivolous, deliberately lackluster buildings in his later years—but even these were venerated by the critics, leaving him feeling empty and disgusted. The stakes for those who expect to derive some kind of existential justification and meaning from their work are, of course, particularly high, as Querry explains: "Men with vocations are different from the others. They have more to lose. Behind all of us in various ways lies a spoilt priest." And thus he felt increasingly ashamed and hypocritical about building churches:

> To build a church when you don't believe in a god seems a little indecent, doesn't it? When I discovered I was doing that, I accepted a commission for a city hall, but I didn't believe in politics either. You never saw such an absurd box of concrete and glass as I landed on the poor city square. You see I discovered what seemed only to be a loose threat in my jacket— I pulled it and all the jacket began to unwind.[53]

Formerly a compulsive womanizer, Querry also realizes that he never really loved anyone, and, following the death of his passion for his vocation, soon everything else dies in him, too. "I want nothing," he explains to the superior of the order with whom he lodges near the leprosery, silently adding: "That is my trouble."[54]

Greene establishes an explicit parallel between Querry, the emotional/spiritual cripple, and the lepers, the physical ones, who are being treated for their disease at the hospital by Dr. Colin. Both Querry and the lepers are mutilated outcasts who are defined, above all, by a lack: in the case of the former, the lacuna is god-shaped and of a spiritual nature, while in the case of the latter, what is missing is physical: limbs, fingers, and toes. In both cases, the respective disease needs to burn itself out so that it is no longer contagious before the sufferers can begin to heal. Yet the doctor freely admits that healing the mind is a more challenging task than healing the body, and it is he who explicitly refers to Querry as a "burnt-out case." In a conversation with the cynical and ruthless journalist Parkinson, who travels to the leprosery in search of a sensationalist story and sets in motion the process leading to Querry's demise, Querry explains:

> "You heard what the doctor called me just now—one of the burnt-out cases. They are the lepers who lose everything that can be eaten away before they are cured."
> "You are a whole man as far as one can see," said Parkinson, looking at the fingers resting on the drawing-board.
> "I've come to an end. This place, you might say, is the end. Neither the road nor the river go any further."[55]

Although technically it is the fathers who should be in charge of Querry's spiritual care, it is in fact the friendship with the outspoken atheist Dr. Colin that gradually reawakens his interest in the world and initiates his healing process. Dr. Colin, in contrast to Querry, is at peace with living without faith, content with his materialist worldview. Querry, however, feels the loss of faith acutely, like a phantom limb. Yet gradually, he begins to register the first stirrings of engagement, interest, and empathy. One night, he ventures into the jungle in search of his (aptly named) leper servant Deo Gratias, who has gone missing, and saves the young man's life—an experience that proves to be cathartic. Eventually he is able to work again, yet he has moved on from building conceptually extravagant cathedrals to designing cheap, functional, and much-needed hospitals. In spite of his refusal to be cast in this role, many people around him begin to consider him a kind of saint and role model. A young woman trapped in an unhappy marriage falls in love with him. Rumors spread, and things begin to go wrong.

Just when the doctor pronounces Querry cured, precisely at the moment when his spiritual disease has burned itself out and he starts feeling and caring for others and himself again, and even admits to being happy in his self-imposed exile, external disaster strikes. Enmeshed in a string of unfortunate circumstances, Querry is shot dead by a drunken and enraged husband, who believes that the burned-out man had an affair with his wife. Querry is buried in the local cemetery in the atheists' corner, his grave provocatively devoid of a Christian cross.

The phrase "burnt-out" in Graham Greene's novel, then, has two distinct meanings: on the one hand, it more or less corresponds to the state of mental exhaustion, spiritual disengagement, careless-ness for the future, and cynicism about the value of one's work that the theorists of clinical and occupational burnout were to define a few years later, although Greene's interest is, of course, primarily centered on questions pertaining to faith rather than the world of work. On the other hand, there is a positive, even optimistic dimension to Greene's deployment of the term: as in the case of the lepers, burnout can burn itself out if it is treated correctly by a professional carer. The disease of the mind, just as the diseases of the body, can run its course and ceases to be contagious and harm-ful once it has used up all its fuel, thus allowing its victims to get back to a state of normality—although, more often than not, not without leaving either physical or mental wounds that attest to the severity of the infection.

✳ ✳ ✳

The German novelist Thomas Mann's interest in neurasthenia, nervous exhaustion, and the link between illness and genius more generally has already been analyzed in numerous critical works, in particular in relation to his novel *Buddenbrooks* (1901).[56] However,

Mann's engagement with exhaustion and what could be described as a case of burnout *avant la lettre* in his novella *Death in Venice* (1912) is even more interesting. Although Mann draws primarily on nerve imagery and was clearly inspired by contemporary debates of neurasthenia, one of the main themes of the novella is a burnout-like form of exhaustion, since it is caused, above all, by a specific attitude toward work and pleasure that is damaging to the individual. Mann describes the malign effects of a Protestant work ethic built on repression, which sociologists would now describe as "self-exploitation." Furthermore, the novella illustrates some intriguing parallels between neurasthenia and burnout: although the organic explanations of the diagnoses differ, the former embracing neurological and the latter endocrinological models, both syndromes include a set of comparable symptoms and emphasize, above all, the exhausting effects of too much "brain work" as a core trigger.

Much like Querry in Greene's text, Gustav von Aschenbach, the middle-aged writer who is the main character in *Death in Venice*, is introduced at the beginning of the novella as a burned-out case. The very first adjective that Mann deploys to characterize him is "overstimulated" (*überreizt*), and images of overstretching delicate organisms and overwrought nervous economies permeate the entire novella.[57] In the first paragraph, we learn that Aschenbach's energies are on the wane, that he has overstrained his fragile nervous system with his demanding "brain work," and that he is now unable to find respite on account of his ceaselessly pulsating "productive mechanism in his mind," his *innere Triebwerk*—a term that does, of course, evoke two distinct meanings, one mechanico-physical and the other alluding to the Freudian conception of the precarious psychological economies of repressed drives and desires.[58] Aschenbach's personal ailments are further intensified by the grave threat that seemed to "hang over the peace of Europe" in the first sentence, which indicates an ominous political menace that both aggravates and externalizes the inner turmoil of the writer:

> The morning's writing had overstimulated him: his work had now reached a difficult and dangerous point which demanded

the utmost care and circumspection, the most insistent and precise effort of will, and the productive mechanism in his mind—that *motus animi continuum* which according to Cicero is the essence of eloquence—had so pursued its reverberating rhythm that he had been unable to halt it even after lunch, and he had been unable to find relief through his daily nap which was now so necessary for him as his energies were increasingly wearing out. And so, soon after taking tea, he had left the house hoping that fresh air and movement would restore him and enable him to spend a productive evening.[59]

Aschenbach is haunted by a roving restlessness, unable to relax, and we learn that he originally understands his sudden desire to travel abroad as nothing but a burdensome "necessary health precaution, to be taken from time to time however disinclined to it one might be," a necessary measure to replenish his depleted bodily and spiritual energy reservoirs.[60] Mann makes it obvious that these ideas reflect Aschenbach's limited perspective on the matter and subtly suggests an alternative interpretation of his character's desire to travel. Through the abundance of death imagery early in the novella, as well as through Aschenbach's telling name (it translates as "river of ashes"), Mann indicates that his actions may be driven by a powerful yet unconscious death wish, a desire not to replenish his energies but in fact to exhaust them once and for all in order to find eternal, not just temporary, respite from the vicissitudes of life.

Aschenbach's sense of identity rests, above all, on his achievement, his iron discipline, and his self-denial—his favorite word is "tenacity" (*durchhalten*). We learn that he is plagued by an ominously "growing weariness," which he fears and conceals from others:

True, [serving his work] was a duty he loved, and by now he had almost even learned to love the enervating daily struggle between his proud, tenacious, tried and tested will and that growing weariness which no one must be allowed to suspect nor his finished work betray by any tell-tale sign of failure or lassitude. Nevertheless, it would be sensible, he decided, not to span the bow too far and willfully stifle a desire that had erupted in him with such vivid force.[61]

As a tribute to his lifelong service to *Geist*, "he had curbed and cooled his feelings; for he knew that feeling is apt to be content with high-spirited approximations and with work that falls short of supreme excellence."[62] However, his twin strategy of repression and intellectualization, which has served Aschenbach well until his fiftieth year, finally demands its levy and results in a mental and physical state of being that is reminiscent of contemporary descriptions of burnout. Not only does he suffer from a deep and chronic form of exhaustion, but he loses his ability to work, becomes disengaged, and even grows cynical about the merit of his works.

Aschenbach's uncompromising subscription to the achievement principle and the sacrifice of feelings, pleasure, and leisure for his profession is not just a recent development; it has defined him all his life. We learn that he has always done violence to his natural inclinations and physical constitution and has lived a life that he was not built to endure, which he could maintain only by a "heroic" act of discipline and repression. Famously, an observer tells us that he lived his life with his fist firmly closed:

Ever since his boyhood the duty to achieve—and to achieve exceptional things—had been imposed on him from all sides, and thus he had never known youth's idleness, its carefree negligent ways. When in his thirty-fifth year he fell ill in Vienna, a subtle observer remarked of him on a social occasion: "You see, Aschenbach has always only lived like *this*"— and the speaker closed the fingers of his left hand tightly into a fist—and never like *this*"—and he let his open hand hang comfortably down along the back of the chair. It was a correct observation; and the morally courageous aspect of the matter was that Aschenbach's native constitution was by no means robust, that the constant harnessing of his energies was something to which he had been called, but not really born.

The description of his self-discipline as a brave, honorable act shows that Aschenbach considers his work ethic and his sacrifices to be markers of moral superiority, even spiritual supremacy. It is significant in this context that he likens himself to Saint Sebastian. He thinks of the image of Saint Sebastian, "who clenches his teeth in proud shame and stands calmly on as the swords and spears pass through his body," as an apt emblem of the writer. His reflection on the saint culminates in a hymn to humans' perpetual battle with weakness and exhaustion, and he wonders "if there is any other heroism at all but the heroism of weakness? In any case, what other heroism could be more in keeping with the times?"[63]

The following passages explain Aschenbach's success as a writer and reveal why his literary works strike a chord with the experiences of so many of his contemporaries:

> The public does not know why it grants the accolade of fame to a work of art. . . . [T]he real reason for their applause is something imponderable, a sense of sympathy. Hidden away among Aschenbach's writings was a passage directly asserting that nearly all the great things that exist owe their existence to a defiant despite; it is despite grief and anguish, despite poverty, loneliness, bodily weakness, vice and passion and a thousand inhibitions, that they have come into being at all. But this was more than an observation, it was an experience, it was positively the formula of his life and his fame, the key to his work.[64]

This passage, rendered like the rest of the novella in free indirect discourse punctuated by interventions that systematically blur the boundaries between Aschenbach's and the narrator's perspectives, can be read as a meta-comment that sums up insights that Aschenbach has not yet fully grasped and that offers a poetological key to the appeal of Mann's novella as a whole: the reason that readers appreciate Aschenbach's writings is that they not only can identify with but also sympathize with the experiences he describes. Significantly, the main experience shared by Aschenbach and his readers is not related to sexually deviant desires (another theme of the text) but is manifest in the perpetual battle to overcome weakness (both spiritual and physical in nature). In other words, he articulates a kind of burnout pride, the idea that his perpetual struggle with physical and emotional work-induced exhaustion renders him somehow morally superiority. Just like Beard and many contemporary theorists of burnout, he elevates work-related exhaustion and our battles with it to something heroic, even sublime—a praiseworthy act of willpower, the victory of mind over matter, the spirit over the flesh:

> Gustav Aschenbach was the writer who spoke for all those who work on the brink of exhaustion, who labour and are heavy-laden, who are worn out already but still stand upright, all those moralists of achievement who are slight of stature and scanty of resources, but who yet, by some ecstasy of the will and by wise husbandry, manage at least for a time to force their work into a semblance of greatness. There are many such, they are the heroes of our age. And they all recognized themselves in his work, they found that it confirmed them and raised them on high and celebrated them; they were grateful for this, and they spread his name far and wide.[65]

It is those who fight on at the brink of exhaustion, who, in spite of everything, manage to keep going owing to the triarchy of discipline, willpower, and wise management of their limited energy capital—it is they, the men and women out of gas, who are the true "heroes of our age."

And yet—and this is where Mann's famous irony strikes—the overall structure and final development of the novella does, of course, radically undermine Aschenbach's philosophy, his hymn to the Protestant work ethic, tenacity, and repression. In fact, it is precisely his attitude toward work that is the cause of Aschenbach's undoing—the repressed returns with a cruel vengeance to undo his sustained efforts at *durchhalten* with a single erotic blow. Mann's novella can therefore be read as a *Zeitkritik*, and one that still strikes a powerful chord with present anxieties about work–life balance, a warning against the veneration of the "moralists of achievement" and the kind of radically repressive work ethic with which Aschenbach identifies so strongly, and that also seems to resonate so powerfully with his contemporaries. The over-valuation of achievement and productivity, and his disregard for the demands of his body, lead not only to exhaustion but to *Lebensmüdigkeit*. Aschenbach's perceived heroic and morally superior self-discipline is harshly ridiculed in the end, when we see him reclining in a deck chair at the beach, succumbing unashamedly to his voyeuristic obsession, dressed up in too youthful clothes, his uncanny makeup and hair dye dripping down his sagging cheeks.

Mann appears to embrace the materialist idea of the dangers of depleting one's limited energy resources, while also acknowledging more complex psychoanalytical ideas about the dangers of repression (and, of course, also the dangers of unrepressing, as all hell breaks loose when Aschenbach relaxes his fist). Yet he radically critiques the simplistic narrative that posits the cultural, social, and individual supremacy of the moralist of achievement, the idea that there is something honorable in burning out and working oneself, quite literally, to death.

Aschenbach's exhaustion, just like burnout, functions as a bridge between individual suffering and wider sociocultural developments. Mann, too, deploys exhaustion as a tool for diagnosing deeper cultural ailments. Anticipating Sigmund Freud's argument in *Civilization and Its Discontents*, he suggests that the price we pay not only for sublimating but also for exhausting our energies in the name of work, and also art, culture, and civilization, may be not only too high but ultimately not sustainable in the long run. Aschenbach's tale is, above all, a cautionary one with which many burned-out cases may well be able to identify: by staking every-thing on work, and by subscribing to cultural assumptions that ultimately celebrate self-exploitation and work-induced exhaustion even while they appear to be warning against their adverse effects, we risk not just the waning of our engagement and our productivity but in fact our very desire to live.

Epilogue

THE FUTURE

As we have seen, the history of exhaustion reveals that concerns about its effects on the mind and the body of the individual, as well as on the wider social community, are by no means a modern phenomenon. The mental, physical, and spiritual symptoms of states of exhaustion have been theorized since classical antiquity and appear, under different names and labels, as common denominators in an ever-shifting historical regime of exhaustion-related syndromes. They include the physical symptoms of fatigue, weakness, and lethargy; the mental symptoms of weariness, disillusionment, hopelessness, lack of engagement, cognitive impairment, and irritability; and behaviors such as restlessness and the avoidance of activity, effort, and challenges. The ways in which the etiology of states of exhaustion is understood in different historical epochs not only illustrate the impact of changing medical and psychological paradigms—from humoral to nerve- and reflex-centered, from biological to psychoanalytical, from endocrinological to immunological, and from hereditary-genetic to psychosocial—but also illuminate prevalent assumptions about conceptions of subjectivity, responsibility, willpower, and the role of human agency in managing and maintaining both our physical and our mental health.

Moreover, since the symptoms of chronic states of exhaustion are predominantly subjective experiences and almost impossible to measure empirically, and especially given that there is as yet no scientifically accepted Western model of human energy, the narratives constructed around exhaustion are to a large extent dependent on metaphors. Theorists describing the interaction of mind, body, and society can very rarely provide evidence in the form of empirically quantifiable data. And even if such data is available— for example, as MRI scans or measurements of specific hormone levels in the brain—the ways in which the data is interpreted tend to be driven by specific assumptions and agendas, as is evident in the powerful influence of the pharmacological industry on the development and marketing of biochemical cures for depression.

Yet the metaphors deployed in exhaustion theories are not just particularly telling with regard to wider medical and ideological assumptions; they are also reality-generating. Metaphors not only are all we have in this field of inquiry (in that we cannot simply translate them into a set of "hard" facts with a definitive basis in material reality) but also shape the ways in which sufferers perceive, interpret, and narrativize their symptoms. Illness beliefs and mental visualizations of inner processes shape our experiences. The exhausted who believe that their weariness is caused by a surplus of black bile and black fumes clouding their judgment will experience their symptoms in a way that differs from those who believe that it is the result of a sinful attitude toward the divine good, or the movement of the planets, or loss and intrapsychological battles, or permanent cognitive overstimulation resulting from new technologies and a faster pace of life, or immunological dysfunction, or a deficit in serotonin levels, or the inhuman demands of a radically restructured world of work governed by the dictates of growth, competitiveness, and relentless acceleration.

Moreover, similes that compare the body to a tepid bowl of milk on which flies settle, a worn-out machine, an empty battery, an overdrawn account, a country with weak defenses invaded by hostile enemy forces, a plant slowly being sucked dry by a suffocating parasite, or an overloaded computer program also shape the cures that are administered by medical and other practitioners. These range from increasing to decreasing cognitive stimulation; from occupational therapy to absolute rest; from electro-, to hydro-, to hypnotherapy; from various dietary regimes to orphic dancing; from psychopharmacological drugs to mindfulness exercises; and from the talking cure to campaigning for legislative changes to protect the twenty-first-century workforce from physical and mental exploitation. The metaphors with which states of exhaustion are described thus have very real experiential and social consequences.

All exhaustion theories address either implicitly or explicitly questions of responsibility, agency, and willpower. In some accounts (most notably theological ones centered on the notion of sin but also more recent neoliberal ones that attempt to redirect responsibility for the management of the subject's physical and mental well-being to the individual), exhaustion is represented primarily as a form of weakness and lack of willpower, and even as a grave spiritual or characterological failing manifest in a bad mental attitude. Some theorists firmly believe in the organic causes of exhaustion, such as a surplus of black bile that wreaks havoc with the bodily humoral economy, a lack of nerve power, the chronic overstrain of the cognitive system by too many external stimuli, the weakening of the immune system by viral infections, or various forms of biochemical imbalance. Within this category, the exhausted individual may be seen either as an innocent victim afflicted by parasitical external agents or as at least partly responsible for the state of exhaustion by having engaged in energy-depleting behaviors, such as working too hard, eating the wrong food, worrying too much, not getting enough rest and sleep, or overindulging in sexual activities.

Other exhaustion theorists allow for the possibility that character traits, individual mental states and attitudes, as well as wider cultural psychosocial pressures can trigger bodily responses: they assume that qualities such as optimism, engagement, contentedness, and resilience, and also insights into our psychological patterns and desires, translate directly into the amount of energy that we have at our disposal. Whether exhaustion is theorized as pertaining to the will, the mind, the body, or wider social developments shapes the ways in which the exhausted are perceived and, as a consequence, treated. The exhausted may be perceived as innocent victims deserving care and support or dismissed as shirkers and slackers; they may be categorized as mentally or physically ill; or they may be considered casualties of wider socio-political developments and technological transformations.

While it is possible to detect historically specific theorizations of the agents that cause exhaustion, and a tendency to look back nostalgically to other historic periods and to relate the depletion of human energies to specific technological and sociocultural changes, it is also possible to diagnose the recurrent production of theories about the loss of energy as expressions of timeless anxieties that concern the natural process of aging, the dangers of the waning of engagement, and death. These anxieties are increasingly commercially exploited not only by the cosmetics industry promising cures that halt and even reverse the physical signs of aging but also by the rapidly growing wellness industry and the manufacturers of the ever-expanding array of energy drinks, energy supplements, stimulants, neuro-enhancers, and mood-lifters.

Whether our own age really is the most exhausted is impossible either to prove or to disprove. It is, however, highly unlikely. Even the quantifiable proliferation of discourses on exhaustion, or the rapid increase in the number of people who are being diagnosed with exhaustion-related syndromes, is not necessarily an indicator that our own subjective experiences of exhaustion are more numerous or more intense than those in earlier periods. It might simply be more acceptable now to articulate and to seek remedies for one's feelings of stress, weariness, and hopelessness. It is impossible to measure and compare the exact amount of energy spent and effort experienced by an office worker in the twenty-first century with that of a factory worker in the nineteenth century, a farmer plowing his fields in the early modern period, or a mother of ten starving children in the Middle Ages. Moreover, the discourses on the chronic forms of exhaustion that cannot be explained in terms of illness or extreme physical exertion that have been the subject of this study tend to focus on the experiences of predominantly middle- and upper-class "brain workers," with a concentration not so much on the effects of external threats—such as viral infections, wars, hunger, violence, or hard physical labor—but on psychosocial stressors.

A frequently repeated argument of the exhaustion theorists, especially in the modern period, is that the technologies that have made our lives physically easier, that have accelerated travel and communication, and that should help us save both time and energy come with their own set of new psychophysical pressures, shaping both our public and our private lives in new, insidious ways, thereby undoing their beneficial effects. It is, of course, important not just to accept technological progress and economic growth as values in themselves, and to keep asking critical questions about the wider cultural and psychological effects of social and technological change. Exhaustion theories have traditionally functioned as vehicles for precisely such forms of cultural critique. At the same time, it is also worth remembering that, as Frank Kermode put it:

> We think of our own crisis as pre-eminent, more worrying, more interesting than other crises. . . . It is commonplace to talk about our historical situation as uniquely terrible and in a way privileged, a cardinal point in time. But can it really be so? It seems doubtful that our crisis . . . is one of the important differences between us and our predecessors. Many of them felt as we do. If the evidence looks good to us, so it did to them.[1]

Kermode neatly sums up a strategy that most cultural commentators tend to deploy, which entails a nostalgic glorification of the past paired with an ahistorical exaggeration of the perceived evils of one's own time. It is the case, however, that our own age is characterized by a new worry—one that did not concern our ancestors. This worry relates to the exhaustion of our planetary raw materials caused by the rapidly increasing energy needs of a fast-growing world population and our careless habits of consumption. In the nineteenth century and especially in the final decades of the twentieth and the first part of the twenty-first centuries, fears about exhaustion, sustainability, and the depletion of limited energy reserves have become truly apocalyptic in that they have been lifted to the planetary level and beyond; that is, they are no longer limited just to the mind, body, or society but have been extended to incorporate our environment—the ground beneath our feet and sky above our heads.

The English cleric Thomas Robert Malthus (1766–1834) articulated concerns about potential discrepancies between food supplies and the rising nutritional demands of a growing population at the end of the eighteenth century. The nineteenth century, moreover, saw the emergence of the second law of thermodynamics and associated apocalyptic anxieties about a "great cosmological exhaustion" brought about by irreversible energy loss, entropy, and the heat death of the universe.[2] The German physician and physicist Hermann von Helmholtz (1821–1894), for example, assumed that all energy would gradually dissipate, that all natural processes would eventually cease, and that the universe would thus soon be condemned "to a state of eternal rest."[3]

Concerns about the effects of climate change, human-made environmental disasters, and rapidly depleting planetary resources such as fossil fuels, freshwater, and rain forests have been articulated and taken increasingly seriously since the 1970s and 1980s. These fears have been backed up with ever more solid scientific research, and the findings of research into climate change have become much more alarming and urgent in recent years. A study published in February 2015 by the Stockholm Resilience Centre, for example, suggests that our current globalized form of neoliberal capitalism—a system based on consumption and the relentless extraction and depletion of natural resources—has already brought about irreversible changes to Earth's biosphere, having thrown it into a state of imbalance.[4] The researchers found that together with rapid population growth and the vastly increased needs for energy and freshwater that follow from it, it is primarily growth-oriented, consumption-based neoliberal capitalism rolled out on a global scale that is responsible for unprecedentedly accelerated changes in Earth's systems over the past sixty years. These include, above all, climate change and stratospheric ozone depletion as a result of unremittingly high carbon emissions.

Temperatures have already risen by 1.5°F (0.8°C) in the past few decades and, if carbon emissions are not curbed with immediate effect, will continue to rise rapidly.[5] Predictions vary, but a temperature rise of 7.2°F (4°C) by the end of the twenty-first century (a calculation that many scientists see as a realistic estimate) will have various dramatic knock-on consequences, including the melting of the ice sheets and glaciers, rising sea levels, and the disappearance not only of low-lying island states but also of numerous major coastal cities. The extinction of species, the loss of biodiversity, and the acidification of the oceans will accelerate dramatically; many crops will no longer grow; and heat waves and tornados will wreak havoc across the globe, putting the very survival of our species at risk. Even the World Bank (neither left-leaning in its politics nor generally particularly concerned with ecological matters) warned in one of its recent reports that we are "on track for a 4°C warmer world [by the end of the century] marked by extreme heat waves, declining global food stocks, loss of ecosystems and biodiversity, and life-threatening sea level rise," cautioning that "there is also no certainty that adaptation to a 4°C world is possible."[6] Kevin Anderson, professor of energy and climate change and deputy director of the Tyndall Centre for Climate Change Research, warns in equally unambiguous terms: "It is fair to say that among climate change researchers there is a widespread view that a 4°C future is incompatible with any reasonable characterisation of an organised, equitable and civilised global community. 4°C is also beyond what many people think we can adapt to."[7]

Will Steffen, director of the Australian National University's Climate Change Institute, who led the "Planetary Boundaries" study conducted by the Stockholm Resilience Centre, has found that of nine vital processes that underpin life on Earth, four have now officially exceeded "safe" levels: human-driven climate change, loss of biosphere integrity, land-system change such as deforestation, and the high level of phosphorus and nitrogen flowing into our oceans as a result of excessive fertilizer use:

> The climate system is a manifestation of the amount, distribution, and net balance of energy at Earth's surface; the biosphere regulates material and energy flows in the Earth system and increases its resilience to abrupt and gradual change. Anthropogenic perturbation levels of four of the

Earth system processes/features (climate change, biosphere integrity, biogeochemical flows, and landsystem change) exceed the proposed Planetary Boundaries.[8]

The effects of human activities on the major Earth systems, he argues, have grown so dramatically since the mid-twentieth century that they threaten the stability of the 11,700-year-long Holocene epoch, ushering in what in effect amounts to a new, "Anthropocene" geological epoch.[9] Human-driven changes such as the pumping of carbon dioxide, other greenhouse gases, aerosols, and fertilizers both into the atmosphere and into the oceans have dramatically destabilized the energy balance of the planetary biosphere. In an interview with the *Guardian*, Steffen states:

> When economic systems went into overdrive, there was a massive increase in resource use and pollution. It used to be confined to local and regional areas but we're now seeing this occurring on a global scale. . . . It's clear the economic system is driving us towards an unsustainable future and people of my daughter's generation will find it increasingly hard to survive. History has shown that civilisations have risen, stuck to their core values and then collapsed because they didn't change. That's where we are today.[10]

In *This Changes Everything: Capitalism vs. the Climate*, the Canadian writer Naomi Klein argues that "climate change has become an existential crisis for the human species," urging that climate change must be treated as a true planetary emergency, akin to September 11, the banking crisis, humanitarian catastrophes, and acute flooding.[11] Numerous scientists agree that if the planet's remaining reserves of coal, gas, and oil really were to be extracted and depleted, contributing to the rapidly accelerated rate of planetary energy consumption that we have seen since the 1950s, which has already done irreversible damage to Earth's biosphere, the exhaustion of these reserves might well lead to the extinction of the human species.

In June 2015, climate change scientists received support from an unlikely ally. In his encyclical aptly titled "On Care for Our

Common Home," Pope Francis I takes a candid and fierce stance against unfettered consumerism and climate change. While, unsurprisingly, not particularly worried about population growth, he deems the depletion and pollution of our planetary resources the greatest challenges facing humanity over the coming decades. Moreover, Francis argues that the exhaustion of raw materials is based on the immoral exploitation of the poorer nations, which suffer the consequences of climate change much more acutely than the richer nations, whose greedy consumerism drives this process.[12] The rich nations therefore owe an "ecological debt" to the poorer ones.

He reminds us that humankind has been granted dominion over Earth in order to "till it and keep it"—not to exploit and destroy it.[13] To till it means to make it fruitful, to enhance its power to yield nourishment, while to keep it entails caring for and protecting it—the stark opposite of exhausting it. According to Francis, the suicidal destruction of our common home thus qualifies as a sin on four counts: against the poor, against ourselves, against future generations, and against God's creation. Harrowed by greed, over-consumption, exploitation, and wastefulness, Earth now "groans in travail";[14] Earth and the poor cry together.

In his 180-page essay, Pope Francis touches on many of the topics discussed in the preceding chapters, but, in stark contrast to his spiritually and physically exhausted predecessor Benedict XVI, he presents concrete solutions to the problems he raises and appears hopeful that a better future is possible. He not only castigates the depletion and pollution of Earth's raw materials, the loss of biodiversity, and the ways in which they are linked to global inequality and poverty but also addresses the underlying social, spiritual, and psychological factors that are responsible for these sinful activities in the first place. Like George M. Beard and other nineteenth-century theorists of neurasthenia, as well as contemporary burnout specialists, he bemoans the rapid acceleration of historical change and the general "rapidification" of life's pace. He also criticizes the belief in technological and scientific progress as ends in themselves and complains about the information overload caused by social media and other communication technologies, which generate "a sort of mental pollution," melancholic dissatisfaction, and social isolation.

The insidious "globalization of the technocratic paradigm," he asserts, is spiritually empty; markets and a desire for economic growth should not be allowed to dictate politics in the exclusive way they currently do, as they encourage "rampant individualism," "compulsive consumerism," our "throwaway society," and a "self-centred culture of instant gratification." He urges us to embrace a "new lifestyle" to overcome this collective and sinful selfishness. All of us should gradually phase out the use of fossil fuels and embrace the principle of the common good, to ensure justice for future generations and the poorer nations; limit the consumption of nonrenewable energy and assist poorer countries to support programs of sustainable development; embrace a new attitude of humility and gratitude; and tackle unethical consumerism by boycotting tainted products and by shopping more ethically, and thus reshape the out-of-control markets. Finally, he also urges his flock to remember to honor the Sabbath, the law of weekly rest that exists to counter physical and spiritual exhaustion—to celebrate a contemplative and communal form of rest that is designed to sensitize and respiritualize us, and to urge us regularly to reflect on the purpose of our existence.

✳ ✳ ✳

While, as we have seen, it is far from being the case that our own age is the only one to have been preoccupied with exhaustion, concerns about exhaustion at a planetary and cosmic scale first emerged in the nineteenth century and have grown ever more intense and urgent in the past few decades. The rhetoric of our age is unique in that anxieties about exhaustion, sustainability, and resilience no longer concern only the mind, body, or society but our very habitat. Might this particularly apocalyptic exhaustion discourse, then, for the first time in human history really correspond to an empirically measurable reality? There is certainly a growing body of evidence to suggest that the threat to our planetary resources and the consequent exhaustion of our very biosphere are very real indeed.

NOTES

INTRODUCTION

1. Quoted in Dagmar Heuberger, "Das ist das historische Vorbild für den Rücktritt des Papsts," *Aargauer Zeitung*, February 12, 2013, http://www.aargauerzeitung .ch/international/das-ist-das-historische-vorbild-fuer-den-ruecktritt-des-papstes -126050271 (accessed February 17, 2015) (my translation).

2. See, for example, Nick Squires, "Pope's Final Address: God Was Asleep on My Watch," *Telegraph*, February 27, 2013, http://www.telegraph.co.uk/news/worldnews /the-pope/9896792/Popes-final-address-God-was-asleep-on-my-watch.html (accessed June 15, 2015).

3. See, for example, Naomi Klein, *This Changes Everything: Capitalism vs. the Climate* (New York: Simon & Schuster, 2014).

4. See, for example, Will Steffen et al., "Planetary Boundaries: Guiding Human Development on a Changing Planet," *Science*, February 13, 2015, http://dx.doi .org/10.1126/science.1259855 (accessed March 7, 2015).

5. See, for example, Stephen Emmott, *Ten Billion* (London: Penguin, 2013); and Danny Dorling, *Population 10 Billion* (London: Constable, 2013).

6. World Health Organization, "Depression," fact sheet, no. 369, October 2012, http://www.who.int/mediacentre/factsheets/fs369/en/ (accessed January 13, 2015).

7. Centers for Disease Control and Prevention (CDC), "Chronic Fatigue Syndrome (CFS)," February 14, 2013, http://www.cdc.gov/cfs/causes/risk-groups.html (accessed January 13, 2015).

8. See, for example, Sighard Neckel and Greta Wagner, eds., *Leistung und Erschöpfung. Burnout in der Wettbewerbsgesellschaft* (Frankfurt am Main: Suhrkamp, 2013); and Wilhelm Schaufeli, Michael P. Leiter, and Christina Maslach, "Burnout: 35 Years of Research and Practice," *Career Development International* 14, no. 3 (2009): 206.

9. See, for example, Slavoj Žižek, *Living in the End Times* (London: Verso, 2011).

10. For a discussion of the different symptoms and definitions of a range of fatigue syndromes, see Johanna Dörr and Ulf Nater, "Erschöpfungssyndrome—Eine Diskussion verschiedener Begriffe, Definitionsansätze und klassifikatorischer Konzepte," *Psychotherapie, Psychosomatic, medizinische Psychologie* 63, no. 2 (2013): 69–76.

11. See, for example, George Lakoff and Mark Johnson, *Metaphors We Live By* (Chicago: University of Chicago Press, 2003). Lakoff and Johnson demonstrate not only that our conceptual system is largely metaphorical in nature but also that concepts structure what we perceive and even how we perceive phenomena, thus substantially shaping our everyday reality. Darian Leader and David Corfield provide some compelling evidence for the power of metaphors to affect the ways in which we experience and interpret bodily symptoms, in *Why Do People Get Ill?* (London: Hamish Hamilton, 2007).

12. See, for example, Alain Ehrenberg, *The Weariness of the Self: Diagnosing the History of Depression in the Contemporary Age*, trans. David Homel et al. (Montreal: McGill-Queen's University Press, 2010).

13. Edward Shorter, *From Paralysis to Fatigue: A History of Psychosomatic Illness in the Modern Era* (New York: Free Press, 1992), 267–94.

14. Ibid., 2, x.

1. HUMORS

1. There are now various other lines of investigation, of course, such as research on the genetics of depression, hormonal abnormalities, the link between depression and stress, and the use of brain imaging to detect microscopic abnormalities in brain structure and functioning.

2. For more general literature on Galen, see, for example, Christopher Gill, *Naturalistic Psychology in Galen and Stoicism* (Oxford: Oxford University Press, 2010); Christopher Gill, Tim Whitmarsh, and John Wilkins, eds., *Galen and the World of Knowledge* (Cambridge: Cambridge University Press, 2009); and R. J. Hankinson, ed., *The Cambridge Companion to Galen* (Cambridge: Cambridge University Press, 2008).

3. For an overview of the historical transformations of the concept and the ways in which the condition was theorized from classical antiquity to the present day, see Jennifer Radden, introduction to *The Nature of Melancholy: From Aristotle to Kristeva*, ed. Jennifer Radden (Oxford: Oxford University Press, 2000), 3–51. See also Matthew Bell, *Melancholia: The Western Malady* (Cambridge: Cambridge University Press, 2014); and Clark Lawlor, *From Melancholia to Prozac: A History of Depression* (Oxford: Oxford University Press, 2012).

4. Aristotle, *Problems*, trans. W. S. Hett (Cambridge, Mass.: Harvard University Press, 1957), 2:155.

5. John Cassian, *The Monastic Institutes*, trans. Edgar C. S. Gibson, in *A Select Library of Nicene and Post-Nicene Fathers of the Christian Church*, ed. Henry Wace

and Philip Schaff (New York: Christian Literature, 1894), 2nd ser., 11:183–641; Sieg-fried Wenzel, *The Sin of Sloth: Acedia in Medieval Thought and Literature* (Chapel Hill: University of North Carolina Press, 1967); Werner Post, *Acedia—Das Laster der Trägheit. Zur Geschichte der siebten Todsünde* (Freiburg: Herder, 2011).

6. See, for example, Marsilio Ficino, *Three Books on Life: A Critical Edition and Translation with Introduction and Notes*, trans. Carol B. Kaske and John R. Clark Medieval & Renaissance Texts & Studies, vol. 57 (Tempe, Ariz.: Medieval & Renais-sance Texts & Studies, 1998); Robert Burton, *The Anatomy of Melancholy* (Oxford: Oxford University Press, 1989); and Johann Wolfgang von Goethe, *The Sorrows of Young Werther*, trans. Michael Hulse (London: Penguin, 1989).

7. Radden, introduction to Radden, *Nature of Melancholy*, 25; Emil Kraepelin, *Manic Depressive Illness*, trans. Mary Barclay, ed. George Robinson [from 8th ed. of *Textbook of Psychiatry*, 1909–1915] (Edinburgh: Livingstone, 1920).

8. Sigmund Freud, "Mourning and Melancholia," in *The Standard Edition of the Complete Psychological Works of Sigmund Freud*, ed. and trans. James Strachey (Lon-don: Vintage, 2001), 14:243–58; Melanie Klein, *Love, Guilt and Reparation and Other Works, 1921–1945* (London: Hogarth Press, 1975).

9. Frederick Goodwin and Kay Renfield Jamison, *Manic-Depressive Illness* (New York: Oxford University Press, 1990).

10. For a recent biography of Galen, see Susan P. Mattern, *The Prince of Medicine: Galen in the Roman Empire* (Oxford: Oxford University Press, 2013).

11. Galen, "The Pulse for Beginners," in *Selected Works*, trans. P. N. Singer (Oxford: Oxford University Press, 1997), 339–41.

12. For an analysis of the symptoms of depression, see Alain Ehrenberg, *The Weariness of the Self: Diagnosing the History of Depression in the Contemporary Age*, trans. David Homel et al. (Montreal: McGill-Queen's University Press, 2010); and the discussion of the *DSM-V* and *ICD-10* definitions of depression in chapter 9 of this book. For a discussion of the parallels between ancient melancholia and modern depression, see also Stanley W. Jackson, *Melancholia and Depression: From Hippo-cratic Times to Modern Times* (New Haven, Conn.: Yale University Press, 1990).

13. Galen, *On the Affected Parts*, ed. and trans. Rudolph E. Siegel (London: Karger, 1976), 92–93.

14. Ibid., 90.

15. Ibid.

16. Ibid., 92, 93.

17. Pbreluigi Donini, "Psychology," in Hankinson, *Cambridge Companion to Galen*, 185–88.

18. Galen, *On the Affected Parts*, 93.

19. Galen also discusses this idea in his treatise *On the Doctrines of Hippocrates and Plato* and in his late pamphlet *The Faculties of the Soul Follow the Mixtures of the Body*. See Donini, "Psychology," 184.

20. Galen, "The Soul's Dependence on the Body," in *Selected Works*, 155.

21. In some texts Galen goes even further, suggesting that the soul is in fact identical to the organs in which it is seated and, in particular, that the soul might be identical to the cerebral *pneuma*. See Donini, "Psychology," 201.

22. Galen, "Soul's Dependence on the Body," 160.

23. See chaps. 2, 4, and 8.

24. Donani, "Psychology," 196.

25. Apollonius of Rhodes, *Jason and the Golden Fleece*, trans. Richard Hunter (Oxford: Oxford University Press, 1993), 75.

26. Glenn R. Bugh, introduction to *The Cambridge Companion to the Hellenistic World*, ed. Glenn R. Bugh (Cambridge: Cambridge University Press, 2006), 1–8. For other texts on Apollonius, see Theodore D. Papanghelis and Antonios Rengakos, eds., *Brill's Companion to Apollonius Rhodius*, 2nd rev. ed. (Leiden: Brill, 2008).

27. Níta Krevans and Alexander Sens, "Language and Literature," in Bugh, *Cambridge Companion to the Hellenistic World*, 201.

28. Apollonius of Rhodes, *Jason and the Golden Fleece*, 14, 33, 50–51.

29. Ibid., 56.

30. Ibid., 78, 113, 128–29.

31. Ibid., 135.

32. Ibid., 136, 51, 31.

33. Ibid., 97.

34. In 1907, the American psychologist William James wrote a short pamphlet called *The Energies of Men*, which, just like the *Argonautica*, illustrates the powerful impact that ideas can have on our physical and mental energy levels.

35. Darian Leader and David Corfield, *Why Do People Get Ill?* (London: Hamish Hamilton, 2007).

36. Placebo studies, for example, have shown that injections have a higher placebo effect than pills, and that large pills work better than smaller pills, but that very small pills are more effective than average-size ones. All this suggests that belief, suggestion, symbolism, and representation play a significant role in the body's reaction to certain stimuli. See ibid., 109.

37. Leader and Corfield cite various studies that show that "the fewer one's social relationships, the shorter one's life expectancy and the more devastating the impact of infectious diseases. Surprising as it may seem, this is statistically a greater risk factor than smoking or obesity, and even after taking these latter variables into account, it makes someone two and a half times more likely to die than someone of the same age and economic status who has a network of social relations" (ibid., 155).

38. Ibid., 207.

39. Ibid., 237.

40. Ibid., 239. Here, Corfield and Leader specifically refer to a study by J. Kiecolt-Glaser et al., "Slowing of Wound Healing by Psychological Stress," *Lancet* 346 (1995): 1194–96.

41. Mindfulness meditation, in contrast, has been shown to boost immune response. See Leader and Corfield, *Why Do People Get Ill?*, 285.

2. SIN

1. The following account of the history of acedia in the Middle Ages is indebted to two excellent studies on the subject: Siegfried Wenzel, *The Sin of Sloth: Acedia in Medieval Thought and Literature* (Chapel Hill: University of North Carolina Press, 1967); and Werner Post, *Acedia—Das Laster der Trägheit. Zur Geschichte der siebten Todsünde* (Freiburg: Herder, 2011).

2. For more information on Evagrius Ponticus, see, for example, A. M. Casiday, *Evagrius Ponticus: The Early Church Fathers* (London: Routledge, 2006); and George Tsakiridis, *Evagrius Ponticus and Cognitive Science: A Look at Moral Evil and the Thoughts* (Eugene, Ore.: Wipf and Stock, 2010).

3. Andrew Solomon, *The Noonday Demon: An Anatomy of Depression* (London: Vintage, 2002).

4. Quoted in Wenzel, *Sin of Sloth*, 5.

5. Ibid., 14.

6. Ibid., 5.

7. John Cassian, *The Monastic Institutes*, trans. Edgar C. S. Gibson, in *A Select Library of Nicene and Post-Nicene Fathers of the Christian Church*, ed. Henry Wace and Philip Schaff (New York: Christian Literature, 1894), 2nd ser., 11: 266.

8. Ibid., 267.

9. Ibid., 267–68.

10. Ibid., 268.

11. Ibid., 269.

12. Ibid., 271. See Thessalonians 3:11.

13. Cassian, *Monastic Institutes*, 271.

14. Ibid., 274, 275.

15. Wenzel, *Sin of Sloth*, 22.

16. However, the current "Catechism of the Catholic Church" still lists the sins in Latin as *superbia, avaritia, invidia, ira, luxuria, gula,* and *pigritia seu acedia* (laziness or acedia).

17. Wenzel, *Sin of Sloth*, 30–31.

18. Ibid., 32.

19. Hugh of Saint Victor, *On the Sacraments of the Christian Faith (De Sacramentis)*, trans. Roy J. Deferrari (Cambridge, Mass.: Mediaeval Academy of America, 1951), 375.

20. Ibid., 376.

21. Ibid., 375.

22. Quoted in Wenzel, *Sin of Sloth*, 34.

23. Saint Thomas Aquinas, *Summa Theologiae: A Concise Translation*, ed. Timothy McDermott (London: Eyre & Spottiswoode, 1989), 365.

24. Ibid.

25. Ibid.

26. Ibid., 269.

27. Ibid., 270.

28. Rowena Mason, "David Cameron Calls on Obese to Accept Help or Risk Losing Benefits," *Guardian*, February 14, 2015, http://www.theguardian.com/politics /2015/feb/14/david-cameron-obese-addicts-accept-help-risk-losing-benefits (accessed February 18, 2015).

29. Geoffrey Chaucer, "The Parson's Tale," in *The Canterbury Tales*, trans. Eugene J. Crook (1993), http://english.fsu.edu/canterbury/parson.html (accessed March 2, 2015) (translation slightly revised).

30. Dante, *The Divine Comedy*, trans. Allen Mandelbaum (New York: Knopf, 1995), 71, 59, 60, 66; Dante, *The Divine Comedy*, vol. 1, *Inferno*, Italian text with translation and comment by John D. Sinclair (Oxford: Oxford University Press, 1961), 40.

31. Dante, *Divine Comedy*, 69.

32. Ibid., 89; Dante, *Inferno*, 104.

33. Wolf-Günther Klostermann, "Acedia und Schwarze Galle: Bemerkungen zu Dante, Inferno VII, 115ff.," *Romanische Forschungen*, 76, nos. 1–2 (1964): 183–94.

34. Ibid.

35. Dante, *Divine Comedy*, 161; Dante, *Inferno*, 296.

36. Dante, *Divine Comedy*, 232; Dante, *The Divine Comedy*, vol. 2, *Purgatorio*, Italian text with translation and comment by John D. Sinclair (Oxford: Oxford University Press, 1961), 60.

37. Dante, *Divine Comedy*, 233; Dante, *Purgatorio*, 60–62.

38. Dante, *Divine Comedy*, 233–34.

39. See, for example, Jenny Law's research project "The Active Patient: Energy, Desire and Active Recoveries," http://theactivepatient.wordpress.com (accessed December 13, 2014).

40. Dante, *Divine Comedy*, 668–69nn.

41. Ibid., 300–301.

42. Ibid., 301.

43. Ibid.; Dante, *Purgatorio*, 236.

44. Guy P. Raffa, *The Complete Danteworlds: A Reader's Guide to the Divine Comedy* (Chicago: University of Chicago Press, 2009), 178–79.

45. Dante, *Divine Comedy*, 272; Dante, *Purgatorio*, 160.

3. SATURN

1. Marsilio Ficino, *Three Books on Life: A Critical Edition and Translation with Introduction and Notes*, ed. Carol V. Kaske and John R. Clark, Medieval & Renaissance Texts & Studies, vol. 57 (Tempe, Ariz.: Medieval & Renaissance Texts & Studies, 1998), 103, 397.

2. Quoted in Kaske and Clark, introduction to ibid., 20. The general information on Ficino presented in this chapter draws on Kaske and Clark's detailed introductory survey.

3. Ibid., 31.

4. Ibid., 22.

5. Ibid., 41.

6. Ficino, *Three Books on Life*, 111.

7. Ibid., 113.

8. Ibid.

9. Ibid., 115.

10. See, for example, Simon Critchley and Jamieson Webster, *The Hamlet Doctrine: Knowing Too Much, Doing Nothing* (New York: Verso, 2013), 65–66.

11. Walter Benjamin, *The Origin of German Tragic Drama*, trans. John Osborne (London: NLB, 1977), 156.

12. G. F. Hegel, *Aesthetics: Lectures on Fine Art*, trans. T. M. Knox (Oxford: Clarendon Press, 1975), 2:1226.

13. Ficino, *Three Books on Life*, 117–18.

14. Ibid., 123–24, 127, 131.

15. Ibid., 135–37.

16. Ibid., 149.

17. Kaske and Clark, introduction to Ficino, *Three Books on Life*, 48–49.

18. Ficino, *Three Books on Life*, 331, 359.

19. Ibid., 251, 249.

20. Ibid., 251, 255, 253, 367.

21. Ibid., 369, 371.

22. W. G. Sebald, *The Rings of Saturn*, trans. Michael Hulse (London: Vintage, 2002), 43; W. G. Sebald, *Die Ringe des Saturn. Eine englische Wallfahrt* (Frankfurt am Main: Fischer, 1997), 58.

23. Sebald, *Rings of Saturn*, 54.

24. Ibid., 19, 42.

25. Ibid., 68.

26. Ibid., 78–79.

27. Ibid., 94–95, 150–51.

28. See, for example, Lars von Trier, "Longing for the End of All," interview with Niels Thorson, http://melancholiathemovie.com (accessed October 30, 2014).

29. Sigmund Freud, "Mourning and Melancholia," in *The Standard Edition of the Complete Psychological Works of Sigmund Freud*, ed. and trans. James Strachey (London: Vintage, 2001), 14:243–58.

30. Quoted in Andrew Solomon, *The Noonday Demon: An Anatomy of Depression* (London: Vintage, 2002), 433–34; Shelley E. Taylor, *Positive Illusions: Creative Self-Deception and the Healthy Mind* (New York: Basic Books, 1989), 7, 213.

4. SEXUALITY

1. I explore the theorization of the so-called perversions in more detail in my previous monograph, *Modernism and Perversion: Sexual Deviance in Sexology and Literature, 1850–1930* (Basingstoke: Palgrave Macmillan, 2011).

2. For an account of sexual perversions in the premodern, presexological era, see, for example, Julie Peakman, "Sexual Perversion in History: An Introduction," in *Sexual Perversions, 1670–1890*, ed. Julie Peakman (New York: Palgrave Macmillan, 2009), 1–49, and other essays in that collection. See also Faramerz Dabhoiwala, *The Origins of Sex: A History of the First Sexual Revolution* (London: Allen Lane, 2012).

3. Quoted in Patricia Simons, *The Sex of Men in Premodern Europe: A Cultural History* (Cambridge: Cambridge University Press, 2011), 165, 168.

4. Fernanda Alfieri, "Urge Without Desire? Confession Manuals, Moral Casuistry, and the Features of *Concupiscencia* Between the Fifteenth and Eighteenth Centuries," in *Bodies, Sex and Desire from the Renaissance to the Present Day*, ed. Kate Fisher and Sarah Toulalan (Basingstoke: Palgrave Macmillan, 2011), 159.

5. Simons, *Sex of Men in Premodern Europe*, 165.

6. Marsilio Ficino, *Three Books on Life. A Critical Edition and Translation with Introduction and Notes*, ed. Carol V. Kaske and John R. Clark, Medieval & Renaissance Texts & Studies, vol. 57 (Tempe, Ariz.: Medieval & Renaissance Texts & Studies, 1998), 124.

7. Saint Thomas Aquinas, *Summa Theologiae*, trans. Thomas Gilby, vol. 43, *Temperance* (London: Blackfriars in conjunction with Eyre & Spottiswoode, 1968), 2a2ae, ques. 154, art. 11, 245, 249.

8. Thomas W. Laqueur, *Solitary Sex: A Cultural History of Masturbation* (New York: Zone Books, 2003), 278.

9. *Onania; or, the Heinous Sin of Self-Pollution, and All its Frightful Consequences, in Both Sexes, Considered, with Spiritual and Physical Advice to Those Who Have Already Injur'd Themselves by This Abominable Practice. To which is Subjoin'd, A Letter from a Lady to the Author, [very curious] concerning the Use and Abuse of the Marriage-Bed, with the Author's Answer*, 4th ed. (London: N. Crouch, n.d.), 1.

10. Ibid., 8–9.

11. Samuel-Auguste Tissot, *Onanism: Or, a Treatise upon the Disorders Produced by Masturbation: Or, the Dangerous Effects of Secret and Excessive Venery*, trans. A. Hume, based on 3rd rev. ed. (London: Wilkinson, 1767), vii–viii.

12. See, for example, Joachim Radkau, "The Neurasthenic Experience in Imperial Germany: Expeditions into Patient Records and Side-Looks into General History," in *Cultures of Neurasthenia from Beard to the First World War*, ed. Marijke Gijswijt-Hofstra and Roy Porter (Amsterdam: Rodopi, 2001), 207–8.

13. Sigmund Freud, "On the Grounds for Detaching a Particular Syndrome from Neurasthenia Under the Description 'Anxiety Neurosis' (1895 [1894])," in *The Standard Edition of the Complete Psychological Works of Sigmund Freud*, ed. and trans. James Strachey (London: Vintage, 2001), 3:85–117.

14. Quoted in ibid., 200.

15. Malcolm Macmillan, *Freud Evaluated: The Complete Arc* (Cambridge, Mass.: MIT Press, 1997), 200.

16. Quoted in Max Nordau, *Degeneration*, trans. George L. Mosse (Lincoln: University of Nebraska Press, 1993), 16.

17. Harry Oosterhuis, *Stepchildren of Nature: Krafft-Ebing, Psychiatry, and the Making of Sexual Identity* (Chicago: University of Chicago Press, 2000), 52–53, 107.

18. Vernon A. Rosario, *The Erotic Imagination: French Histories of Perversity* (New York: Oxford University Press, 1997), 88.

19. Ibid., 40.

20. The authorship of this story is contested. Some argue that it was written by Tieck's contemporary Ernst Benjamin Salomo Raupach. See, for example, Heide Crawford, "Ernst Benjamin Salomo Raupach's Vampire Story 'Wake Not the Dead,'" *Journal of Popular Culture* 45, no. 6 (2012): 1189–1205.

21. Karl Marx, *Capital: A Critique of Political Economy*, trans. Ben Fowkes (Harmondsworth: Penguin, 1976), 1:342.

22. Tzvetan Todorov presents this argument in *The Fantastic: A Structural Approach to a Literary Genre*, trans. Richard Howard (Ithaca, N.Y.: Cornell University Press, 1975), 157–74.

23. Richard Dyer, "Children of the Night: Vampirism as Homosexuality, Homosexuality as Vampirism," in *Sweet Dreams: Sexuality, Gender and Popular Fiction*, ed. Susannah Radstone (London: Lawrence and Wishart, 1988), 60. On vampirism and homosexuality, see also Christopher Craft, "'Kiss Me with Those Red Lips:' Gender and Inversion in Bram Stoker's Dracula," *Representations* 8 (1984): 107–33.

24. J. Sheridan Le Fanu, "Carmilla," in *In a Glass Darkly* (Oxford: Oxford University Press, 1993), 261–65, 274.

25. Ibid., 281.

26. Ibid., 282.

27. Ibid.

5. NERVES

1. Edgar Allan Poe, "The Fall of the House of Usher," in *The Collected Tales and Poems of Edgar Allan Poe* (New York: Modern Library, 1992), 235.

2. George Cheyne, *The English Malady: or, A Treatise of Nervous Diseases of All Kinds, as Spleen, Vapours, Lowness of Spirits, Hypochondriacal, and Hysterical Distempers, etc.*, 6th ed. (London: G. Strahan and J. Leake, 1735), 16, 5.

3. Ibid., 7, 8, 15, 17.

4. Ibid., ii.

5. Ibid., 325–26.

6. The rest cure and, particularly, its gender-political dimension are discussed in detail in chap. 7.

7. Tom Lutz, *American Nervousness, 1903: An Anecdotal History* (Ithaca, N.Y.: Cornell University Press, 1991), 32.

8. Janet Oppenheim, *"Shattered Nerves": Doctors, Patients, and Depression in Victorian England* (New York: Oxford University Press, 1991), 81.

9. Joachim Radkau, *Das Zeitalter der Nervosität. Deutschland zwischen Bismarck und Hitler* (Munich: Carl Hanser Verlag, 1998).

10. George M. Beard, *A Practical Treatise on Nervous Exhaustion (Neurasthenia): Its Symptoms, Nature, Sequences, Treatment* (New York: Wood, 1880); George M. Beard, *American Nervousness: Its Causes and Consequences. A Supplement to Nervous Exhaustion (Neurasthenia)* (New York: Putnam, 1881).

11. Beard, *American Nervousness*, vi, 5, 7.

12. Oscar Wilde to Robert Ross, February 1900, in *More Letters of Oscar Wilde*, ed. Rupert Hart-Davis (London: Murray, 1985), 184.

13. For general discussions of neurasthenia, see, for example, Andreas Killen, *Berlin Electropolis: Shock, Nerves, and German Modernity* (Berkeley: University of California Press, 2006); Radkau, *Das Zeitalter der Nervosität*; Marijke Gijswijt-Hofstra and Roy Porter, eds., *Cultures of Neurasthenia from Beard to the First World War* (Amsterdam: Rodopi, 2001); Volker Roelcke, *Krankheit und Kulturkritik. Psychiatrische Gesellschaftsdeutungen im bürgerlichen Zeitalter, 1790–1914* (Frankfurt am Main: Campus, 1999); Simon Wessely, "Neurasthenia and Fatigue Syndromes," in *A History of Clinical Psychiatry: The Origins and History of Psychiatric Disorders*, ed. German E. Berrios and Roy Porter (London: Athlone, 1995), 509–32; Tom Lutz, "Neurasthenia and Fatigue Syndromes," in ibid., 533–44; Edward Shorter, *From Paralysis to Fatigue: A History of Psychosomatic Illness in the Modern Era* (New York: Free Press, 1992); Lutz, *American Nervousness, 1903*; Oppenheim, *"Shattered Nerves"*; F. Gosling, *Before Freud: Neurasthenia and the American Medical Community, 1870–1910* (Urbana: University of Illinois Press, 1987); and Elaine Showalter, *The Female Malady: Women, Madness and English Culture, 1830–1980* (London: Virago, 1987). For reflections on neurasthenia and literature, see Maximilian Bergengruen, Klaus Müller-Wille, and Caroline Pross, eds., *Neurasthenie. Die Krankheit der Moderne und die moderne Literatur* (Freiburg im Breisgau: Rombach, 2010).

14. Beard, *American Nervousness*, vi.

15. On the connection among sleep, technology, and brain work in the late nineteenth and early twentieth centuries, see Lee Scrivner's important study, *Becoming Insomniac: How Sleeplessness Alarmed Modernity* (Basingstoke: Palgrave Macmillan, 2014).

16. Beard, *American Nervousness*, 91, 26.

17. Ibid., 9–10.

18. Oppenheim, *"Shattered Nerves,"* 85.

19. However, the ways in which neurasthenia was defined and diagnosed differed from country to country. Gijswijt-Hofstra and Porter's anthology *Cultures of Neurasthenia: From Beard to the First World War* provides a good comparative overview of the more subtle national differences, which also had repercussions with regard to the race, gender, and class dimensions of the diagnosis. In England and Germany, for example, the diagnosis was soon "democratized" and not just the reserve of middle- and upper-class people.

20. Franz Kafka, *The Diaries of Franz Kafka, 1910–1913*, ed. Max Brod (London: Secker & Warburg, 1948), 287.

21. Heinrich Mann, "Doktor Biebers Versuchung," in *Haltlos: Sämtliche Erzählungen* (Frankfurt am Main: Fischer, 1995), 1:522 (my translation).

22. Wilhelm Erb, *Über die wachsende Nervosität unserer Zeit* (Heidelberg: Hörning, 1884), 20 (my translation).

23. Karl Kraus, *Half-Truths and One-and-a-Half Truths: Selected Aphorisms*, trans. Harry Zohn (Chicago: University of Chicago Press, 1990), 112.

24. Freiherr Richard von Krafft-Ebing, *Über Gesunde und Kranke Nerven*, 4th rev. and exp. ed. (Tübingen: Verlag der H. Laupp'schen Buchhandlung, 1898), 2–4 (my translation).

25. Ibid., 7–8, 17, 115.

26. Max Nordau, *Entartung*, 3rd ed., vol. 1 (Berlin: Duncker, 1896).

27. Krafft-Ebing, *Über Gesunde und Kranke Nerven*, 9.

28. Ibid., 10.

29. Ibid., 27.

30. Joris-Karl Huysmans, *Against Nature (À rebours)*, trans. Margaret Mauldon (Oxford: Oxford University Press, 2009), 3, 7.

31. Ibid., 22; Joris-Karl Huysmans, *À rebours* (Paris: Flammarion, 2004), 62.

32. Huysmans, *Against Nature*, 14; Huysmans, *À rebours*, 52.

33. Huysmans, *Against Nature*, 38; Huysmans, *À rebours*, 82.

34. Huysmans, *Against Nature*, 20; Huysmans, *À rebours*, 60.

35. Huysmans, *Against Nature*, 26.

36. Ibid., 117; Huysmans, *À rebours*, 175.

37. Huysmans, *Against Nature*, 118.

38. Ibid., 156.

39. Ibid., 162–63; Huysmans, *À rebours*, 228.

40. Huysmans, *Against Nature*, 91; Huysmans, *À rebours*, 144.

41. Huysmans, *Against Nature*, 177.

42. Ibid., 145–46.

43. Marcel Proust, *In Search of Lost Time*, trans. C. K. Scott Moncrieff and Terence Kilmartin, rev. D. J. Enright, vol. 1, *Swann's Way* (London: Vintage, 2002), 43.

44. *ICD-10* (Version 2010), http://apps.who.int/classifications/icd10/browse/2010/en#/F48.0 (accessed February 23, 2015).

45. Radkau, *Das Zeitalter der Nervosität*, 440.

46. Killen, however, challenges this account in his illuminating study *Berlin Electropolis*. He argues that in Germany it was primarily processes related to the welfare state and, in particular, to social insurance practices that were responsible for the changing attitude toward neurasthenia after the First World War, when the vast number of shell-shocked and neurasthenic veterans was deemed to pose a serious financial threat to the system.

47. Wessely, "Neurasthenia and Fatigue Syndromes," 509–32; Lutz, "Neurasthenia and Fatigue Syndromes," 533–44.

48. Chronic fatigue syndrome is discussed in detail in chap. 10.

49. Tsung-Yi Lin, "Neurasthenia Revisited: Its Place in Modern Psychiatry," *Culture, Medicine and Psychiatry* 13, no. 2 (1989): 105–29.

50. T. Suzuki, "The Concept of Neurasthenia and Its Treatment in Japan," *Culture, Medicine and Psychiatry* 13, no. 2 (1989): 187–202.

6. CAPITALISM

1. Ivan Goncharov, *Oblomov*, trans. Natalie Duddington (New York: Knopf, 1992).

2. Ibid., 181.

3. Ibid., 196, 205, 207.

4. Ibid., 463, 563, 577.

5. For a detailed discussion of Freud's theories of exhaustion, and in particular his notion of the death drive, see chap. 8.

6. Anson Rabinbach, *The Human Motor: Energy, Fatigue and the Origins of Modernity* (Berkeley: University of California Press, 1990), 72.

7. Max Weber, *Die Protestantische Ethik und der Geist des Kapitalismus*, ed. Dirk Kaesler (Munich: Beck, 2004).

8. Joachim Radkau, *Max Weber: A Biography*, trans. Patrick Camiller (Cambridge: Polity, 2011).

9. Marianne Weber to Helene Weber, 1900, quoted in ibid., 149.

10. Max Weber to Robert Michels, 1908, quoted in ibid., 152.

11. Max Weber to Robert Michels, 1909, quoted in ibid.

12. Ibid., 83.

13. This parable circulates in different versions on the Internet (it is also sometimes called "The Mexican Fisherman and the Harvard MBA"). Ironically, it often features in investment-banking and entrepreneurial self-help manuals, with a slightly different ending. I have retold it here in my own words.

14. Weber, *Die Protestantische Ethik*, 146, 157, 181, 194.

15. Ibid., 190–91, 183–84. See also Max Weber, *The Protestant Ethic and the Spirit of Capitalism*, trans. Talcott Parsons and Anthony Giddens, https://www.marxists.org/reference/archive/weber/protestant-ethic/index.htm (accessed February 24, 2015) (translation slightly modified).

16. Rabinbach, *Human Motor*, 58.

17. Thomas Mann, *Buddenbrooks. Verfall einer Familie* (Frankfurt am Main: Fischer, 2007), 320 (my translation).

18. Thomas Mann, *Buddenbrooks*, trans. H. T. Lowe-Porter (London: Vintage, 1999), 496 (translation modified); Mann, *Buddenbrooks. Verfall einer Familie*, 614–15.

19. Joseph Stiglitz, *The Price of Inequality: How Today's Divided Society Endangers Our Future* (New York: Norton, 2012).

20. Thomas Pikkety, *Capital in the Twenty-First Century*, trans. Arthur Goldhammer (Cambridge, Mass.: Harvard University Press, 2014).

21. Adair Turner, *Economics After the Crisis: Objectives and Means* (Cambridge, Mass.: MIT Press, 2012).

22. Kate Pickett and Richard Wilkinson, *The Spirit Level: Why More Equal Societies Almost Always Do Better* (London: Penguin, 2009); Richard Layard, *Happiness: Lessons from a New Science* (London: Penguin, 2005); Bruno S. Frey and Alois Stutzer, *Happiness and Economics: How the Economy and Institutions Affect Human Well-Being* (Princeton, N.J.: Princeton University Press, 2001).

7. REST

1. Exodus 20:8–11.

2. Silas Weir Mitchell, *Wear and Tear: Or, Hints for the Overworked*, 5th rev. ed. (Philadelphia: Lippincott, 1887), 12–13.

3. Ibid., 18–19.

4. Charlotte Perkins Gilman, "The Yellow Wallpaper," in *The Yellow Wall-Paper and Other Stories*, ed. Robert Shulman (Oxford: Oxford University Press, 1998), 3.

5. Ibid., 5.

6. For different interpretations of this story, see, for example, Judith Allen, *The Feminism of Charlotte Perkins Gilman: Sexualities, Histories, Progressivism* (Chicago: University of Chicago Press, 2009); and Jeffrey Berman, "The Unrestful Cure: Charlotte Perkins Gilman and 'The Yellow Wallpaper,'" in *The Captive Imagination: A Casebook on The Yellow Wallpaper*, ed. Catherine Colden (New York: Feminist Press, 1992), 211–41.

7. Silas Weir Mitchell, *Fat and Blood and How to Make Them*, ed. Michael S. Kimmel (1882; repr., New York: Altamira Press, 2004), 9, 13, 25.

8. Charlotte Perkins Gilman, *The Living of Charlotte Perkins Gilman: An Autobiography* (New York: Harper & Row, 1975), 96.

9. Hermione Lee, *Virginia Woolf* (London: Vintage, 1997), 182–86.

10. Quoted in ibid., 184.

11. Ibid., 186.

12. Virginia Woolf, *On Being Ill*, with an introduction by Hermione Lee (Ashfield, Mass.: Paris Press, 2002), xxviii.

13. Mitchell, *Wear and Tear*, 8, 9, 33, 56.

14. Ibid., 36, 57, 43.

15. Ibid., 32.

16. Mitchell, *Fat and Blood*, 32.

17. Lisa Appignanesi, *Mad, Bad and Sad: A History of Women and the Mind Doctors from 1800 to the Present* (London: Virago, 2008); Elaine Showalter, *The Female Malady: Women, Madness and English Culture, 1830–1980* (London: Virago, 1987).

18. Freiherr Richard von Krafft-Ebing, *Über Gesunde und Kranke Nerven*, 4th rev. and exp. ed. (Tübingen: Verlag der H. Laupp'schen Buchhandlung, 1898), 57–58 (my translation).

19. Quoted in Darwin Correspondence Project, http://www.darwinproject.ac.uk/darwins-letters (accessed February 24, 2015).

20. Brian Dillon, *The Hypochondriacs: Nine Tormented Lives* (New York: Faber and Faber, 2009), 79–88.

21. Quoted in Darwin Correspondence Project.

22. Alan Derickson, *Dangerously Sleepy: Overworked Americans and the Cult of Manly Wakefulness* (Philadelphia: University of Pennsylvania Press, 2014). On the gradual erosion of sleep under the conditions of modernity, see also, for example, Lee Scrivner, *Becoming Insomniac: How Sleeplessness Alarmed Modernity* (Basingstoke: Palgrave Macmillan, 2014); and Roger Ekirch, "The Modernization of Western Sleep: Or, Does Insomnia Have a History?," *Past and Present* 226 (2015): 149–92.

23. Quoted in "Why Do We Sleep, Anyway?," December 8, 2007, http://healthysleep.med.harvard.edu/healthy/matters/benefits-of-sleep/why-do-we-sleep (accessed February 24, 2015).

24. Quoted in ibid.

25. A. Roger Ekirch, *At Day's Close: Night in Times Past* (New York: Norton, 2006).

26. Jonathan Crary, *24/7: Late Capitalism and the Ends of Sleep* (London: Verso, 2013).

8. THE DEATH DRIVE

1. Sigmund Freud, "On the Grounds for Detaching a Particular Syndrome from Neurasthenia Under the Description 'Anxiety Neurosis'" (1895 [1894]), in *The Standard Edition of the Complete Psychological Works of Sigmund Freud*, ed. and trans. James Strachey (London: Vintage, 2001), 3:85–117.

2. Sigmund Freud, "Sexuality in the Aetiology of the Neuroses" (1898), in ibid., 3:274; Sigmund Freud, "Die Sexualität in der Ätiologie der Neurosen" (1898), in *Studienausgabe, Sexualleben*, ed. Alexander Mitscherlich, Angela Richards, and James Strachey (Frankfurt am Main: Fischer, 1982), 5:25.

3. Sigmund Freud, "Introductory Lectures on Psycho-Analysis (1916–1917 [1915–1917]): Part III. General Theory of the Neuroses (1917 [1916–1917]). Lecture XXIV: The Common Neurotic State," in *Standard Edition*, 16:378–91.

4. Sigmund Freud, "'Civilized' Sexual Morality and Modern Nervous Illness" (1908), in *Standard Edition*, 9:187.

5. Ibid., 204.

6. Sigmund Freud, *Civilization and Its Discontents*, in *Standard Edition*, 21:57–145.

7. Ibid., 84–85.

8. Ibid., 89, 115, 87–88, 104.

9. Ibid., 145.

10. Sigmund Freud, "Instincts and Their Vicissitudes" (1915), in *Standard Edition*, 14:109–40.

11. Ibid., 121–22; Freud, "Triebe und Triebschicksale" (1915), in *Studienausgabe, Psychologie des Unbewußten*, 3:85.

12. Freud, "Instincts and Their Vicissitudes," 123.

13. Sigmund Freud, "Beyond the Pleasure Principle" (1920), in *Standard Edition*, 18:7, 34, 53, 51.

14. Sigmund Freud, "Jenseits des Lustprinzips" (1920), in *Studienausgabe, Psychologie des Unbewußten*, 3:239, 240, 237.

15. Sigmund Freud, "The Ego and the Id" (1923), in *Standard Edition*, 19:25.

16. Freud, "Beyond the Pleasure Principle," 69.

17. Ibid., 55–56. The parenthetical reference is to Barbara Low, *Psycho-Analysis: A Brief Account of the Freudian Theory* (New York: Harcourt, Brace and Howe, 1920), 73.

18. Freud, "Beyond the Pleasure Principle," 40–41; Freud, "Jenseits des Lustprinzips," 250.

19. Freud, *Civilization and Its Discontents*, 123.

20. For a discussion of the rise of the depression diagnosis, see Alain Ehrenberg, *The Weariness of the Self: Diagnosing the History of Depression in the Contemporary Age*, trans. David Homel et al. (Montreal: McGill-Queen's University Press, 2010).

21. Sigmund Freud, "Mourning and Melancholia" (1917 [1915]), in *Standard Edition*, 14:244.

22. Ibid., 246 (my emphasis).

23. Ibid., 253.

24. On the idea of giving up as a form of giving in, see Joyce McDougall, *Theatres of the Body: A Psychoanalytical Approach to Psychosomatic Illness* (London: Free Association Books, 1989).

25. Herman Melville, "Bartleby, the Scrivener," in *Billy Budd, Sailor, and Selected Tales*, ed. Robert Milder (Oxford: Oxford University Press, 1998), 4, 6, 7, 10.

26. Ibid., 21.

27. Ibid., 40.

28. Ibid., 10, 11, 19.

29. Ibid., 22, 33, 32.

30. Ibid., 31.

31. Pierre Janet, *Les obsessions et la psychasthénie* (Paris: Félix Alcan, 1903), 1:vii, xiii–ix, 501–2 (my translation).

32. Ibid., 2:viii. He defines the *fonctions du réel* as "fonctions les plus élevées, qui permettent l'adaptation psychologique de l'être à son milieu physique et surtout à son milieu social" (the highest functions, which permit the human being's psychological adaptation to its physical and especially its social environment).

33. Ibid., 1:737–38.

34. Quoted in W. S. Taylor, "Pierre Janet: 1859–1947," *American Journal of Psychology* 60 (1947): 643.

35. Primo Levi, *The Drowned and the Saved*, trans. Raymond Rosenthal (New York: Summit Books, 1988), 98.

36. Primo Levi, *If This Is a Man / The Truce*, trans. Stuart Wolf (London: Everyman's Library, 2000), 102.

37. Ibid., 106.

38. Ibid., 105.

9. DEPRESSION

1. Sigmund Freud, "Mourning and Melancholia" (1917 [1915]), in *The Standard Edition of the Complete Psychological Works of Sigmund Freud*, ed. and trans. James Strachey (London: Vintage, 2001), 14:246, 244.

2. Ibid., 253.

3. Alain Ehrenberg, *The Weariness of the Self: Diagnosing the History of Depression in the Contemporary Age*, trans. David Homel et al. (Montreal: McGill-Queen's University Press, 2010), 42.

4. See, for example, Edward Shorter, *Before Prozac: The Troubled History of Mood Disorders in Psychiatry* (Oxford: Oxford University Press, 2008); and Edward Shorter, *How Everyone Became Depressed: The Rise and Fall of the Nervous Breakdown* (New York: Oxford University Press, 2013).

5. Ehrenberg, *Weariness of the Self*, 79–83.

6. World Health Organization, "Depression," fact sheet, no. 369, October 2012, http://www.who.int/mediacentre/factsheets/fs369/en/ (accessed January 9, 2015).

7. Elizabeth Wurtzel, *Prozac Nation: Young and Depressed in America. A Memoir* (London: Quartet Books, 1995), 263–64.

8. Ibid., 99, 303.

9. Ibid., 228, 257.

10. Ibid., 258–59, 286.

11. Ibid., 292.

12. American Psychiatric Association, *Diagnostic and Statistical Manual of Mental Disorders*, 5th ed. (Arlington, Va.: APA, 2013), 163, 162, 163–64.

13. World Health Organization, *International Statistical Classification of Diseases and Related Health Problems*, 10th ed., http://apps.who.int/classifications/apps/icd/icd10online2003/fr-icd.htm?gf30.htm+ (accessed January 9, 2015).

14. Andrew Solomon, *The Noonday Demon: An Anatomy of Depression* (London: Vintage, 2002), 18–19.

15. Ibid., 19.

16. Ibid., 15.

17. Roland Barthes, *How to Live Together: Novelistic Simulations of Some Everyday Spaces*, trans. Kate Briggs (New York: Columbia University Press, 2012), 21–23.

18. See, for example, Ben Goldacre, *Bad Pharma: How Drug Companies Mislead Doctors and Harm Patients* (London: Faber and Faber, 2013); Ethan Watters, *Crazy Like Us: The Globalization of the American Psyche* (New York: Free Press, 2010); Irving Kirsch, *The Emperor's New Drugs: Exploding the Antidepressant Myth* (New York: Basic Books, 2010); Darian Leader, *The New Black: Mourning, Melancholia and Depression* (London: Penguin, 2009); Shorter, *Before Prozac*; and Allan V. Horwitz and Jerome C. Wakefield, *The Loss of Sadness: How Psychiatry Transformed Normal Sorrow into Depressive Disorder* (New York: Oxford University Pres, 2007).

19. Ehrenberg, *Weariness of the Self*, 219 (Ehrenberg's emphasis).

20. Ibid., 229.

21. Franz Kafka, *Briefe an Milena* (Frankfurt am Main: Fischer, 1998), 290–91 (my translation).

22. Ehrenberg, *Weariness of the Self*, 4, 190.

23. Ibid., 233.

10. MYSTERY VIRUSES

1. Gary Holmes at the Centers for Disease Control and Prevention coined the term "chronic fatigue syndrome" in 1988.

2. For an analysis of the debates concerning the symptoms, epidemiology, and therapeutics of the condition, see Simon Wessely, Matthew Hotopf, and Michael Sharpe, *Chronic Fatigue and Its Syndromes*, rev. ed. (Oxford: Oxford University Press, 1999).

3. See Edward Shorter's argument on the pivotal role of the popular press in the emergence and spread of CFS in *From Paralysis to Fatigue: A History of Psychosomatic Illness in the Modern Era* (New York: Free Press, 1992), 314–20, as well as Wessely, Hotopf, and Sharpe, *Chronic Fatigue and Its Syndromes*, 322–48.

4. See, for example, Shorter, *From Paralysis to Fatigue*; and Richard L. Kradin, *Pathologies of the Mind/Body Interface: Exploring the Curious Domain of the Psychosomatic Disorders* (New York: Routledge, 2013).

5. Shorter, *From Paralysis to Fatigue*, 308–9.

6. Ibid., 311.

7. Two of the most influential patient stories of the 1980s were Sue Finlay, "An Illness Doctors Don't Recognize," *Observer*, June 1, 1986; and Hillary Johnson, "Journey into Fear," *Rolling Stone*, July 30, 1987. The *Observer* received fourteen thousand requests from readers for an ME fact sheet that it offered to supply after the publication of Finlay's article.

8. Wessely, Hotopf, and Sharpe, *Chronic Fatigue and Its Syndromes*, 133–34.

9. In the 1990s, Anthony David and Simon Wessely challenged the World Health Organization's clinical descriptors of CFS (*ICD-10*), which allowed for its classification either under neurology as "post viral fatigue" or under psychiatry as "neurasthenia." They argued for its reclassification as a psychiatric condition, causing much outrage among those with the condition. The WHO admitted that it had opted for this solution to recognize the fundamental divide that existed in the medical establishment about the syndrome, so that both camps would be able to use a diagnosis. See Anthony David and Simon Wessely, "Chronic Fatigue, ME and ICD-10," *Lancet* 342, no. 8881 (1993): 1247–48; and Wessely, Hotopf, and Sharp, *Chronic Fatigue and Its Syndromes*, 221.

10. See, for example, Wessely, Hotopf, and Sharp, *Chronic Fatigue and Its Syndromes*, 416.

11. Stephen T. Holgate, Anthony L. Komaroff, Dennis Mangan, and Simon Wessely, "Chronic Fatigue Syndrome: Understanding a Complex Illness," *Nature* 12 (2011): 539–44.

12. Nasim Marie Jafry, *The State of Me* (London: Friday Project, 2008), 75.

13. Ibid., 470–71, 250.

14. Ibid., 85, 241–42, 244.

15. Ibid., 247–49.

16. Ibid., 153–54.

17. Nasim Marie Jafry, "velo-gubbed-legs," http://velo-gubbed-legs.blogspot.co.uk /search/label/blinkered%20medics (accessed October 31, 2014).

18. Wessely, Hotopf, and Sharp, *Chronic Fatigue and Its Syndromes*, 416.

19. Elaine Showalter, *Hystories: Hysterical Epidemics and Modern Media* (New York: Columbia University Press, 1998).

20. Shorter, *From Paralysis to Fatigue*, 277, 304–5.

21. Ibid., 305, 307, 317.

22. Ibid., 320, 322–23.

23. ME Association, "What Is ME/CFS?," http://www.meassociation.org.uk/about /what-is-mecfs/; Centers for Disease Control and Prevention, Chronic Fatigue Syndrome (CFS), http://www.cdc.gov/cfs/causes/risk-groups.html (both accessed January 13, 2015).

24. Wessely, Hotopf, and Sharp, *Chronic Fatigue and Its Syndromes*, 283.

25. "In Search of a Cause," *Awake*, August 1992, quoted in ibid., 333.

26. Wessely, Hotopf, and Sharp, *Chronic Fatigue and Its Syndromes*, 336.

27. Quoted in ibid., 286.

28. Shorter, *From Paralysis to Fatigue*, 314.

29. K. Flett, "Why ME?," *Arena*, March 1990, quoted in Wessely, Hotopf, and Sharp, *Chronic Fatigue and Its Syndromes*, 332.

30. Darian Leader and David Corfield, *Why Do People Get Ill?* (London: Hamish Hamilton, 2007), 42.

31. Wessely, Hotopf, and Sharp, *Chronic Fatigue and Its Syndromes*, 339–40.

32. Ibid., 227, 289.

33. Ibid., 285–86.

34. Leader and Corfield, *Why Do People Get Ill?*, 136, 50, 20, 323.

35. Shorter, *From Paralysis to Fatigue*, 2, x.

11. BURNOUT

1. Anson Rabinbach, *The Human Motor: Energy, Fatigue, and the Origins of Modernity* (Berkeley: University of California Press, 1992), 233.

2. See, for example, World Health Organization, *Investing in Mental Health* (Geneva: WHO, 2003), http://www.who.int/mental_health/media/investing_mnh. pdf (accessed February 6, 2015). A recent survey estimates that stress-related absenteeism and sick leave cost the British economy £6.5 billion in 2013. See Natasha Shearer, "As Work Related Stress Costs UK Economy Nearly £6.5bn Each Year, What Steps Should Businesses and Employees be Taking?," *Huffington Post*, July 5, 2013, http://www.huffingtonpost.co.uk/natasha-shearer/work-related-stress-business _b_3545476.html (accessed February 6, 2015).

3. Patrick Kury, *Der Überforderte Mensch. Eine Wissensgeschichte vom Stress zum Burnout* (Frankfurt am Main: Campus, 2012), 271.

4. Ibid.

5. Ibid., 82.

6. Walter B. Cannon, *The Wisdom of the Body* (London: Kegan Paul, Trench, Trübner, 1932), 286.

7. Hans Selye, *Stress Without Distress* (London: Hodder and Stoughton, 1975), 27, 29, 28.

8. Ibid., 38.

9. Ibid., 38–39.

10. See also Hans Selye, *The Physiology and Pathology of Exposure to Stress: A Treatise Based on the Concepts of the General-Adaptation-Syndrome and the Diseases of Adaptation* (Montreal: Acta, 1950), 774, 787.

11. Selye, *Stress Without Distress*, 40.

12. Selye, *Physiology and Pathology of Exposure to Stress*, 787.

13. Selye, *Stress Without Distress*, 40.

14. Ibid., 40–41.

15. Hans Selye, *The Stress of Life: Revised Edition* (New York: McGraw-Hill, 1976), 457–58.

16. Ibid., 460–61.

17. Kury, *Der Überforderte Mensch*, 89–108, 223–66.

18. Lennart Levi, foreword to *Emotional Stress: Physiological and Psychological Reactions. Medical, Industrial and Military Implications*, ed. Lennart Levi (Basel: Karger, 1967), 9.

19. Lennart Levi, preface to *Society, Stress and Disease*, vol. 1, *The Psychosocial Environment and Psychosomatic Diseases*, ed. Lennart Levi (London: Oxford University Press, 1971), xi.

20. Lennart Levi, "The Human Factor—and the Inhuman," in ibid., 3.

21. Lennart Levi, preface to *Society, Stress and Disease*, vol. 4, *Working Life* (London: Oxford University Press, 1981), xi, xii.

22. Ibid., xi.

23. Levi, "Human Factor," 3–4.

24. See, for example, the essays in Sighard Neckel and Greta Wagner, eds., *Leistung und Erschöpfung. Burnout in der Wettbewerbsgesellschaft* (Frankfurt am Main: Suhrkamp, 2013), especially Neckel and Wagner, "Einleitung: Leistung und Erschöpfung," 7–26.

25. See, for example, Hartmut Rosa, *Social Acceleration: A New Theory of Modernity*, trans. Jonathan Trejo-Mathys (New York: Columbia University Press, 2013); and Jonathan Crary, *24/7: Capitalism and the End of Sleep* (London: Verso, 2013).

26. See, for example, Ehrenberg, *Weariness of the Self*; Luc Boltanski and Eve Chiapello, *The New Spirit of Capitalism*, trans. Gregory Elliott (London: Verso, 2005); and Richard Sennett, *The Corrosion of Character: The Personal Consequences of Work in the New Capitalism* (New York: Norton, 1998).

27. On the "subjectivization" of work, see, for example, Ulrich Bröckling, *Das unternehmerische Selbst. Soziologie einer Subjektivierungsform* (Frankfurt am Main: Suhrkamp, 2007); and G. Günter Voß and Hans J. Pongratz, "Der Arbeitskraftunternehmer. Eine neue Grundform der Ware Arbeitskraft?," *Kölner Zeitschrift für Soziologie und Sozialpsychologie* 1 (1998): 131–58.

28. Herbert J. Freudenberg, "Staff Burn-Out," *Journal of Social Issues* 30 (1974): 159–64.

29. Wilhelm Schaufeli, "Past Performance and Future Perspectives on Burnout Research," *SA Journal of Industrial Psychology* 29, no. 4 (2003): 1–15.

30. Quoted in ibid., 2.

31. Quoted in Wilhelm Schaufeli, Michael P. Leiter, and Christina Maslach, "Burnout: 35 Years of Research and Practice," *Career Development International* 14, no. 3 (2009): 206.

32. Ibid., 214.

33. Jonathon R. B. Halbesleben, preface to *Handbook of Stress and Burnout in Health Care*, ed. Jonathon R. B. Halbesleben (New York: Nova Science, 2008), viii.

34. Marjan J. Gorgievsky and Stevan E. Hobfoll, "Work Can Burn Us Out or Fire Us Up: Conservation of Resources in Burnout and Engagement," in ibid., 10.

35. Halbesleben, preface to Halbesleben, *Handbook of Stress and Burnout in Health Care*, viii, xi.

36. Gorgievsky and Hobfoll, "Work Can Burn Us Out or Fire Us Up," 9, 11.

37. Sebastian Beck, "Die Müdigkeit der Rastlosen," in *Süddeutsche Zeitung*, March 14 and 15, 2009 (my translation).

38. The Austrian writer Kathrin Röggla has written a powerful and deeply unsettling, partly interview-based and partly fictionalized, account of the ways in which "management-speak" and the metaphors that twenty-first-century workers live by not just insidiously shape their conceptual view of the world and themselves but structure every aspect of their lived experiences. See Kathrin Röggla, *wir schlafen nicht* (Frankfurt am Main: Fischer, 2006).

39. Kury, *Der Überforderte Mensch*, 272–73.

40. See, for example, Andrew Procter and Elizabeth Procter, *The Essential Guide to Burnout: Overcoming Excess Stress* (Oxford: Lion Hudson, 2013).

41. Ibid., 41.

42. Ibid., 47.

43. Ibid., 181.

44. Steve Bagi, *Pastorpain: My Journey in Burnout* (Palm Beach, Australia: Actuate Consulting, 2008), 18, 8.

45. Donna Andronicus, *Coping with Burnout* (London: Sheldon Press, 2007), 10, 11.

46. Miriam Meckel, *Brief an Mein Leben: Erfahrungen mit einem Burnout* (Reinbek bei Hamburg: Rowohlt, 2010), 174, 172, 179–80 (all translations mine).

47. Greta Wagner, conversation with the author, February 4, 2015, Canterbury, England.

48. Meckel, *Brief an Mein Leben*, 31–33, 69–70.

49. Ibid., 73, 92, 93, 216–17.

50. James J. Bono, "Science, Discourse, and Literature: The Role/Rule of Metaphor in Science," in *Literature and Science: Theory and Practice*, ed. Stuart Peterfreund (Boston: Northeastern University Press, 1990), 75.

51. Graham Greene, *A Burnt-Out Case* (London: Vintage, 2004), 8, 42.

52. Ibid., 36.

53. Ibid., 101, 105.

54. Ibid., 8.

55. Ibid., 99, 101.

56. See, for example, Thomas Sprecher, ed., *Literatur und Krankheit im Fin-de-Siècle. Thomas Mann im Europäischen Kontext*, Die Davoser Literaturtage 2000 (Frankfurt am Main: Klostermann, 2002), especially the essays by Volker Roelcke, "Psychiatrische Kulturkritik um 1900 und Umrisse ihrer Rezeption im Frühwerk Thomas Manns," 95–113; Helmut Koopmann, "Krankheiten der Jahrhundertwende im Frühwerk Thomas Manns," 115–30; and Manfred Dierks, "Krankheit und Tod im frühen Werk Thomas Manns," 11–32. See also Manfred Dierks, "Buddenbrooks als Europäischer Nervenroman," *Thomas Mann Jahrbuch* 15 (2002): 135–52; and Joachim Radkau, "Neugier der Nerven. Thomas Mann als Interpret des nervösen Zeitalters," *Thomas Mann Jahrbuch* 9 (1996): 29–53.

57. Thomas Mann, *Death in Venice and Other Stories*, trans. David Luke (London: Vintage, 1998), 197; Thomas Mann, *Der Tod in Venedig und andere Erzählungen* (Frankfurt am Main: Fischer, 1954), 7.

58. Mann, *Death in Venice*.

59. Ibid. (translation modified).

60. Ibid., 200.

61. Ibid., 201 (translation slightly modified).

62. Ibid.

63. Ibid., 203, 205.

64. Ibid., 204–5.

65. Ibid., 205–6.

EPILOGUE

1. Frank Kermode, *The Sense of an Ending: Studies in the Theory of Fiction* (Oxford: Oxford University Press, 1968), 94–95.

2. Anson Rabinbach, *The Human Motor: Energy, Fatigue, and the Origins of Modernity* (Berkeley: University of California Press, 1992), 62.

3. Quoted in ibid.

4. Will Steffen et al., "Planetary Boundaries: Guiding Human Development on a Changing Planet," *Science*, February 13, 2015, http://dx.doi.org/10.1126/science.1259855 (accessed March 7, 2015).

5. See, for example, Bill McKibben, "Global Warming's Terrifying New Math: Three Simple Numbers That Add Up to Global Catastrophe—and That Make Clear Who the Real Enemy Is," *Rolling Stone*, July 19, 2012, http://www.rollingstone.com /politics/news/global-warmings-terrifying-new-math-20120719 (accessed March 8, 2015).

6. Quoted in Naomi Klein, "Don't Look Away Now: The Climate Crisis Needs You," *Guardian*, March 6, 2015, http://www.theguardian.com/environment/2015/mar /06/dont-look-away-now-the-climate-crisis-needs-you (accessed March 9, 2015).

7. Kevin Anderson, "To Meet International Commitments on '*Avoiding Dangerous Climate Change*,' Wealthy Nations Must Reduce Emissions by over 10% Each Year," *Svenska Dagbladet*, November 7, 2012, http://kevinanderson.info/blog/wp-content /uploads/2012/11/Opinion-Piece-by-Anderson-for-SvD-Swedish-Daily-Newspaper -Nov-2012.pdf (accessed March 8, 2015).

8. Steffen et al., "Planetary Boundaries."

9. Ibid.

10. Oliver Milman, "Rate of Environmental Degradation Puts Life on Earth at Risk, Say Scientists," *Guardian*, January 15, 2015, http://www.theguardian.com /environment/2015/jan/15/rate-of-environmental-degradation-puts-life-on-earth -at-risk-say-scientists (accessed March 7, 2015).

11. Naomi Klein, *This Changes Everything: Capitalism vs. the Climate* (New York: Simon & Schuster, 2014).

12. Pope Francis I, "On Care for Our Common Home" [encyclical letter], released June 18, 2015, http://w2.vatican.va/content/francesco/en/encyclicals/documents/papa -francesco_20150524_enciclica-laudato-si.html (accessed July 2, 2015).

13. Genesis 2:15.

14. Romans 8:22.

BIBLIOGRAPHY

Allen, Judith. *The Feminism of Charlotte Perkins Gilman: Sexualities, Histories, Progressivism*. Chicago: University of Chicago Press, 2009.

American Psychiatric Association, *Diagnostic and Statistical Manual of Mental Disorders*. 5th ed. Arlington, Va.: APA, 2013.

Anderson, Kevin. "To Meet International Commitments on '*Avoiding Dangerous Climate Change*,' Wealthy Nations Must Reduce Emissions by over 10% Each Year." *Svenska Dagbladet,* November 7, 2012. http://kevinanderson.info/blog/wp-content/uploads/2012/11/Opinion-Piece-by-Anderson-for-SvD-Swedish-Daily-Newspaper-Nov-2012.pdf.

Andronicos, Donna. *Coping with Burnout*. London: Sheldon Press, 2007.

Apollonius of Rhodes. *Jason and the Golden Fleece*. Translated by Richard Hunter. Oxford: Oxford University Press, 1993.

Appignanesi, Lisa. *Mad, Bad and Sad: A History of Women and the Mind Doctors from 1800 to the Present*. London: Virago, 2008.

Aquinas, Saint Thomas. *Summa Theologiae*. Translated by Thomas Gilby. Vol. 43, *Temperance*. London: Blackfriars in conjunction with Eyre & Spottiswoode, 1968.

——. *Summa Theologiae: A Concise Translation*. Edited by Timothy McDermott. London: Eyre & Spottiswoode, 1989.

Aristotle. *Problems*. Translated by W. S. Hett. Vol. 2. Cambridge, Mass.: Harvard University Press, 1957.

Bagi, Steve. *Pastorpain: My Journey in Burnout*. Palm Beach, Australia: Actuate Consulting, 2008.

Barthes, Roland. *How to Live Together: Novelistic Simulations of Some Everyday Spaces*. Translated by Kate Briggs. New York: Columbia University Press, 2012.

Beard, George M. *American Nervousness: Its Causes and Consequences. A Supplement to Nervous Exhaustion (Neurasthenia).* New York: Putnam, 1881.

——. *A Practical Treatise on Nervous Exhaustion (Neurasthenia): Its Symptoms, Nature, Sequences, Treatment.* New York: Wood, 1880.

Beck, Sebastian. "Die Müdigkeit der Rastlosen." *Süddeutsche Zeitung*, March 14 and 15, 2009.

Bell, Matthew. *Melancholia: The Western Malady.* Cambridge: Cambridge University Press, 2014.

Benjamin, Walter. *The Origin of German Tragic Drama.* Translated by John Osborne. London: NLB, 1977.

Bergengruen, Maximilian, Klaus Müller-Wille, and Caroline Pross, eds. *Neurasthenie. Die Krankheit der Moderne und die moderne Literatur.* Freiburg im Breisgau: Rombach, 2010.

Berman, Jeffrey. "The Unrestful Cure: Charlotte Perkins Gilman and 'The Yellow Wallpaper.'" In *The Captive Imagination: A Casebook on The Yellow Wallpaper*, edited by Catherine Colden, 211–41. New York: Feminist Press, 1992.

Boltanski, Luc, and Eve Chiapello. *The New Spirit of Capitalism.* Translated by Gregory Elliott. London: Verso, 2005.

Bono, James J. "Science, Discourse, and Literature: The Role/Rule of Metaphor in Science." In *Literature and Science: Theory and Practice*, edited by Stuart Peterfreund, 59–90. Boston: Northeastern University Press, 1990.

Bröckling, Ulrich. *Das unternehmerische Selbst. Soziologie einer Subjektivierungsform.* Frankfurt am Main: Suhrkamp, 2007.

Bugh, Glenn R. Introduction to *The Cambridge Companion to the Hellenistic World*, edited by Glenn R. Bugh, 1–8. Cambridge: Cambridge University Press, 2006.

Burton, Robert. *The Anatomy of Melancholy.* Oxford: Oxford University Press, 1989.

Cannon, Walter B. *The Wisdom of the Body.* London: Kegan Paul, Trench, Trübner, 1932.

Casiday, A. M. *Evagrius Ponticus: The Early Church Fathers.* Oxford: Routledge, 2006.

Cassian, John. *The Monastic Institutes.* Translated by Edgar C. S. Gibson. In *A Select Library of Nicene and Post-Nicene Fathers of the Christian Church*, edited by Henry Wace and Philip Schaff, 2nd ser., 11:183–641. New York: Christian Literature, 1894.

Centers for Disease Control and Prevention. Chronic Fatigue Syndrome (CFS). http://www.cdc.gov/cfs/causes/risk-groups.html.

Chaucer, Geoffrey. "The Parson's Tale." In *The Canterbury Tales.* Translated into modern English by Eugene J. Crook, 1993. http://english.fsu.edu/canterbury/parson. html.

Cheyne, George. *The English Malady: or, A Treatise of Nervous Diseases of all Kinds, as Spleen, Vapours, Lowness of Spirits, Hypochondriacal, and Hysterical Distempers, etc.* 6th ed. London: G. Strahan and J. Leake, 1735.

Craft, Christopher. "'Kiss Me with Those Red Lips': Gender and Inversion in Bram Stoker's Dracula." *Representations* 8 (1984): 107–33.

Crary, Jonathan. *24/7: Late Capitalism and the Ends of Sleep.* London: Verso, 2013.

Crawford, Heide. "Ernst Benjamin Salomo Raupach's Vampire Story 'Wake Not the Dead.'" *Journal of Popular Culture* 45, no. 6 (2012): 1189–1205.

Critchley, Simon, and Jamieson Webster. *The Hamlet Doctrine: Knowing Too Much, Doing Nothing.* New York: Verso, 2013.

Dabhoiwala, Faramerz. *The Origins of Sex: A History of the First Sexual Revolution.* London: Allen Lane, 2012.

Dante Alighieri. *The Divine Comedy.* Italian text with translation and comment by John D. Sinclair. Vol. 1, *Inferno.* Oxford: Oxford University Press, 1961.

——. *The Divine Comedy.* Italian text with translation and comment by John D. Sinclair. Vol. 2, *Purgatorio.* Oxford: Oxford University Press, 1961.

——. *The Divine Comedy.* Translated by Allen Mandelbaum. New York: Knopf, 1995.

Darwin, Charles. Darwin Correspondence Project. http://www.darwinproject.ac.uk/darwins-letters.

David, Anthony, and Simon Wessely. "Chronic Fatigue, ME and ICD-10." *Lancet* 342, no. 8881 (1993): 1247–48.

Derickson, Alan. *Dangerously Sleepy: Overworked Americans and the Cult of Manly Wakefulness.* Philadelphia: University of Pennsylvania Press, 2014.

Dierks, Manfred. "Buddenbrooks als Europäischer Nervenroman." *Thomas Mann Jahrbuch* 15 (2002): 135–52.

——. "Krankheit und Tod im frühen Werk Thomas Manns." In *Literatur und Krankheit im Fin-de-Siècle. Thomas Mann im Europäischen Kontext,* edited by Thomas Sprecher, 11–32. Die Davoser Literaturtage 2000. Frankfurt am Main: Klostermann, 2002.

Dillon, Brian. *The Hypochondriacs: Nine Tormented Lives.* New York: Faber and Faber, 2009.

Donini, Pierluigi. "Psychology." In *The Cambridge Companion to the Hellenistic World,* edited by Glenn R. Bugh, 184–209. Cambridge: Cambridge University Press, 2006.

Dorling, Danny. *Population 10 Billion.* London: Constable, 2013.

Dörr, Johanna, and Ulf Nater. "Erschöpfungssyndrome—Eine Diskussion verschiedener Begriffe, Definitionsansätze und klassifikatorischer Konzepte." *Psychotherapie, Psychosomatic, medizinische Psychologie* 63, no. 2 (2013): 69–76.

Dyer, Richard. "Children of the Night: Vampirism as Homosexuality, Homosexuality as Vampirism." In *Sweet Dreams: Sexuality, Gender and Popular Fiction,* edited by Susannah Radstone, 47–72. London: Lawrence and Wishart, 1988.

Ehrenberg, Alain. *The Weariness of the Self: Diagnosing the History of Depression in the Contemporary Age.* Translated by David Homel et al. Montreal: McGill-Queen's University Press, 2010.

Ekirch, A. Roger. *At Day's Close: Night in Times Past.* New York: Norton, 2006.

——. "The Modernization of Western Sleep: Or, Does Insomnia Have a History?" *Past and Present* 226 (2015): 149–92.

Emmott, Stephen. *Ten Billion.* London: Penguin, 2013.

Erb, Wilhelm. *Über die wachsende Nervosität unserer Zeit.* Heidelberg: Hörning, 1884.

Ficino, Marsilio. *Three Books on Life: A Critical Edition and Translation with Introduction and Notes.* Edited by Carol V. Kaske and John R. Clark. Medieval & Renaissance Texts & Studies, vol. 57. Tempe, Ariz.: Medieval & Renaissance Texts & Studies, 1998.

Finlay, Sue. "An Illness Doctors Don't Recognize." *Observer*, June 1, 1986.

Freud, Sigmund. "Beyond the Pleasure Principle" (1920). In *The Standard Edition of the Complete Psychological Works of Sigmund Freud*, edited and translated by James Strachey, 18:1–64. London: Vintage, 2001.

——. "'Civilized' Sexual Morality and Modern Nervous Illness" (1908). In *Standard Edition*, 9:177–204.

——. "Die Sexualität in der Ätiologie der Neurosen" (1898). In *Studienausgabe, Sexualleben*. Edited by Alexander Mitscherlich, Angela Richards, and James Strachey, 5:11–35. Frankfurt am Main: Fischer, 1982.

——. "The Ego and the Id" (1923). In *Standard Edition*, 19:1–66.

——. "Instincts and Their Vicissitudes" (1915). In *Standard Edition*, 14:109–40.

——. "Introductory Lectures on Psycho-Analysis (1916–1917 [1915–1917]): Part III. General Theory of the Neuroses (1917 [1916–1917]). Lecture XXIV: The Common Neurotic State." In *Standard Edition*, 16:378–91.

——. "Jenseits des Lustprinzips" (1920). In *Studienausgabe, Psychologie des Unbewußten*, 3:213–72.

——. "Mourning and Melancholia" (1917). In *Standard Edition*, 14:243–58.

——. "On the Grounds for Detaching a Particular Syndrome from Neurasthenia Under the Description 'Anxiety Neurosis'" (1895 [1894]). In *Standard Edition*, 3:85–117.

——. "Sexuality in the Aetiology of the Neuroses" (1898). In *Standard Edition*, 3:259–85.

——. "Triebe und Triebschicksale" (1915). In *Studienausgabe, Psychologie des Unbewußten*, 3:75–102.

Freudenberg, Herbert J. "Staff Burn-Out." *Journal of Social Issues* 30 (1974): 159–64.

Frey, Bruno S., and Alois Stutzer. *Happiness and Economics: How the Economy and Institutions Affect Human Well-Being.* Princeton, N.J.: Princeton University Press, 2001.

Galen. *On the Affected Parts.* Edited and translated by Rudolph E. Siegel. London: Karger, 1976.

——. *Selected Works.* Translated by P. N. Singer. Oxford: Oxford University Press, 1997.

Gijswijt-Hofstra, Marijke, and Roy Porter, eds. *Cultures of Neurasthenia from Beard to the First World War.* Amsterdam: Rodopi, 2001.

Gill, Christopher. *Naturalistic Psychology in Galen and Stoicism.* Oxford: Oxford University Press, 2010.

Gill, Christopher, Tim Whitmarsh, and John Wilkins, eds. *Galen and the World of Knowledge.* Cambridge: Cambridge University Press, 2009.

Gilman, Charlotte Perkins. *The Living of Charlotte Perkins Gilman: An Autobiography.* New York: Harper & Row, 1975.

——. "The Yellow Wallpaper." In *The Yellow Wall-Paper and Other Stories*. Edited by Robert Shulman, 3–19. Oxford: Oxford University Press, 1998.

Goethe, Johann Wolfgang von. *The Sorrows of Young Werther*. Translated by Michael Hulse. London: Penguin, 1989.

Goldacre, Ben. *Bad Pharma: How Drug Companies Mislead Doctors and Harm Patients*. London: Faber and Faber, 2013.

Goncharov, Ivan. *Oblomov*. Translated by Natalie Duddington. New York: Knopf, 1992.

Goodwin, Frederick, and Kay Renfield Jamison. *Manic-Depressive Illness*. New York: Oxford University Press, 1990.

Gorgievsky, Marjan J., and Stevan E. Hobfoll. "Work Can Burn Us Out or Fire Us Up: Conservation of Resources in Burnout and Engagement." In *Handbook of Stress and Burnout in Health Care*, edited by Jonathon R. B. Halbesleben, 7–22. New York: Nova Science, 2008.

Gosling, F. *Before Freud: Neurasthenia and the American Medical Community, 1870–1910*. Urbana: University of Illinois Press, 1987.

Greene, Graham. *A Burnt-Out Case*. London: Vintage, 2004.

Halbesleben, Jonathon R. B. Preface to *Handbook of Stress and Burnout in Health Care*, edited by Jonathon R. B. Halbesleben, vii–xi. New York: Nova Science, 2008.

Hankinson, R. J., ed. *The Cambridge Companion to Galen*. Cambridge: Cambridge University Press, 2008.

Hegel, G. F. *Aesthetics: Lectures on Fine Art*. Translated by T. M. Knox. 2 vols. Oxford: Clarendon Press, 1975.

Heuberger, Dagmar. "Das ist das historische Vorbild für den Rücktritt des Papsts." In *Aargauer Zeitung*, February 12, 2013. http://www.aargauerzeitung.ch/international/das-ist-das-historische-vorbild-fuer-den-ruecktritt-des-papstes-126050271.

Holgate, Stephen T., Anthony L. Komaroff, Dennis Mangan, and Simon Wessely. "Chronic Fatigue Syndrome: Understanding a Complex Illness." *Nature* 12 (2011): 539–44.

Horwitz, Allan V., and Jerome C. Wakefield, *The Loss of Sadness: How Psychiatry Transformed Normal Sorrow into Depressive Disorder*. New York: Oxford University Pres, 2007.

Hugh of Saint Victor. *On the Sacraments of the Christian Faith (De Sacramentis)*. Translated by Roy J. Deferrari. Cambridge, Mass.: Mediaeval Academy of America, 1951.

Huysmans, Joris-Karl. *À rebours*. Paris: Flammarion, 2004.

——. *Against Nature (A rebours)*. Translated by Margaret Mauldon. Oxford: Oxford University Press, 2009.

Jackson, Stanley W. *Melancholia and Depression: From Hippocratic Times to Modern Times*. New Haven, Conn.: Yale University Press, 1990.

Jafry, Nasim Marie. *The State of Me*. London: Friday Project, 2008.

——. "velo-gubbed-legs." http://velo-gubbed-legs.blogspot.co.uk/search/label/blinkered%20medics.

James, William. *The Energies of Men*. Milton Keynes, Eng.: Read Books, 2011.

Janet, Pierre. *Les obsessions et la psychasthénie*. 2 vols. Paris: Félix Alcan, 1903.

Johnson, Hillary. "Journey into Fear." *Rolling Stone*, July 30, 1987.

Kafka, Franz. *Briefe an Milena*. Frankfurt am Main: Fischer, 1998.

——. *The Diaries of Franz Kafka, 1910–1913*. Edited by Max Brod. London: Secker & Warburg, 1948.

Karjalainen, Antti. *International Statistical Classification of Diseases and Related Health Problems (ICD)*. 10th ed. Geneva: World Health Organization, 1999. http://apps.who.int/classifications/apps/icd/icd10online2003/fr-icd.htm?gf30.htm+.

Kaske, Carol V., and John R. Clark. Introduction to *Three Books on Life: A Critical Edition and Translation with Introduction and Notes*, by Marsilio Ficiono. Edited by Carol V. Kaske and John R. Clark, 3–90. Medieval & Renaissance Texts & Studies, vol. 57. Tempe, Ariz.: Medieval & Renaissance Texts & Studies, 1998.

Kermode, Frank. *The Sense of an Ending: Studies in the Theory of Fiction*. Oxford: Oxford University Press, 1968.

Kiecolt-Glaser, J. K., P. T. Marucha, W. B. Malarkey, A. M. Mercado, and R. Glaser. "Slowing of Wound Healing by Psychological Stress." *Lancet* 346 (1995): 1194–96.

Killen, Andreas. *Berlin Electropolis: Shock, Nerves, and German Modernity*. Berkeley: University of California Press, 2006.

Kirsch, Irving. *The Emperor's New Drugs: Exploding the Antidepressant Myth*. New York: Basic Books, 2010.

Klein, Melanie. *Love, Guilt and Reparation and Other Works, 1921–1945*. London: Hogarth Press, 1975.

Klein, Naomi. "Don't Look Away Now: The Climate Crisis Needs You." *Guardian*, March 6, 2015. http://www.theguardian.com/environment/2015/mar/06/dont-look-away-now-the-climate-crisis-needs-you.

——. *This Changes Everything: Capitalism vs. the Climate*. New York: Simon & Schuster, 2014.

Klostermann, Wolf-Günther. "Acedia und Schwarze Galle: Bemerkungen zu Dante, Inferno VII, 115ff." *Romanische Forschungen* 76, nos. 1–2 (1964): 183–94.

Koopmann, Helmut. "Krankheiten der Jahrhundertwende im Frühwerk Thomas Manns." In *Literatur und Krankheit im Fin-de-Siècle. Thomas Mann im Europäischen Kontext*, edited by Thomas Sprecher, 115–30. Die Davoser Literaturtage 2000. Frankfurt am Main: Klostermann, 2002.

Kradin, Richard L. *Pathologies of the Mind/Body Interface: Exploring the Curious Domain of the Psychosomatic Disorders*. New York: Routledge, 2013.

Kraepelin, Emil. *Manic Depressive Illness*. Translated by Mary Barclay, edited by George Robinson [from 8th edition of *Textbook of Psychiatry*, 1909–1915]. Edinburgh: Livingstone, 1920.

Krafft-Ebing, Freiherr Richard von. *Über Gesunde und Kranke Nerven*. 4th rev. and exp. ed. Tübingen: Verlag der H. Laupp'schen Buchhandlung, 1898.

Kraus, Karl. *Half-Truths and One-and-a-Half Truths: Selected Aphorisms*. Translated by Harry Zohn. Chicago: University of Chicago Press, 1990.

Krevans, Níta, and Alexander Sens. "Language and Literature." In *The Cambridge Companion to the Hellenistic World*, edited by Glenn R. Bugh, 186–207. Cambridge: Cambridge University Press, 2006.

Kury, Patrick. *Der Überforderte Mensch. Eine Wissensgeschichte vom Stress zum Burnout*. Frankfurt am Main: Campus, 2012.

Lakoff, George, and Mark Johnson. *Metaphors We Live By*. Chicago: University of Chicago Press, 2003.

Laqueur, Thomas W. *Solitary Sex: A Cultural History of Masturbation*. New York: Zone Books, 2003.

Law, Jenny. "The Active Patient: Energy, Desire and Active Recoveries." http://theactivepatient.wordpress.com.

Lawlor, Clark. *From Melancholia to Prozac: A History of Depression*. Oxford: Oxford University Press, 2012.

Layard, Richard. *Happiness: Lessons from a New Science*. London: Penguin, 2005.

Le Fanu, J. Sheridan. "Carmilla." In *In a Glass Darkly*. Oxford: Oxford University Press, 1993.

Leader, Darian. *The New Black: Mourning, Melancholia and Depression*. London: Penguin, 2009.

Leader, Darian, and David Corfield. *Why Do People Get Ill?* London: Hamish Hamilton, 2007.

Lee, Hermione. *Virginia Woolf*. London: Vintage, 1997.

Levi, Lennart. Foreword to *Emotional Stress: Physiological and Psychological Reactions. Medical, Industrial and Military Implications*, edited by Lennart Levi, 9–10. Basel: Karger, 1967.

——. "The Human Factor—and the Inhuman." In *Society, Stress and Disease*. Vol. 1, *The Psychosocial Environment and Psychosomatic Diseases*, edited by Lennart Levi, 3–4. London: Oxford University Press, 1971.

——. Preface to *Society, Stress and Disease*. Vol. 1, *The Psychosocial Environment and Psychosomatic Diseases*, edited by Lennart Levi, xi. London: Oxford University Press, 1971.

——. Preface to *Society, Stress and Disease*. Vol. 4, *Working Life*, xi–xiii. London: Oxford University Press, 1981.

Levi, Primo. *The Drowned and the Saved*. Translated by Raymond Rosenthal. New York: Summit Books, 1988.

——. *If This Is a Man / The Truce*. Translated by Stuart Wolf. London: Everyman's Library, 2000.

Lin, Tsung-Yi. "Neurasthenia Revisited: Its Place in Modern Psychiatry." *Culture, Medicine and Psychiatry* 13, no. 2 (1989): 105–29.

Lutz, Tom. *American Nervousness, 1903: An Anecdotal History*. Ithaca, N.Y.: Cornell University Press, 1991.

——. "Neurasthenia and Fatigue Syndromes." In *A History of Clinical Psychiatry: The Origins and History of Psychiatric Disorders*, edited by German E. Berrios and Roy Porter, 533–44. London: Athlone, 1995.

Macmillan, Malcolm. *Freud Evaluated: The Complete Arc.* Cambridge, Mass.: MIT Press, 1997.

Mann, Heinrich. "Doktor Biebers Versuchung." In *Haltlos: Sämtliche Erzählungen,* 1:494–550. Frankfurt am Main: Fischer, 1995.

Mann, Thomas. *Buddenbrooks.* Translated by H. T. Lowe-Porter. London: Vintage, 1999.

——. *Buddenbrooks. Verfall einer Familie.* Frankfurt am Main: Fischer, 2007.

——. *Death in Venice and Other Stories.* Translated by David Luke. London: Vintage, 1998.

——. *Der Tod in Venedig und andere Erzählungen.* Frankfurt am Main: Fischer, 1954.

Marx, Karl. *Capital: A Critique of Political Economy.* Translated by Ben Fowkes. Vol. 1. Harmondsworth: Penguin, 1976.

Mason, Rowena. "David Cameron Calls on Obese to Accept Help or Risk Losing Benefits." *Guardian,* February 14, 2015. http://www.theguardian.com/politics/2015 /feb/14/david-cameron-obese-addicts-accept-help-risk-losing-benefits.

Mattern, Susan P. *The Prince of Medicine: Galen in the Roman Empire.* Oxford: Oxford University Press, 2013.

McDougall, Joyce. *Theatres of the Body: A Psychoanalytical Approach to Psychosomatic Illness.* London: Free Association Books, 1989.

McKibben, Bill. "Global Warming's Terrifying New Math: Three Simple Numbers That Add Up to Global Catastrophe—and That Make Clear Who the Real Enemy Is." *Rolling Stone,* July 19, 2012. http://www.rollingstone.com/politics/news/global -warmings-terrifying-new-math-20120719.

ME Association. "What Is ME/CFS?" http://www.meassociation.org.uk/about/what -is-mecfs/.

Meckel, Miriam. *Brief an Mein Leben: Erfahrungen mit einem Burnout.* Reinbek bei Hamburg: Rowohlt, 2010.

Melville, Herman. "Bartleby, the Scrivener." In *Billy Budd, Sailor, and Selected Tales,* edited by Robert Milder, 1–41. Oxford: Oxford University Press, 1998.

Milman, Oliver. "Rate of Environmental Degradation Puts Life on Earth at Risk, Say Scientists." *Guardian,* January 15, 2015. http://www.theguardian.com/environment /2015/jan/15/rate-of-environmental-degradation-puts-life-on-earth-at-risk-say- scientists.

Mitchell, Silas Weir. *Fat and Blood and How to Make Them.* Edited by Michael S. Kimmel. 1882. Reprint, New York: Altamira Press, 2004.

——. *Wear and Tear: Or, Hints for the Overworked.* 5th rev. ed. Philadelphia: Lippincott, 1887.

Neckel, Sighard, and Greta Wagner, "Einleitung: Leistung und Erschöpfung." In *Leistung und Erschöpfung. Burnout in der Wettbewerbsgesellschaft,* edited by Sighard Neckel and Greta Wagner, 7–26. Frankfurt am Main: Suhrkamp, 2013.

——, eds. *Leistung und Erschöpfung. Burnout in der Wettbewerbsgesellschaft.* Frankfurt am Main: Suhrkamp, 2013.

Nordau, Max. *Degeneration.* Translated by George L. Mosse. Lincoln: University of Nebraska Press, 1993.

——. *Entartung.* 3rd ed. 2 vols. Berlin: Duncker, 1896.

Onania; or, the Heinous Sin of Self-Pollution, and All Its Frightful Consequences, in Both Sexes, Considered, with Spiritual and Physical Advice to Those Who Have Already Injur'd Themselves by This Abominable Practice. To which is Subjoin'd, A Letter from a Lady to the Author, [very curious] concerning the Use and Abuse of the Marriage-Bed, with the Author's Answer. 4th ed. London: Crouch, n.d.

Oosterhuis, Harry. *Stepchildren of Nature: Krafft-Ebing, Psychiatry, and the Making of Sexual Identity.* Chicago: University of Chicago Press, 2000.

Oppenheim, Janet. *"Shattered Nerves": Doctors, Patients, and Depression in Victorian England.* New York: Oxford University Press, 1991.

Papanghelis, Theodore D., and Antonios Rengakos, eds. *Brill's Companion to Apollonius Rhodius.* 2nd rev. ed. Leiden: Brill, 2008.

Peakman, Julie. "Sexual Perversion in History: An Introduction." In *Sexual Perversions, 1670–1890,* edited by Julie Peakman, 1–49. New York: Palgrave Macmillan, 2009.

Pickett, Kate, and Richard Wilkinson. *The Spirit Level: Why More Equal Societies Almost Always Do Better.* London: Penguin, 2009.

Pikkety, Thomas. *Capital in the Twenty-First Century.* Translated by Arthur Goldhammer. Cambridge, Mass.: Harvard University Press, 2014.

Poe, Edgar Allan. "The Fall of the House of Usher." In *The Collected Tales and Poems of Edgar Allan Poe,* 231–45. New York: Modern Library, 1992.

Pope Francis I. "On Care for Our Common Home" [encyclical letter], released June 18, 2015. http://w2.vatican.va/content/francesco/en/encyclicals/documents/papa-francesco_20150524_enciclica-laudato-si.html.

Post, Werner. *Acedia—Das Laster der Trägheit. Zur Geschichte der siebten Todsünde.* Freiburg: Herder, 2011.

Procter, Andrew, and Elizabeth Procter. *The Essential Guide to Burnout: Overcoming Excess Stress.* Oxford: Lion Hudson, 2013.

Proust, Marcel. *In Search of Lost Time.* Translated by C. K. Scott Moncrieff and Terence Kilmartin, revised by D. J. Enright. Vol. 1, *Swann's Way.* London: Vintage, 2002.

Rabinbach, Anson. *The Human Motor: Energy, Fatigue, and the Origins of Modernity.* Berkeley: University of California Press, 1990.

Radden, Jennifer. Introduction to *The Nature of Melancholy: From Aristotle to Kristeva,* edited by Jennifer Radden, 3–51. Oxford: Oxford University Press, 2000.

Radkau, Joachim. *Das Zeitalter der Nervosität. Deutschland zwischen Bismarck und Hitler.* Munich: Carl Hanser Verlag, 1998.

——. *Max Weber: A Biography.* Translated by Patrick Camiller. Cambridge: Polity, 2011.

——. "The Neurasthenic Experience in Imperial Germany: Expeditions into Patient Records and Side-Looks into General History." In *Cultures of Neurasthenia from Beard to the First World War*, edited by Marijke Gijswijt-Hofstra and Roy Porter, 199–218. Amsterdam: Rodopi, 2001.

——. "Neugier der Nerven. Thomas Mann als Interpret des nervösen Zeitalters." *Thomas Mann Jahrbuch* 9 (1996): 29–53.

Raffa, Guy P. *The Complete Danteworlds: A Reader's Guide to the Divine Comedy.* Chicago: University of Chicago Press, 2009.

Roelcke, Volker. *Krankheit und Kulturkritik. Psychiatrische Gesellschaftsdeutungen im bürgerlichen Zeitalter, 1790–1914.* Frankfurt am Main: Campus, 1999.

——. "Psychiatrische Kulturkritik um 1900 und Umrisse ihrer Rezeption im Frühwerk Thomas Manns." In *Literatur und Krankheit im Fin-de-Siècle. Thomas Mann im Europäischen Kontext*, edited by Thomas Sprecher, 95–113. Die Davoser Literaturtage 2000. Frankfurt am Main: Klostermann, 2002.

Röggla, Kathrin. *wir schlafen nicht.* Frankfurt am Main: Fischer, 2006.

Rosa, Hartmut. *Social Acceleration: A New Theory of Modernity.* Translated by Jonathan Trejo-Mathys. New York: Columbia University Press, 2013.

Rosario, Vernon A. *The Erotic Imagination: French Histories of Perversity.* New York: Oxford University Press, 1997.

Schaffner, Anna Katharina. *Modernism and Perversion: Sexual Deviance in Sexology and Literature, 1850–1930.* Basingstoke: Palgrave Macmillan, 2011.

Schaufeli, Wilhelm. "Past Performance and Future Perspectives on Burnout Research." *SA Journal of Industrial Psychology* 29, no. 4 (2003): 1–15.

Schaufeli, Wilhelm, Michael P. Leiter, and Christina Maslach. "Burnout: 35 Years of Research and Practice." *Career Development International* 14, no. 3 (2009): 204–20.

Scrivner, Lee. *Becoming Insomniac: How Sleeplessness Alarmed Modernity.* Basingstoke: Palgrave Macmillan, 2014.

Sebald, W. G. *Die Ringe des Saturn. Eine englische Wallfahrt.* Frankfurt am Main: Fischer, 1997.

——. *The Rings of Saturn.* Translated by Michael Hulse. London: Vintage, 2002.

Selye, Hans. *The Physiology and Pathology of Exposure to Stress: A Treatise Based on the Concepts of the General-Adaptation-Syndrome and the Diseases of Adaptation.* Montreal: Acta, 1950.

——. *The Stress of Life: Revised Edition.* New York: McGraw-Hill, 1976.

——. *Stress Without Distress.* London: Hodder and Stoughton, 1975.

Sennett, Richard. *The Corrosion of Character: The Personal Consequences of Work in the New Capitalism.* New York: Norton, 1998.

Shearer, Natasha. "As Work Related Stress Costs UK Economy Nearly £6.5bn Each Year, What Steps Should Businesses and Employees Be Taking?" *Huffington Post*, July 5, 2013. http://www.huffingtonpost.co.uk/natasha-shearer/work-related-stress-business_b_3545476.html.

Shorter, Edward. *Before Prozac: The Troubled History of Mood Disorders in Psychiatry.* Oxford: Oxford University Press, 2008.

——. *From Paralysis to Fatigue: A History of Psychosomatic Illness in the Modern Era.* New York: Free Press, 1992.

——. *How Everyone Became Depressed: The Rise and Fall of the Nervous Breakdown.* New York: Oxford University Press, 2013.

Showalter, Elaine. *The Female Malady: Women, Madness and English Culture, 1830–1980.* London: Virago, 1987.

——. *Hystories: Hysterical Epidemics and Modern Media.* New York: Columbia University Press, 1998.

Solomon, Andrew. *The Noonday Demon: An Anatomy of Depression.* London: Vintage, 2002.

Squires, Nick. "Pope's Final Address: God Was Asleep on My Watch." *Telegraph*, February 27, 2013. http://www.telegraph.co.uk/news/worldnews/the-pope/9896792/Popes-final-address-God-was-asleep-on-my-watch.html.

Steffen, Will, et al. "Planetary Boundaries: Guiding Human Development on a Changing Planet." *Science*, February 13, 2015. http://dx.doi.org/10.1126/science.1259855.

Stiglitz, Joseph. *The Price of Inequality: How Today's Divided Society Endangers Our Future.* New York: Norton, 2012.

Suzuki, T. "The Concept of Neurasthenia and Its Treatment in Japan." *Culture, Medicine and Psychiatry* 13, no. 2 (1989): 187–202.

Taylor, Shelley E. *Positive Illusions: Creative Self-Deception and the Healthy Mind.* New York: Basic Books, 1989.

Taylor, W. S. "Pierre Janet: 1859–1947." *American Journal of Psychology* 60 (1947): 637–45.

Tissot, Samuel-Auguste. *Onanism: Or, a Treatise upon the Disorders Produced by Masturbation: Or, the Dangerous Effects of Secret and Excessive Venery.* Translated by A. Hume, based on 3rd rev. ed. London: Wilkinson, 1767.

Todorov, Tzvetan. *The Fantastic: A Structural Approach to a Literary Genre.* Translated by Richard Howard. Ithaca, N.Y.: Cornell University Press, 1975.

Trier, Lars von. "Longing for the End of All." Interview with Niels Thorson. http://melancholiathemovie.com.

Tsakiridis, George. *Evagrius Ponticus and Cognitive Science: A Look at Moral Evil and the Thoughts.* Eugene, Ore.: Wipf and Stock, 2010.

Turner, Adair. *Economics After the Crisis: Objectives and Means.* Cambridge, Mass.: MIT Press, 2012.

Voß, G. Günter, and Hans J. Pongratz. "Der Arbeitskraftunternehmer. Eine neue Grundform der Ware Arbeitskraft?," *Kölner Zeitschrift für Soziologie und Sozialpsychologie* 1 (1998): 131–58.

Watters, Ethan. *Crazy Like Us: The Globalization of the American Psyche.* New York: Free Press, 2010.

Weber, Max. *The Protestant Ethic and the Spirit of Capitalism.* Translated by Talcott Parsons and Anthony Giddens. https://www.marxists.org/reference/archive/weber/protestant-ethic/index.htm.

——. *Die Protestantische Ethik und der Geist des Kapitalismus.* Edited by Dirk Kaesler. Munich: Beck, 2004.

Wenzel, Siegfried. *The Sin of Sloth: Acedia in Medieval Thought and Literature.* Chapel Hill: University of North Carolina Press, 1967.

Wessely, Simon. "Neurasthenia and Fatigue Syndromes." In *A History of Clinical Psychiatry: The Origins and History of Psychiatric Disorders,* edited by German E. Berrios and Roy Porter, 509–32. London: Athlone, 1995.

Wessely, Simon, Matthew Hotopf, and Michael Sharpe. *Chronic Fatigue and Its Syndromes.* Rev. ed. Oxford: Oxford University Press, 1999.

Wilde, Oscar. *More Letters of Oscar Wilde.* Edited by Rupert Hart-Davis. London: Murray, 1985.

Woolf, Virginia. *On Being Ill.* Introduction by Hermione Lee. Ashfield, Mass.: Paris Press, 2002.

World Health Organization. "Depression." Fact sheet, no. 369. October 2012. http://www.who.int/mediacentre/factsheets/fs369/en/.

——. *Investing in Mental Health.* Geneva: WHO, 2003. http://www.who.int/mental_health/media/investing_mnh.pdf.

Wurtzel, Elizabeth. *Prozac Nation: Young and Depressed in America. A Memoir.* London: Quartet Books, 1995.

Žižek, Slavoj. *Living in the End Times.* London: Verso, 2011.

INDEX

acedia: Cassian on, 34–38; Chaucer on, 43; in *The Divine Comedy*, 44–51; Evagrius on, 32–34; Hugh of Saint Victor on, 39–40; melancholia redefined as, 17, 31; modern, 180; as sin, 32; sociocultural context of, 197; symptoms and indicators of, 31; as term (etymology, definitions), 32, 38; Thomas Aquinas on, 40–42; work as antidote to, 36–38

adaptation energy, 205–9, 212. *See also* energy (human); stress

adrenaline, 205, 221

aestheticism, in *Against Nature*, 101–5

Against Nature (Huysman), 101–5

agency: acedia and, 33–34, 40–42, 46; Ficino on, 63; neoliberal and conservative views on, 42–43, 195–96, 220, 235; questions pertaining to, 11; sin vs. vice and, 39. *See also* personal responsibility; willpower

aging, 206, 236

agrarian societies, 117, 133. *See also* natural rhythms

Allen, Woody, 85

American Nervousness (Beard), 91. *See also* Beard, George M.

Anderson, Kevin, 239

Andronicus, Donna, 219

anhedonia, 180

animal spirits, 8, 86, 166. *See also* life energy

antibiotics, 196

Antichrist (Trier; film), 68

antidepressants, 12, 171–75, 179–80, 183

Antirrhetikos (Evagrius), 32–34

anxiety, 22, 29–30, 107, 151, 236. *See also* nervousness

apathy, 6, 31, 40–41, 43, 48–49, 52. *See also* inaction and paralysis; willpower

Apollonius of Rhodes, 22–29

appetite, loss of, 25, 26–27, 104, 176. *See also* diet

Argonautica (Apollonius), 23–29

Aristotle: Ficino and, 54; on melancholia, 17, 18, 127; on semen, 73; on sleep, 145–46; on sullenness, 46

asceticism, 123–24. *See also* Protestant work ethic

asthenic nervous diseases, 89–90

astrology, 53–55, 62–63. *See also* Ficino, Marsilio; Sebald, W. G.

automation, 211–12. *See also* factory work; technology

autonomy (freedom), as cause of depression, 181–83

Avicenna, 73, 76

bacterial-infection model, 200

Bagi, Steve, 218–19

balance: homeostasis, 204; in humoral theory, 15–16, 59–60, 204–5 (*see also* humoral theory); of nerve force, 93–94, 99; of work and rest, 143, 144 (*see also* rest). *See also* brain: chemical imbalance in

Barr, Y. M., 186

Barthes, Roland, 180

"Bartleby, the Scrivener" (Melville), 161–65

battery, as metaphor, 218–19

Baudelaire, Charles, 103

Beard, George M.: economic metaphors of, for nerve force, 6, 93–94; Freud and, 107, 151; on neurasthenia, 91–95, 105–6, 117, 177; sociocultural context of, 108–9, 139, 197

Beck, Sebastian, 216

belief, and illness, 193, 199–201, 234. *See also* chronic fatigue syndrome

Benedict XVI (pope), 1–2, 45

Benjamin, Walter, 57

Berufspflicht (duty to one's calling), 120–21

"Beyond the Pleasure Principle" (Freud), 116, 155–59

biomedical research, 15, 22, 192, 201, 244n.1

bipolar disorder, 28–29. See also *Argonautica*

black bile: Ficino on, 56–57, 59–60; in humoral theory, 16, 18–19, 46, 235 (*see also* humoral theory)

black moods, 19

blistering, 16

blood: bloodletting and leeching, 12, 16, 18; Ficino on, 55, 56, 59; Galen on, 16, 18, 19, 22, 46; Mitchell on, 137–38; stress response and, 205, 217, 218. *See also* vampires and vampirism

body: effect of, on mind/soul, 16–22, 246n.21; homeostasis and, 204; as machine, 87, 206, 218–19, 222; mind's effect on (Apollonius), 22–29; mind's effect on (Ficino), 56–57; mind's effect on (scientific), 29–30; sleep and, 145–46 (*see also* sleep); stress response of, 204–6, 218 (*see also* stress). *See also* brain; energy (human); immune system; nerves

Boltanski, Luc, 220

Bono, James J., 222

brain: as battery, 90; chemical imbalance in, 15, 21, 116, 172, 181 (*see also* antidepressants; medication; serotonin); as computer, 219–23; and melancholia, 18–19, 56; mental illness as disease of, 198; neurotransmitters in, 15, 172, 221; overstimulation and overwork of, 134–35, 139–40, 144 (*see also* rest: rest cure); sleep and, 145, 146. *See also* "brain work"; cognitive impairment; mind

"brain work": burnout and, 227; exhaustion theories and, 9, 236; Freud on, 150; gender ideology and, 140–42 (*see also* women); limited by Darwin, 144; melancholia and, 17, 55–57; neurasthenia and, 92–94, 104, 105, 134, 136, 203. *See also* acedia; creativity; genius

Brown, John, 89–90

Brunonian theory, 89–90

Buddenbrooks (T. Mann), 125–27
burnout: causes of, 9, 204, 212–13 (*see also* stress); defined by its opposites, 180; definitions of, 213–16; economic and social costs of, 38, 216–17; frequent diagnosis of, 4; individual experiences with, 218–23; in literature, 223–32; symptoms of, 6, 213–14, 215, 223; treatment suggestions for, 217–18; twenty-first-century discourses on, 203–4, 216, 217, 220; valorization of, 95, 218, 231
Burnt-Out Case, A (Greene), 223–26
Byron, Lord, 81

Calvin, John, 123
Cameron, David, 43
candida, 196
Cannon, Walter B., 204
Canterbury Tales, The (Chaucer), 43
Capital (*Das Kapital*; Marx), 80
Capital in the Twenty-First Century (Pikkety), 129
capitalism: age of greed and, 195–96; burnout as economic problem of, 38, 216–17; climate change and, 238, 240; disenchantment with (capitalism fatigue), 128–31; Francis I on, 241–42; in literature, 114, 125–27, 164 (*see also specific works*); Mitchell on, 140; modern preoccupation with exhaustion and, 9; natural rhythms disrupted by, 117, 133–34, 147–48; nerve force, energy likened to capital, 93–94, 99, 119, 139–40; psychological costs of, 117–18, 131 (see also *Buddenbrooks*; burnout); stress and, 210–12; traditionalism vs., 121–22, 254n.13; vampirism as metaphor for, 80; Weber on, 120–24. *See also* work
Carmilla (Le Fanu), 80–84
Cassian, Saint John, 34–38, 177

catastrophes, in *Melancholia*, 69–70
Celestine V (pope), 2, 45
Centers for Disease Control and Prevention (CDC), 187, 195
Chaucer, Geoffrey, 43
Cheyne, George, 61, 87–89, 108–9
Chiapello, Eve, 220
childhood, desire to return to, 113–14
China, 66, 108. See also *qi*
Christian theology. *See* acedia; *Canterbury Tales, The*; *Divine Comedy, The*; Francis I; religion; sin
Chronic Fatigue and Its Syndromes (Wessely), 196. *See also* Wessely, Simon
chronic fatigue immune dysfunction syndrome (CFIDS). *See* chronic fatigue syndrome
chronic fatigue syndrome (CFS): coexisting physical conditions of, 187; controversy over psychological aspects of, 189–94, 198–99, 201; Darwin and, 143; depression and, 191, 199; diagnostic criteria of, 186, 259n.9; dietary restrictions with, 61; emergence of, as diagnosis, 184–85; frequent diagnosis of, 4, 195; individual experiences with, 187–91; sociocultural developments and, 195–98; suspected causes of, 184–87, 191–94, 196–99; symptoms of, 5, 184–87, 188–89; terms for, 184, 259n.1; treatment of, 187
civilization: decline of, 23–24, 103; degeneration theory and, 77–79 (*see also* degeneration theory); Freud on sexual drive and, 151–54; nervous weakness and, in *Buddenbrooks*, 125–27; neurasthenia as disease of, 92, 95–100, 105, 117. *See also* capitalism; sociocultural developments; technology; work

Civilization and Its Discontents (Freud), 151–54, 158–59

"'Civilized' Sexual Morality and Modern Nervous Illness" (Freud), 151–52

climate change, 3, 238–41

cognitive behavioral theory, 17, 40

cognitive behavioral therapy (CBT), 12, 181, 191, 192, 222–23

cognitive impairment: as acedia symptom, 31, 35–36; as burnout symptom, 221; as chronic fatigue syndrome symptom, 184, 186; clouded judgment and, 19; as depression symptom, 176–77; difficulty concentrating and, 21, 35–36, 107, 146, 176–77, 184, 186, 221; as exhaustion symptom, 21, 233; lack of sleep and, 145, 146; as melancholia symptom, 59; as neurasthenia symptom, 107

coldness: of feet, 6, 91; of heart, 26, 43; in humoral theory, 16, 19; in Le Fanu, 83; melancholia and, 56, 59; Saturn associated with, 54, 55; as stressor, 205

colonial oppression, Freud on, 154

"Common Neurotic State, The" (Freud), 151

concentration, difficulty with, 21, 35–36, 107, 146, 176–77, 184, 186, 221

concentration camps, 167–68

conservation of resources (COR) theory, 214–15

contrapasso, law of, 45

Corfield, David, 29, 199–200, 244n.11, 246n.37

cortisol, 217

Crary, Jonathan, 147–49

creativity, 17, 54, 127. *See also* "brain work"

cruelty, human, 66, 67

culture(s): decline of, 23–24, 77–79, 103 (*see also* degeneration theory); Ehrenberg on depression and,

181–83; Freud on, 153–55, 159; "lateness" of, and ennui/decadence, 5; stress and, 210–12. *See also* agrarian societies; civilization; sociocultural developments; technology

Dante Alighieri, 44–51

darkness, and melancholia, 18–19

Darwin, Charles, 94, 142–44

David, Anthony, 259n.9

Dead in Love, The (Gautier), 80

death: adaptation energy depletion and, 206, 207; death drive (death wish), 69, 115–16, 150, 157–65, 167–68, 178 (*see also* suicide and suicidal thoughts); fear of, 13, 236; in literature, 65–66, 82; "too tired to die," 170, 174

Death in Venice (T. Mann), 226–32

decadence, 101–5

decay, in *The Rings of Saturn*, 64–65

Degeneration (Nordau), 78, 94

degeneration theory, 77–79, 94–95, 100, 105. See also *Against Nature*

demons and demonic possession, 10, 32–33, 34

depression: antidepressants and, 12, 171–75, 179–80, 183; atypical, 173; autonomy (freedom) as cause of, 181–83; behavioral symptoms of, 6, 18, 25, 175, 176–77, 181–83; biomedical research on, 15, 22, 244n.1; bipolar disorder and, 28–29; burnout and, 216; as chemical imbalance in brain, 15, 21, 172, 181 (*see also* antidepressants); chronic fatigue syndrome and, 191, 199; debate over causes of, treatments for, 181–82; diet and exercise and, 20; economic and social costs of, 38; exhaustion as symptom of, 3, 5, 6, 175–77; frequent diagnosis of, 3–4, 108, 172; genetic predisposition to, 19; individual experiences with, 169–70, 173–75,

177–80 (*see also specific individuals*);
mental/emotional symptoms of, 6,
159, 176–77, 180, 181–83; modern epidemic of, 9; negative attention and
memory biases and, 19; neurasthenia
and, 107–8 (*see also* neurasthenia);
"noonday demon" and, 33, 177–80;
official diagnoses of, 176–77; psychological treatments for (*see* cognitive
behavioral therapy; psychoanalytic
theory and psychoanalysis; psychotherapy); as realistic worldview,
68, 70–71, 180; rise of, as diagnosis,
107–8, 170; statistics for, 172. *See
also* acedia; despair; despondency;
melancholia; *specific symptoms*
Descartes, René, 86
Desert Fathers, 32. *See also* Evagrius
Ponticus
despair, 24–29, 39–40, 43. *See also*
depression; despondency
despondency, 20, 24–29. *See also*
depression; despair
*Diagnostic and Statistical Manual of
Mental Disorders* (*DSM*), 106, 176–77
diet, 12; melancholia and, 19–20, 60–61;
nervous weakness and, 88–89; neurasthenia and, 104; refusal of nourishment, 25, 26–27 (*see also* appetite,
loss of); Sebald's description of fish
and chips and, 64; vegetarian, 88, 89
digestive disorders, 76, 91, 104
Divine Comedy, The (Dante), 44–51
Dracula (Stoker), 80
Dr. Bieber's Temptation (H. Mann),
96–97, 98
dreams, 146
Drowned and the Saved, The (P. Levi),
167
*DSM. See Diagnostic and Statistical
Manual of Mental Disorders*
Dürer, Albrecht, 58
Dyer, Richard, 81

eccentrics, 65
economic metaphors. *See* metaphors
and similes: economic, for energy,
nerve force
education, of women, 139–40
ego, 39, 46, 150, 156–57, 159–61, 165,
170–71. *See also* Freud, Sigmund
Ehrenberg, Alain, 58, 171, 181–83,
220
Ekirch, Roger, 146–47
élan vital, 8, 166. *See also* life energy
electricity, 87, 90
electrotherapy, 12, 90, 119
Eliot, T. S., 109–10
emetics, 12, 16
emotional exhaustion, 5. *See also*
burnout; depression; melancholia;
neurasthenia
encephalomyelitis, 185. *See also* chronic
fatigue syndrome
endocrinology, 205, 207–8, 217, 218
energy (generally), 238. *See also* thermodynamics, second law of
energy (human): adaptation energy, 212;
in astrological doctrine, 53; burnout
and, 218–19; concentration camp
survival and, 167–68; in COR theory,
215; depressives' lack of, 173–74,
176–79, 183; in *The Divine Comedy*,
44–45, 47–51; energy conservation
theory (sleep) and, 145; Ficino on,
61–63; Freud on, 150–61, 165, 171;
Janet's energy-insufficiency model,
165–66, 257n.32; as limited resource,
6–7; as opposite of exhaustion, 8;
rarely defined or quantified, 167;
scientific model of, lacking, 8, 234;
sexual activities and, 73, 75–77,
81–82, 151–52; stress and, 205–9, 217;
Western vs. Eastern models of, 8,
108, 208. *See also* chronic fatigue
syndrome; exhaustion; life energy;
nerve force

English Malady, The (Cheyne), 87–89
environment, concerns about, 31, 196, 237–42
epistemes, 198
Epstein, Michael, 186
Epstein-Barr virus (EBV), 186
Erb, Wilhelm, 97–98, 151
Essential Guide to Burnout, The (Procter and Procter), 217–18
Evagrius Ponticus, 32–34, 38
evolutionary biology, 94. *See also* degeneration theory
exercise, 12, 20, 60–61
exhaustion: core cultural values and, 12, 124; core symptoms of diagnoses related to, 5, 21, 177, 223 (*see also specific symptoms and diagnoses*); defined by its opposites, 7–8; definition of, 4–8; economic and social costs of, 38, 216–17; historical changes in perception of dominant symptoms of, 9–11, 12, 233–34; historical explanations of, 11–12 (*see also specific diagnoses and theories*); as key theme in *Argonautica*, 28–29 (see also *Argonautica*); mental or social causation theories of, 235–36 (*see also* acedia; chronic fatigue syndrome; depression; Freud, Sigmund; neurasthenia; personal responsibility; sin); opposites of, 7–8; one's own era as most exhausted, 8–9, 88–89, 148, 236, 237; organic causation theories of, 235–36 (*see also* brain: chemical imbalance in; chronic fatigue syndrome; depression; humoral theory; nerves; neurasthenia; viruses); primordial fears and, 13; as result of stress response, 205–7; sexual activities and, 60, 73–74, 75, 84 (*see also* sex and sexuality); as term (origins, etymology, associations), 6–8. *See also* mental

exhaustion; physical exhaustion; spiritual exhaustion; *specific symptoms, diagnoses, and topics*

factory work, 117–18, 202–3, 211–12
faith: acedia and, 17, 38, 40 (*see also* acedia); desire for, 104; lukewarm, 45. See also *Divine Comedy, The*; religion
"Fall of the House of Usher, The" (Poe), 85
Fat and Blood and How to Make Them (Mitchell), 137
fatigue: acedia and, 35 (*see also* acedia); psychasthenia and, 165–66; saturnine disposition and, 54; "science" of, 202–3; as symptom of depression/melancholia, 59, 176 (*see also* depression; melancholia); as warning signal, 133–34. *See also* chronic fatigue syndrome; weariness
Fatigue (Mosso), 203
fear, 20, 46, 52, 54, 67, 91. *See also* anxiety
Ferenczi, Sándor, 77
feudalism, in *Oblomov*, 112–13
fibromyalgia, 185. *See also* chronic fatigue syndrome
Ficino, Marsilio, 52–63, 71, 73–74, 127, 177, 197. *See also* melancholia; Saturn
fiction, 13–14. *See also specific works*
fisherman, parable of, 121–22, 254n.13
food. *See* diet
Foucault, Michel, 198, 220
Francis I (pope), 240–42
freedom (autonomy), and depression, 181–83
frenzy, 54
Freud, Sigmund: on agency and willpower, 42; on death drive, 116, 150, 157–59, 160–61, 165; dual-drive theory of, 8, 155–59, 160–61, 165; influence of, 170; on Janet's model, 166; on life drive, 8, 150, 157–58, 165;

on melancholia, 17, 46, 159–61, 170–71; on sexuality and sexual behavior, 77, 78, 107, 150–55, 160, 165
Freudenberger, Herbert J., 213

Galen of Pergamum: on "animal spirits" and nerves, 8, 86; Ficino and, 52, 53, 54, 61; humoral theory of, 15–22, 46; on melancholia, 16–22, 46, 177; on seminal expulsion, 73; on soul/spirit, 20–22, 57, 246n.21
Galvani, Luigi, 87
Gautier, Théophile, 80
gender. See women
genes and heredity: adaptation energy and, 207; degeneration theory and, 77–78, 94–95, 100; depression and, 19; Janet on energy levels and, 166; neurasthenia and, 100, 105
genius, 17, 54, 127. See also creativity
Gilman, Charlotte Perkins, 135–38, 139, 144
Goncharov, Ivan, 111–16, 131
Gorgievsky, Marjan J., 214–15
Gothic, 79. See also vampires and vampirism
Greece, ancient, 8, 23–24. See also Argonautica; Aristotle; Galen of Pergamum; Hippocrates; humoral theory
Greene, Graham, 223–26
Gregory I the Great (pope), 38
Gregory XII (pope), 45
grief. See sadness
Griesinger, Wilhelm, 198

Hamlet (Shakespeare), 57
happiness, 129–30, 152–53
Harvey, William, 222
headache, 104, 107, 186
Hegel, G. F., 57
Helmholtz, Hermann von, 238
heredity. See genes and heredity

Hippocrates, 15, 20, 46, 53, 74
Hobfoll, Stevan E., 214–15
Holocaust, 67, 167–68
homeostasis, 204
homosexuality, vampires associated with, 80–84
hopelessness: as acedia symptom, 31, 33, 43; as depression symptom, 176–77; in literature, 24–29, 48–49, 66, 67; as melancholia symptom, 52, 59; as neurasthenia symptom, 91
hormones. See endocrinology
Hugh of Saint Victor, 39–40, 41
human energy. See energy (human)
human-services sector, 213–14
humoral theory, 15–22, 46, 55–56, 59–60, 72–74, 204–5. See also Ficino, Marsilio; Galen of Pergamum; melancholia
Huysman, Joris-Karl, 101–5
hydrotherapy, 12, 90, 119, 143–44
hypersensitivity, 87
hypochondria, 87, 98, 108, 125, 143
hysteria, 10, 87, 92, 140–41, 185, 193
Hystories (Showalter), 193

ICD-10. See International Classification of Diseases
id, 150, 156–57, 161, 165. See also Freud, Sigmund
identity and work, 13, 118, 120, 228–29
idleness, 36–37, 43. See also apathy; inaction and paralysis; lethargy; rest
If This Is a Man (P. Levi), 167–68
Imipramine, 172
immune system, 30, 196, 197, 235, 246n.41
inaction and paralysis: in literature, 25, 26, 57 (see also apathy); Paul on, 36; Sebald and, 64, 67
industrialization, 117–18, 133–34, 202–3. See also capitalism; technology; work

inequality, 128–30
inferiority, sense of, 160, 170–71, 181–83.
   See also worthlessness, sense of
information overload, 220–23
In Search of Lost Time (Proust), 98, 106
insomnia, 91, 104, 107, 147, 176. *See also*
   sleep
"Instincts and Their Vicissitudes"
   (Freud), 155–56
intellectual patients. *See* "brain work";
   creativity; genius; *specific individuals
   and fictional works*
International Classification of Diseases
   (*ICD-10*), 106–7, 176–77, 215–16,
   259n.9
Iproniazid, 171–72
irritability: as acedia symptom, 31, 32,
   33; in "Bartleby, the Scrivener," 161,
   163; as exhaustion symptom, 5; as
   melancholia symptom, 17, 21; nerves
   and, 87, 91; as neurasthenia symptom, 6, 91–92, 100, 107, 177 (see also
   Against Nature)

Jafry, Nasim Marie, 187–92
James, Henry, 96
James, William, 246n.34
Janet, Pierre-Marie-Félix, 165–66
Japan, 108
Jason and the Golden Fleece, 22–29
Johnson, Mark, 244n.11

Kafka, Franz, 96, 182
Kermode, Frank, 237
Klein, Naomi, 240
Kline, Nathan, 172
Klosterman, Wolf-Günther, 46
Knox, John, 123
Krafft-Ebing, Richard von: degeneration
   theory and, 94; dietary suggestions
   of, 61; Freud and, 107, 151; influenced
   by Darwin, 142; on neurasthenia,
   98–100, 105–6, 117, 177; sociocultural

context of, 108–9; on women and
   work, 141
Kraus, Karl, 98
Kuhn, Roland, 171–72
Kury, Patrick, 204

Lakoff, George, 244n.11
languor, 81–83
Laqueur, Thomas, 74–75
Lazarus, Richard S., 210
laziness, 47, 48, 112. *See also* apathy; lethargy; *Oblomov*; sloth
Leader, Darian, 29, 199–200, 244n.11,
   246n.37
lechery, 74. *See also* sex and sexuality
Le Fanu, Sheridan, 80–84
Leiter, Michael, 214
lesbianism, 80–84
lethargy: as acedia symptom, 31, 33,
   35–36 (*see also* acedia); as melancholia symptom, 18, 20, 52, 59 (*see
   also* melancholia); as neurasthenia
   symptom, 6 (*see also* neurasthenia);
   in *Oblomov*, 111–13
Levi, Lennart, 210–12
Levi, Primo, 167–68
Lewis, Matthew, 79
libido. *See* life drive, theories of; sex and
   sexuality
life drive, theories of, 8, 150, 157–58
life energy: nerves and, 86, 87, 90 (*see
   also* nerve force); sexual activities
   and, 73, 75–77, 81–82; vampirism and,
   80, 81–83, 208–9 (*see also* vampires
   and vampirism); Western and Eastern models of, 8, 108, 208. *See also*
   energy (human)
literature, 13–14. *See also specific works*
Lombroso, Cesare, 78
loss, and melancholia, 159–60, 171. *See
   also* sadness
love, 49, 68, 179–80
Lowestoft, England, 65

Luther, Martin, 123

Magic Mountain, The (T. Mann), 98
Mallarmé, Stéphane, 103
Malthus, Thomas Robert, 238
manic depression (bipolar disorder),
28–29. See also *Argonautica*
Mann, Heinrich, 96–97, 98
Mann, Thomas, 98, 125–27, 131, 226–32
Mars, 53–54
Marx, Karl, 117–18
Maslach, Christina, 213–14
masturbation, 60, 72–73, 74–77, 79, 81,
151. *See also* sex and sexuality
meat, 19–20, 88, 89
Meckel, Miriam, 219–23
medical discourses: bacterial-infection
model, 200; on chronic fatigue
syndrome, 184–87, 189, 191–94,
198–99, 201 (*see also* chronic fatigue
syndrome); gender and diagnosis,
137–42; monocausal external-agent
illness models, 200; on nerves,
86–94 (*see also* neurasthenia);
referenced by exhaustion-based
syndromes, 197; on sex and sexuality,
60, 72–73, 75–77, 79, 81–82, 84 (*see
also* sex and sexuality); sociocul-
tural/historical developments and,
11, 95, 108–9, 233; symptoms shaped
by, 10–11, 193, 200–201. *See also
specific diagnoses and topics*
medication, 12, 171–75, 179–80, 183. *See
also* tonics
melancholia: Cheyne on, 87; creativity/
genius and, 17, 54, 127; exhaustion
as symptom of, 5, 17; as fashionable
disease, 96; Ficino on, 55–63 (*see also*
Ficino, Marsilio); Freud on, 17, 46,
159–61, 170–71 (*see also* Freud, Sigmund); Galen on, 15–22, 46 (*see also*
Galen of Pergamum); in literature
and film, 22–29, 63–71, 82; mastur-

bation and, 76; melancholic/satur-
nine temperament, 54, 57, 59–60;
sociohistorical models/explanations
of, 17, 31; symptoms and associated
complaints of, 16–17, 19, 20, 46, 52,
67, 159 (*see also specific symptoms*);
valorization of, 17, 53, 54, 70–71. *See
also* acedia; depression
Melancholia (Trier; film), 67–71, 180
Melencolia I (Dürer), 58
Melville, Herman, 161–65
mental exhaustion, 107, 134–35. See also
Against Nature; cognitive impairment; depression; melancholia;
neurasthenia
mental illness, psychiatric vs. biological origins of, 198. *See also specific
diagnoses*
Mercury, 55
metaphors and similes: body as
machine, 87, 206, 218–19, 222; brain
as computer, 219–23; economic, for
energy, nerve force, 93–94, 99, 119,
139–40, 206–7; energy vampire, 219;
influence of, 6–7, 234–35, 262n.38;
life stages, for stress, 206; military,
in immunological arguments, 197;
vampirism, for capitalism, 80; vine
and oak tree, 177–79
Michels, Robert, 119–20
Middle Ages: demonic possession
in, 10; melancholia redefined as
acedia in, 17, 31 (*see also* acedia);
sloth, concept of, in, 31–32; views on
sexual activity in, 72, 73–74. *See also*
Avicenna; Chaucer, Geoffrey; Dante
Alighieri; Ficino, Marsilio
mind: belief and illness, 10, 193, 199–201,
234 (*see also* chronic fatigue syndrome: controversy over psychological aspects of); body affected by
(Apollonius), 22–29; body affected
by (Ficino), 56–57, 74; body affected

mind (*continued*)
by (scientific), 29–30; body's effect on, 16–22; as computer, 220–22; difficulty concentrating and, 21, 35–36, 107, 146, 176–77, 184, 186, 221; Freud's dual-drive theory of, 155–59; overstimulation, overwork, and, 134–35 (*see also* rest: rest cure); positive thinking and, 29. *See also* brain; cognitive behavioral therapy; depression; mental exhaustion; psychoanalytic theory and psychoanalysis; psychology; psychotherapy
Mitchell, Silas Weir, 61, 90, 134–35, 137–38, 139–41, 197
Modern Times (Chaplin; film), 202
Monastic Institutes, The (Cassian), 34–35. *See also* Cassian, Saint John
monastic life. *See* acedia
Monk, The (Lewis), 79
monogamy, 152
Morel, Bénédict Augustin, 77–78
Morita therapy, 108
Mosso, Angelo, 203
"Mourning and Melancholia" (Freud), 159–60, 170–71
Mrs. Dalloway (Woolf), 139
music, 60, 61–62, 69
myalgic encephalomyelitis (ME). *See* chronic fatigue syndrome

natural resources, depletion of, 3, 237–38, 241. *See also* climate change
natural rhythms, 8–9, 117, 133–34, 146–48, 213
neoliberalism, 42–43, 195–96, 220, 235, 238
nerve force: definition of, 87; lack of, 86, 90, 91, 106; limited supply of, 6, 87, 90, 93–94, 119, 139–40; management (balance) of, 6, 93–94, 99, 119–20. *See also* energy (human); nerves; neurasthenia

nerves: eighteenth- and nineteenth-century beliefs about, 86–94; Galen on, 86; imagery of, 109; twenty-first-century understanding of, 86; weak (nervous weakness), 87–88, 91, 93–94, 99–100, 126–27, 235 (*see also* Cheyne, George; neurasthenia; rest: rest cure). *See also* nerve force; nervous breakdown; nervousness; neurasthenia
"nervous age," 90–91. *See also* nerves; nervousness
nervous breakdown, 109–10, 118–19
nervousness: cultural, 90–91; as disposition, 84–85, 93–94, 104–5 (*see also* neurasthenia); as symptom of exhaustion, 5. *See also* anxiety
neurasthenia: antipathy toward patients/diagnosis of, 98, 193; Beard on, 6, 91–95, 105–6, 107, 108–9, 117, 139 (*see also* Beard, George M.); burnout compared with, 227; chronic fatigue syndrome compared with, 196–97; civilization/technology and, 92, 95, 96–98, 99–100, 105, 117; as diagnosis (definition, origins, influence), 91–92, 106–8, 170, 253n.46, 259n.9; Freud on sexuality and, 150–55; individual experiences with, 96, 109–10, 118–20, 137–39; intellect/class and, 92–93, 104, 105, 136 (*see also* "brain work"); Krafft-Ebing on, 98–100, 105–6, 107, 108–9, 117 (*see also* Krafft-Ebing, Richard von); in literature, 96–98, 101–6, 109–10, 135–37, 139, 226–27; masturbation linked to exhaustion and, 76–77, 151 (*see also* masturbation); national variations of, 108, 252n.19; as organic disorder, 91–92, 105–6; popularity of, 95–99, 106–7, 170; as postexertion malaise, 134; symptoms and associated complaints if, 5, 6, 17,

91, 104, 106–7, 108; types of, 106–7;
valorization of, 92–93, 95; women
and, 135–42. *See also* nerves; nervous
breakdown; psychasthenia; rest: rest
cure
neuro-linguistic programming (NLP),
222–23
neurotransmitters, 15, 172, 221
Nirvana principle, 116, 158. *See also*
Freud, Sigmund: on death drive
"noonday demon," 32–33, 34
Noonday Demon, The (Solomon),
177–80
Nordau, Max, 78, 94
norepinephrine, 15
Nymphomaniac (Trier; film), 68

obesity, 89
Oblomov (Goncharov), 111–16
Obsessions et la psychasthénie, Les
(*Obsession and Pschyasthenia*; Janet),
165–66
occupational therapy, 12, 90
Occupy movement, 130–31
Odysseus, 24
*Onania; or, the Heinous Sin of Self-
Pollution* (anon.), 75
"On Being Ill" (Woolf), 139
"On Care for Our Common Home"
(Francis I), 240–42
On Healthy and Sick Nerves (Krafft-
Ebing), 98–100. *See also* Krafft-
Ebing, Richard von
On the Affected Parts (Galen), 18. *See
also* Galen of Pergamum
"On the Grounds for Detaching a Par-
ticular Syndrome from Neurasthe-
nia Under the Description 'Anxiety
Neurosis'" (Freud), 151
On the Origin of Species (Darwin), 94
*On the Sacraments of the Christian
Faith* (Hugh of Saint Victor), 39–40
Oosterhuis, Harry, 78

Oppenheim, Janet, 94
orphic dancing, 61–62

pain, in chronic fatigue syndrome, 186
paralysis. *See* inaction and paralysis
past, nostalgia for, 8, 9–10, 88–89, 100,
148–49, 209
Pastorpain (Bagi), 218–19
Paul, Saint, 36, 43
personality traits, 16. *See also*
temperament
personal responsibility: acedia and,
41–42; burnout and, 217; depression/
melancholia and, 171, 181–83; desire
for freedom from, 113–14; exhaustion
caused by behavioral choices, 84;
Ficino on, 63; neoliberalism/politi-
cal conservatism and, 42–43, 195–96,
220, 235; for stress management,
206–7. *See also* agency; willpower
pessimism, 52, 70–71, 154–55
phlegm, in humoral theory, 16, 21, 59
physical exhaustion: in chronic fatigue
syndrome, 187–89 (*see also* chronic
fatigue syndrome); in literature and
film, 27–28, 44–45, 47–49, 51, 69; in
neurasthenia, 107 (see also *Against
Nature*; neurasthenia); symptoms of,
5, 44–45, 66–67. *See also* depression;
melancholia
Pikkety, Thomas, 129, 130
placebo effect, 29, 246n.36
planetary resources. *See* natural
resources, depletion of
planets, influence of, 53–54. *See also*
Saturn
Plato, 21, 52
pneuma, 8, 166, 246n.21. *See also* Galen
of Pergamum
Poe, Edgar Allan, 85, 103
Polidori, John, 80
political apathy, 3
popes, resignation of, 1–3, 45

positive thinking, 29

possession, demonic, 10

postexertion malaise, 35

postviral fatigue syndrome (PVFS). *See* chronic fatigue syndrome

Price of Inequality, The (Stiglitz), 128–29

Problemata (Aristotle), 17, 54

Procter, Andrew and Elizabeth, 217

productivity, 13, 202–3. *See also* capitalism; work

Protestant Ethic and the Spirit of Capitalism, The (Weber), 118, 120–24. *See also* Weber, Max

Protestant Reformation, 123–24

Protestant work ethic, 120–24, 227

Proust, Marcel, 96, 98, 106

Prozac, 172–75

Prozac Nation (Wurtzel), 173–75

psychasthenia, 165–66, 257n.32

psychoanalytic theory and psychoanalysis, 39, 107, 116, 181, 189–94. *See also* Freud, Sigmund

psychology: belief and illness, 193, 199–201, 234; chronic fatigue syndrome and, 189–94, 198–99 (*see also* chronic fatigue syndrome); depressives' view as more realistic and, 70–71, 180; psychological tension, 166 (*see also* Janet, Pierre-Marie-Félix); stress research and, 210–12. *See also* brain; cognitive behavioral theory; depression; Freud, Sigmund; Janet, Pierre-Marie-Félix; mind; psychoanalytic theory and psychoanalysis; psychotherapy

Psychopathia Sexualis (Krafft-Ebing), 94. *See also* Krafft-Ebing, Richard von

psychotherapy, 180, 181, 189–94. *See also* cognitive behavioral therapy

qi, 8, 108, 166, 208

Rabinbach, Anson, 118, 124–25, 202–3

Radkau, Joachim, 90–91, 118

raw materials. *See* natural resources, depletion of

recuperation hypothesis, 145–46

religion: acedia and, 17, 38, 40 (*see also* acedia); in *A Burnt-Out Case*, 223–26; desire for lost belief, 104; Freud on, 153; lukewarm faith, 45; and Protestant work ethic, 123–24; Sabbath and, 132–33, 242; on sex and sexuality, 72, 74. *See also Divine Comedy, The*; sin

resources, conservation of (COR) theory, 214–15

resources, natural. *See* natural resources, depletion of

rest: adaption energy and, 207; changing attitudes toward, 123–24 (*see also* Protestant work ethic); chronic fatigue syndrome and, 196–97; as cure for burnout, 217; Darwin on, 143; definition of, 132; desire for, 13, 114–15, 148 (*see also* death: death drive; *Oblomov*); rest cure, 12, 90, 109–10, 135–38, 197; on Sabbath, 132–33, 242. *See also* sleep

restlessness, 6, 17, 33, 35, 36

rhythms. *See* natural rhythms

Rings of Saturn, The (Sebald), 63–67, 71

Röggla, Kathrin, 262n.38

Romantic era, 17, 54

Rosario, Vernon A., 79

Rousseau, Jean-Jacques, 79

ruin(s), in *The Rings of Saturn*, 65–66

Sabbath, 132–33, 242

Sade, Marquis de, 81

sadness (sorrow): acedia and, 39–41, 43, 46, 50–51; melancholia and, 20, 22, 46, 50, 52, 67; saturnine disposition and, 54

Saturn, 53–54, 55, 62–63, 64, 66. *See also* Ficino, Marsilio; Sebald, W. G.; temperament: melancholic (saturnine)

scholars, melancholia of, 55–57. *See also* "brain work"

seasickness, 142–43

Sebald, W. G., 63–67, 71

selective serotonin reuptake inhibitors (SSRUIs), 15, 172. *See also* serotonin

self-discipline, in *Death in Venice*, 228–30

self-hatred (self-loathing), 6, 17, 57, 131, 159–60, 170–71, 173

self-reflexivity, 56–58, 71

Selye, Hans, 204–9

seminal fluid, 60, 73. *See also* sex and sexuality

serotonin, 15, 116, 172, 221. *See also* brain: chemical imbalance in

Seven Deadly Sins, 31, 32, 38, 44, 247n.16. See also *Divine Comedy, The*

sex and sexuality: eighteenth- and nineteenth-century discourses on, 72–79, 81; Freud on, 77, 78, 107, 150–55, 160; homosexuality, 80–84; humoral theory and, 73–74; medieval discourses on, 60, 72–74; premature ejaculation, 91; sexual activity and energy, 60, 73, 75–77, 151–52, 235; sins of, 72, 74, 79 (*see also* masturbation); vampires and homosexuality, 80–84

"Sexuality in the Aetiology of the Neuroses" (Freud), 151

Shakespeare, William, 57

Shorter, Edward, 10, 185, 193–95, 197, 200–201

Showalter, Elaine, 193

sin: acedia and, 17, 32–39, 40–51; in *The Divine Comedy*, 44–51; exhaustion as, 235; rest and nonproductive activity as, 124; Seven Deadly Sins,

31, 32, 38, 247n.16; sexual, 72, 74, 79 (*see also* masturbation); vs. vice, 39

sleep, 145–49; chronic fatigue syndrome and, 186; depression/melancholia and, 20, 60, 174, 176; insomnia, 91, 104, 107, 147, 176; sleepiness, 31, 33, 44, 49, 91

sloth, 31–32, 38, 47–50. *See also* acedia

sluggishness, 33, 43, 46, 54, 59

sociocultural developments: burnout and, 203–4; changes in perception of exhaustion symptoms and, 9–11, 12; chronic fatigue syndrome and, 194–98; core cultural values and exhaustion, 12, 124; medical discourses and, 11, 95, 108–9, 233 (*see also* medical discourses; *specific diagnoses*); nostalgic/conservative/ apocalyptic responses to, 8–10, 88–89, 100, 133, 148–49, 209 (*see also specific individuals*); Protestant Reformation as, 123–24 (*see also* Protestant work ethic); stress and, 210–12; women's emancipation, medical diagnosis, and, 139–42 (*see also* women); work and, 116–17 (*see also* capitalism; technology; work). *See also* civilization; Greece, ancient; Middle Ages

solar affinities, 62

Solomon, Andrew, 33, 177

somatization, 191, 193–94

sorrow. *See* sadness

soul: acedia and, 36 (*see also* acedia); Ficino on, 55–57; Galen on, 20–22, 57, 246n.21

spirit, 55, 63. *See also* acedia; faith; Ficino, Marsilio; soul

spiritual exhaustion, 1–3, 5, 40–41, 44–51, 223–26. *See also* acedia

"Staff Burn-Out" (Freudenberger), 213

Starling, Ernest H., 207

state, responsibility of, 211–12, 220

State of Me, The (Jafry), 187–91. *See also* Jafry, Nasim Marie

Steffen, Will, 239–40

Stiglitz, Joseph, 128–29, 130, 131

stimulants, 12, 90

stimulation therapies, 119. *See also* electrotherapy; hydrotherapy

Stockholm Resilience Centre, 238, 239

stomach, 18, 76, 91, 104. *See also* diet

stress, 30, 203–12, 214–15, 235

Stress of Life, The (Selye), 208. *See also* Selye, Hans

Stress Without Distress (Selye), 209. *See also* Selye, Hans

suicide and suicidal thoughts, 99, 138, 173, 174, 176. *See also* death: death drive

sullenness, 45–46

Summa Theologiae (Thomas Aquinas), 40–42, 74

superego, 39, 150, 159, 160–61, 165, 171, 182. *See also* Freud, Sigmund

Svevo, Italo, 98

Taylor, Shelley E., 70–71

technology: burnout and, 9, 213, 221–22; exhaustion theories on, 237; Francis I on, 241–42; as modern stressor, 211–12; natural rhythms disrupted by, 8–9, 117, 133–34, 146–48, 213; neurasthenia and, 93, 95, 96–98; progress driven by desire to reduce work, 124–25

teeth, 139

temperament: astrological doctrine on, 53–54; melancholic (saturnine), 54, 57, 59–60 (*see also* melancholia); nervous, 84–85, 93–94, 105 (*see also* *Against Nature*; neurasthenia); neurasthenic, 108

thermodynamics, second law of, 90, 238

This Changes Everything (Klein), 240

Thomas Aquinas, Saint, 40–42, 74

Three Books on Life (Ficino), 52–63, 71, 73–74. *See also* Ficino, Marsilio

Three Essays on the Theory of Sexuality (Freud), 78

Tieck, Ludwig, 80, 251n.20

Tissot, Samuel-Auguste, 75–76, 79

tonics, 12, 61, 90

torpor, 31, 40, 54, 59

traditionalism vs. capitalism, 121–22, 254n.13

Treatise on Physical, Intellectual and Moral Degeneracy in the Human Species and the Causes That Produce These Diseased Varieties (Morel), 77–78

treatments, 234–35. *See also* antidepressants; diet; *specific diagnoses, treatments, and therapies*

Trier, Lars von, 67–71, 180

Tristan (T. Mann), 98

Turner, Aidan, 129, 130, 131

24/7 (Crary), 147–49

vampires and vampirism, 79–84, 140, 208–9, 219

"Vampyre, The" (Polidori), 80

vine and oak tree, as metaphor, 177–79

Virgil, in *The Divine Comedy*, 44–46, 47–49, 51

viruses, 184–87, 235. *See also* chronic fatigue syndrome

Wagner, Greta, 220

Wake Not the Dead (Tieck), 80, 251n.20

Waste Land, The (Eliot), 109–10

water cure. *See* hydrotherapy

Wear and Tear (Mitchell), 137, 139–40

"wear-and-tear" principle, 206

weariness, 31, 34–35, 40, 52, 58. *See also* fatigue; spiritual exhaustion

Weariness of the Self, The (Ehrenberg), 58. *See also* Ehrenberg, Alain

Weber, Max, 118–24, 131
Wenzel, Siegfried, 37–38
Wessely, Simon, 191–92, 196, 199, 259n.9
Why Do People Get Ill? (Leader and Corfield), 29, 199–200. *See also* Corfield, David; Leader, Darian
Wilde, Oscar, 81, 91, 96, 101
willpower, 11, 17, 47, 49, 235. *See also* agency; personal responsibility
Wolff, Harold G., 210
women, 137–42. *See also specific individuals*
Woolf, Virginia, 96, 138–39, 144
work: as antidote to acedia, 36–38; burnout and, 9, 95, 202–3, 213–17, 220 (*see also* burnout); changing nature of, 117–18, 120; class, neurasthenia, and, 92–93 (*see also* neurasthenia); desire to avoid responsibility of, 113–14; fatigue and productivity, 13, 202–3, 260n.2; human-services sector and, 213–14; identity and, 13, 118, 120, 228–29; Krafft-Ebing on women and, 141; maximum-results-with-minimum-effort mentality of, 128;

in *Oblomov*, 112–16; Protestant ethic of, 120–24; repetitive labor in, 117–18, 202–3, 211–12; stress and, 203, 210–12, 260n.2 (*see also* burnout); technological progress driven by desire to reduce, 124–25; workers' worldviews shaped by metaphors of, 262n.38. *See also* capitalism; natural rhythms
World Bank, 239
World Health Organization (WHO), 4, 172, 203, 210, 259n.9. See also *International Classification of Diseases*
worthlessness, sense of, 160, 170, 176
wrath, 45
Wurtzel, Elizabeth, 173–75

yeast infection, 196
yellow bile, in humoral theory, 16
"Yellow Wallpaper, The" (Gilman), 135–37. *See also* Gilman, Charlotte Perkins
youth, restoring, 208–9

zeal, 50
Zeno's Conscience (Svevo), 98